Renal Disease in Pregnancy

Renal Disease in Pregnancy

Second Edition

Edited by

Kate Bramham, MBBS, MA, PhD, MRCP
King's College Hospital NHS Foundation Trust, London

Matt Hall, MBBS, MA, MD, FRCP
Nottingham University Hospitals NHS Trust, Nottingham

Catherine Nelson-Piercy, MBBS, MA, FRCP, FRCOG
Guy's and St Thomas' NHS Foundation Trust, London

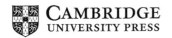

CAMBRIDGE
UNIVERSITY PRESS

CAMBRIDGE
UNIVERSITY PRESS

University Printing House, Cambridge CB2 8BS, United Kingdom

One Liberty Plaza, 20th Floor, New York, NY 10006, USA

477 Williamstown Road, Port Melbourne, VIC 3207, Australia

314–321, 3rd Floor, Plot 3, Splendor Forum, Jasola District Centre, New Delhi – 110025, India

79 Anson Road, #06–04/06, Singapore 079906

Cambridge University Press is part of the University of Cambridge.

It furthers the University's mission by disseminating knowledge in the pursuit of
education, learning, and research at the highest international levels of excellence.

www.cambridge.org
Information on this title: www.cambridge.org/9781107124073
DOI: 10.1017/9781316403839

© Cambridge University Press 2018

First edition published 2008
Second edition published 2018

Printed in the United Kingdom by Clays, St Ives plc

A catalogue record for this publication is available from the British Library.

Library of Congress Cataloging-in-Publication Data
Names: Bramham, Kate, editor. | Hall, Matt, MRCP, editor. | Nelson-Piercy, Catherine, editor.
Title: Renal disease in pregnancy / edited by Kate Bramham, Matt Hall, Catherine Nelson-Piercy.
Other titles: Renal disease in pregnancy (Bramham)
Description: Second edition. | New York, NY : Cambridge University Press, [2018] | Includes
bibliographical references and index.
Identifiers: LCCN 2018012807 | ISBN 9781107124073 (alk. paper)
Subjects: | MESH: Kidney Diseases | Pregnancy Complications | Pregnancy
Classification: LCC RG580.K5 | NLM WQ 260 | DDC 618.3–dc23
LC record available at https://lccn.loc.gov/2018012807

ISBN 978-1-107-12407-3 Hardback

Contents

v

Contributors

Ian Aird, MBChB, DA, FRCOG
Gateshead Fertility Unit, Queen Elizabeth Hospital, Gateshead, UK

Anita Banerjee, MBBS, FHEA, FRCP
Guy's and St Thomas' NHS Foundation Trust, London, UK

Kate Bramham, MBBS, MA, PhD, MRCP
King's College Hospital NHS Foundation Trust, London

Mark Brown MBBS, MD
St. George Hospital & University of NSW Sydney, Australia

Nigel Brunskill, MB ChB, PhD
University of Leicester, Leicester, UK

Sue Carr, MD, MMedSci, FRCP, FAcadMEd
University Hospitals of Leicester NHS Trust, Leicester, UK

Floria Cheng, RN, RM
Imperial College Healthcare NHS Trust, London, UK

Martin Drage, MB BChir, MA, FRCS, PhD
Guy's and St Thomas' NHS Foundation Trust, London, UK

Al Ferraro, MRCP, PhD
Nottingham University Hospitals NHS Trust, Nottingham, UK

Matt Hall, MBBCh, MD, FRCP
Nottingham University Hospitals NHS Trust, Nottingham, UK

Michele Hladunewich, MD, MSc, FRCP(C)
University of Toronto, Toronto, Canada

Louise C. Kenny, MBChB (hons), MRCOG, PhD
University College Cork, Cork, Ireland

Ellen Knox, MBBS, MD, MRCOG
Birmingham Women's and Children's NHS Foundation Trust, UK

Liz Lightstone, PhD, FRCP
Imperial College, London, UK

Graham Lipkin, MD, FRCP
Queen Elizabeth Hospital, Birmingham, UK

Lucy Mackillop, MA (Oxon), FRCP
Oxford University Hospitals NHS Foundation Trust, Oxford, UK

Andrew McCarthy, MRCPI, FRCOG, MD
Imperial College Healthcare, London, UK

Jenny Myers, MRCOG, PhD
University of Manchester, Manchester, UK

Jonathon Olsburgh, PhD FRCS (Urol)
Guy's and St Thomas' NHS Foundation Trust, London, UK

Liam Plant, BSc, MB, FRCPI, FRCPE
University College Cork and Cork University Hospital, Cork, Ireland

Joyce Popoola, PhD, FRCP
St George's University Hospitals NHS Foundation Trust, London, UK

Tracey Salter, BMBCh, MA, MRCP
Epsom and St Helier University Hospitals NHS Trust, Carshalton, UK

Asif Sarwar, MRPharmS
University Hospitals Birmingham NHS Foundation Trust, Birmingham, UK

Nadia Sarween, MBChB, MSc
University Hospitals Birmingham NHS Foundation Trust, Birmingham, UK

Kainat Shahid, MD, FRCP
University of Toronto, Toronto, Canada

Jason Waugh, MBBS, BSc, MRCOG, DA
Newcastle Upon Tyne Hospitals NHS Foundation Trust, Newcastle upon Tyne, UK

Kate Wiles, MSc, MBBS, MRCP
Guy's and St Thomas' Hospital and King's College London, London, UK

David Williams, PhD, FRCP
University College London Hospital, UK

Susan Willis, MD (Res), FRCS (Urol)
Guy's and St Thomas' NHS Foundation Trust, London, UK

Preface

Renal disorders, both newly diagnosed and preexisting or chronic, are some of the most common non-obstetric problems encountered during pregnancy. Furthermore, pregnancy makes major physiological demands on all maternal organs, and certainly the kidney is no exception. In women with a chronic problem these demands may not be adequately catered for, thus compromising pregnancy outcome and even risking further maternal harm. Thus obstetric nephrology is an important component of what is nowadays referred to as maternal or obstetric medicine.

There can be little doubt that this, the second edition of *Renal Disease and Pregnancy*, is timely, as it capitalizes on all of the new information that has accrued since the first edition in 2007. This current volume stems from a Study Day, held on December 3, 2014, where there were presentations from specialists in relevant disciplines and from members of the Study Group of the UK Registry for Rare Kidney Diseases (RaDaR), a 2013 initiative of the UK Renal Association (a professional body for UK renal physicians and scientists), which oversees and liaises with other information-gathering bodies, including the UK Renal Registry (UKRR) and the UK Renal Data Collaboration (UKRDC). In turn, these are all affiliated with the British Renal Association, an umbrella organization for renal health care, to ensure the availability of up-to-date information technologies, the better use of existing knowledge and better collaboration with the NHS and patient organizations, so as to improve the reporting and recording of data and then the subsequent efficient handling and availability of that data. Pregnancy and chronic kidney disease (CKD) is an important item in RaDaR's portfolio, as it has been for the UK Obstetric Surveillance System (UKOSS) [1, 2].

Although it is just over three years since that Study Day, the editors and all contributors have very diligently kept an eye on the expanding literature (with many contributing to it) to ensure that chapters are brimming with up-to-date information, covering most of the situations likely to be encountered by obstetric/renal physicians, obstetricians specializing in maternal medicine and specialist midwives working in the field. This book is also aligned with the 2018 theme for World Kidney Day, "Kidneys and Women's Health."

And now for some relevant history. In 2007 the first edition of this book was a timely reminder of what had been achieved in the preceding 30 years, since a 1976 "turning point" *Lancet* editorial [3] explained the need to revise the advice concerning pregnancy in women with renal disorders that had understandably pervaded the earlier decades, by stating that "children of women with renal disease used to be born dangerously, or not at all – not at all, if their doctors had their way." By 1989, another *Lancet* editorial [4] was applauding the new attitudes and approaches while emphasizing that it was still not a straightforward situation because "the thoughtful doctor still should admit his difficulties," and more so, because "the thoughtful woman demands straight answers to apparently straight questions." Also, in the 1970s and 1980s, there was a reemphasis of the view that clinicians in this field must be cognizant of the marked systemic physiological upheaval of maternal adaptation to pregnancy, with the kidneys and renal tract extensively involved, resulting in new "norms" for renal assessment during pregnancy itself [5, 6]. There was a realization too that there was no room for complacency about the need for further research alongside the need for meticulous recording of clinical and laboratory data.

Much earlier in 1964, this had also been a stance taken by Sir Dugald Baird (1899–1986) in Aberdeen, a pioneer in the development of methods for reliable data acquisition and the use of databases and, interestingly, in the investigation of the renal tract in pregnancy. He was the founding director of the Medical Research Council's Obstetric Medicine Research Unit (OMRU) in the 1950s (perhaps the first time the phrase "obstetric medicine" was coined), with the acronym OMRU becoming world renowned. That Unit "produced" a series of outstanding clinicians and scientists who filled important and influential posts throughout the United Kingdom and indeed, worldwide, including Frank Hytten (1923–2018), an inspiring and innovative human pregnancy physiologist [7]. He always emphasized that the kidney provided a convenient "physiological window" through which to view maternal physiological adaptation to pregnancy and in turn, as mentioned earlier, renal adaptation itself, in health and disease, tested the functional capacity of the kidneys, so prepregnancy status and information were very important [7, 8]. Often forgotten is that Sir Dugald Baird himself in 1964 had pointed out that prepregnancy health was important and that many of the physiological adaptations "occur so early that they cannot be responses to an immediate need but must be fundamental changes necessary to secure the later stages of gestation" and that "their monitoring may give insights not only into the aetiology of the pathological but that any pathological response itself may help us to understand the normal" [7]. Significantly, his interest in the urinary tract was obvious more than two decades earlier [10], at a time when it was also becoming recognized that pregnancy problems, particularly preeclampsia (or toxemia as it was called then), could be superimposed in women who already had hypertension and/or so-called low kidney reserve, perhaps unknowingly, alluding to CKD [11], where it is now known that there can often be a lack of the normal gestational hyperfiltration response, an index of that functional kidney reserve [6].

Of interest, in the 1960s there was starting to be an influence of the work and writings of Homer W. Smith (1895–1962) [12, 13], perhaps the inaugural "Dean of Renal Physiology" and a truly polymathic figure with a tremendous legacy. He played a major role in introducing, popularizing and bringing a rigorous discipline to renal clearance methodology as well as creating broad concepts that defined the properties of glomeruli, renal tubules and the renal circulation. He pioneered the need for very close cooperation and collaboration between physiologists and clinicians and is justly credited to have advanced our knowledge of altered renal function in disease. Famously, in 1956, he wrote, "To a renal physiologist, a pregnant woman is a very interesting phenomenon: I do not know any other way to increase the filtration rate by fifty per cent or better for prolonged periods" [14]. He commented that further renal studies were absolutely essential during pregnancy in health and disease and hinted at the need for consideration to be given to the clinical assessment and care of all pregnant women with underlying medical issues.

By the early 1960s, London physician Cyril G Barnes had "unofficially" established the subspecialty of "obstetric medicine" in the United Kingdom, with his single-authored seminal book (of 302 pages), which pointed out so clearly that medical diseases in pregnant women were a challenge for any clinician! That book ran to many editions [15] and along the way stimulated other eminent physicians and obstetricians to edit books and contribute similarly, with many editions, some chapters being written by colleague specialists [16–18]. Thus, although up-to-date advice was now available, these publications also highlighted the need for formal recognition of and structured training in obstetric medicine, both for physicians and for obstetricians.

Significantly, Cyril Barnes's book was "inherited and further developed and expanded" by his successor, Michael de Swiet, another key figure in this rapidly changing area [17]. Looking back [6], it was apparent that "new" books were also being published by other experts alongside revisions of the earlier ones. Concomitantly, it was also becoming obvious that as obstetric medicine was evolving there was a need for recognition of its individual components too, such as obstetric nephrology.

This somewhat lengthy, but hopefully interesting history, brings us back to this second and outstanding edition of *Renal Disease and Pregnancy*, in which the up-to-date chapters are the fruits of recent research and clinical developments. The editors have ensured that these chapters are in a logical sequence so as to deal in orderly fashion with the many issues likely to be faced by any multidisciplinary team (MDT) caring for women with renal problems. Furthermore, from this book there can now be little doubt that a starting-point emphasis on the basic components of prepregnancy assessment should be analysis of risks and provision of health education and advice, plus any interventions considered helpful, all united under the banner of that much-used word "counseling." The MDT has to decide what is important, so that "active preparation for pregnancy" is tailored to each woman's needs, with her being encouraged to involve her partner, so that all the implications can be discussed, including potential areas of disagreement, even whether infertility treatment, if needed, would be made available.

The patient (and her partner) will want to know, aside from that the MDT wants to discuss, four straightforward issues. Should I get pregnant? Will my pregnancy be complicated? Will I have a live and healthy baby? Will I have problems after my pregnancy? In addition, she needs to understand the risks that are discussed with her and the need to improve her own knowledge, so that she can best use the guidance and support to make any necessary changes in her behavior, attitude and medication(s). Knowledge of, and even understanding the risks, however, may not be sufficient to ensure the patient makes the changes because many other factors influence her behavior. Even when there is an element of self-management (perhaps best exemplified with dialysis and/or diabetes), this will also be affected by the woman's repertoire of beliefs, skills, intuition, motivation and not just her so-called knowledge, however gained. The key is a strong, unwavering, positive, supportive relationship with the MDT that allows prepregnancy advice to be included in the overall care agenda as a goal-orientated process. Thus a "planned pregnancy" is one that is desired well before conception, occurs when contraception is discontinued and where the woman attempts to achieve optimal health beforehand.

During counseling, even if some of the answers are not favorable, a woman, being an autonomous adult, may still choose to plan for (or proceed with) a pregnancy in an effort to reestablish a normal life in the face of chronic illness. Indeed some women may not seek advice until already pregnant. Occasionally, there may be ethical dilemmas regarding the clinician's duty of care for women who ignore advice; interestingly, there are studies that have differentiated "healthy" and "pathological" levels of assumed risk and that have tried to understand the psychology of women who pursue parenthood despite big risks to their own health and the unborn child. This area is superbly covered in this book, incorporating what we need to know about contraception and assisted contraception as well.

Reassuringly, none of the chapters attempts to skim over controversial areas. Dealt with are current knowledge of basic renal physiology and pathophysiology in pregnancy, pregnancy in specific kidney diseases, the role of renal biopsy, the diagnosis

(including multi-marker screening) and the effects of preeclampsia and its long-term postpregnancy sequelae as it can no longer be assumed that it is "a condition cured by delivery." Also covered are the pharmacology and rationalization of the many medications prescribed for these women, acute kidney injury (AKI) and urological problems during pregnancy, as well as the special issues in pregnancy in dialysis patients and renal transplant recipients, both of whom may have significant comorbidities too. Where appropriate the important midwifery issues are well discussed.

There is mention of the current CKD classification and staging that are part of the clinical practice guidelines of the US National Kidney Foundation (NKF) [19–21], endorsed by the UK National Services Framework for Renal Services [22] and now widely adopted in nephrological practice. The cornerstone of this classification is the use of estimated glomerular filtration rate (eGFR) calculated from formulae based on serum creatinine, adjusted for age, gender and race [23]. Nowadays most chemical pathology laboratories are encouraged to report eGFR, so it has become enshrined in nephrological practice and even the lay press [24]. There is some evidence in CKD patients that prepregnancy eGFR has a better sensitivity in detecting subclinical renal dysfunction as compared to serum creatinine alone [25], but this might not be the case for renal transplant recipients [26]. Thus discussions still prevail [23, 27, 28] about the applicability of eGFR, but there can be no doubt that these formulae must not be used in pregnancy [29, 30], as true GFR will be significantly underestimated, so that in any patient, not just those with a renal problem, this could signal to the unwary clinician an exaggerated deterioration in kidney function, prompting totally unnecessary delivery.

The recurrent message throughout this book is that the MDT is the key to judicious decision-making. This will ensure optimal antenatal supervision, with up-to-date technology for fetal surveillance and careful management of delivery and afterward, in a center with all the necessary facilities for dealing with these high-risk patients and their babies. Although other recent publications [31–36] also espouse these views, this soundly edited book, without doubt, further extends and enhances this approach.

Not to be forgotten is that effective monitoring and documentation of maternal and perinatal health and health care are an essential part of obstetric care, aiding the identification of women affected by a chronic disease problem and the evaluation of current service provision and health care planning, so as to focus on future research needs. For instance, there are the UK Obstetric Surveillance System (UKOSS) [1, 2, 37–39], a variety of specific medical registries (which despite their flaws and limitations can be an excellent means of continuous surveillance and storage of data) and, of course, the relatively new Mother and Babies: Reducing Risk through Audits and Confidential Enquiries across the UK (MBRRACE-UK). The latter has shown that among several independent contributing factors associated with maternal death, almost 50 percent of that increased risk was associated with medical comorbidities [38]. Also, as part of the current Safer Maternity Action Plan [40] there is strong emphasis on data collection and plans for better networked maternal medicine involving all the relevant personnel.

With improvements in methods of data acquisition, computer technology and specific registries, another main aim for the future must be enhanced communication between clinicians in MDTs at the "ground level," perhaps comparing cases with patient profiles derived from analyzed national databases and/or registries. Case reports and single-center experiences will continue to supplement evidence-based medicine and help clinicians in practical terms, but there is a crucial need for prospective data too. Renal medicine in the United Kingdom leads the field in electronic patient records and obstetrics is not far behind. Efficiently remedying the comprehensive collection and storage of useful data and their analyses are essential, and this is where RaDaR and UKOSS are so important. Such approaches and initiatives, alongside good basic research, should stimulate quality improvements in patient care and safeguarding, service development, teaching and clinical research. All of this must be meticulously recorded as there is no place for poor documentation or lapses in documentation. Indeed, we should take heed of the Queen in Chapter 1 (Looking Glass House) in Lewis Carroll's *Alice in Wonderland*: "That moment ... the King went on, I shall never forget! You will though, the Queen said, if you don't make a memorandum of it! Alice looked on with great interest as the King took an enormous book out of his pocket, and began writing."

Congratulations to the editors and all contributors. Obstetric nephrology is definitely here to stay. Hope you will all be back for a third edition.

John Davison
January 2018

References

1. The UK Obstetric Surveillance System for rare disorders of pregnancy (Commentary) (2005) *BJOG*, **112**:263–265.

2. Bramham K, Nelson-Piercy C, Gao H, Pierce M, Bush N, Spark P et al. Pregnancy in renal transplant recipients: A UK national cohort study. *Clin J Am Soc Nephrol*, 2013;**8**:290–298.

3. Pregnancy and renal disease (Editorial). *Lancet* 1957;**2**:801–882.

4. Pregnancy and glomerulonephritis (Editorial). *Lancet* 1989;**2**:253–254.

5. Lindheimer MD and Katz AI. *Kidney function and disease in pregnancy*. Philadelphia, PA: Lea & Febiger, 1977.

6. Lindheimer MD, Davison JM, Katz AI. The kidney and hypertension in pregnancy: Twenty exciting years. *Sem Nephrol* 2001;**21**:173–189.

7. Hytten FE, Leitch I. *The physiology of human pregnancy* (2nd edn.). Oxford, London and Edinburgh: Blackwell Scientific Publications, 1971.

8. Davison JM, Hytten FE. Glomerular filtration during and after pregnancy. *J Obstet Gynae Brit Commonw* 1974;**81**:588–595.

9. Baird, D (1971) Foreword to first edition (1964). In Hytten FE, Leitch I (eds.). *The physiology of human pregnancy* (2nd edn.). Oxford, London and Edinburgh: Blackwell Scientific Publications:vii–x.

10. Baird D The upper urinary tract in pregnancy and puerperium, with special reference to pyelitus of pregnancy. *JOG Brit Emp* 1935;**42**:733.

11. Dexter L, Weiss S. *Preeclamptic and eclamptic toxemia of pregnancy*. Boston, MA: Little, Brown and Company, 1941, 8.

12. Gottschalk CW. Homer William Smith: A remembrance. *J Am Soc Nephrol* 1995;**5**:1984–1987.

13. Navar LG. The legacy of Homer W Smith: Mechanistic insights into renal physiology. *J Clin Invest* 2004;**114**: 1048–1050.

14. Smith HW. Summary interpretation of observations of renal hemodynamics in preeclampsia. *Report of First*

Rose Obstetric Research Conference. SJ Foman (ed.). Ohio Ross Laboratories, 1956, 75.

15. Barnes CG. *Medical disorders in obstetric practice* (4th edn.). Oxford, London and Edinburgh: Blackwell Scientific Publications, 1974.

16. Burrow GN, Ferris TF. *Medical complications during pregnancy* (4th edn.). Philadelphia, PA: WB Saunders Company, 1995.

17. De Swiet M. *Medical disorders in obstetric practice* (4th edn.). Oxford: Blackwell Science Ltd., 2002.

18. Barron WM, Lindheimer MD. *Medical disorders during pregnancy* (3rd edn.). St. Louis, MO: Mosby Inc., 2002.

19. National Kidney Foundation K/DOQI Clinical Practice Guidelines for Chronic Kidney Disease: Evaluation, Classification and Stratification. *Am J Kid Dis* 2002;**39**(Suppl 1):S1–S266.

20. National Kidney Foundation Guidelines for Chronic Kidney Disease: Evaluation, Classification and Stratification. *Ann Intern Med* 2003;**139**:137–147.

21. KDIGO. Kidney Disease: Improving Global Outcomes (KDIGO) CKD Work Group. KDIGO 2012 clinical practice guideline for the evaluation and management of chronic kidney disease. *Kid Intl Suppl* 2013;**3**:1–150.

22. Department of Health. Estimating glomerular filtration rate (GFR): Information for laboratories. Available at: www.dh.gov.uk/prod_cons_dh/group s_digitalassets/@dh/@en/documents/digitalasset/d h_4133025.pdf.

23. DeLanaye P, Marcat C. The applicability of eGFR equation to different populations. *Nature Reviews Nephrology* 2013;**9**:513–522.

24. *The Times* (2017) August 1, p. 50.

25. Picolli GB, Fassio F, Attini R, Parisi S, Bidcali M, Ferraresi M et al. Pregnancy in CKD: Whom should we follow and why? *Nephrol Dial Transpl* 2012;**27**(Suppl 3): 111–118.

26. Attia A, Zahran A, Shoker A. Comparison of equations to estimate glomerular filtration rate in post-renal transplant kidney disease patients. *Saudi J Kidney Dis Transpl* 2012;**23**:453–460.

27. Bauer C, Melamed ML, Hosteffer TH. Staging of chronic kidney disease: Time for a course correction. *J Am Soc Nephrol* 2008;**19**:844–846.

28. Nguyen MT, Maynard SE, Kinnear PL. Misapplication of commonly used kidney equations: Renal physiology in practice. *Clin J Am Soc Nephrol* 2009;**4**:528–534.

29. Smith MC, Moran P, Ward MK, Davison JM. Assessment of glomerular filtration rate during pregnancy using the MDRD formula. *BJOG* 2008;**115**:109–112.

30. Smith MC, Moran P, Davison JM. EPI-CKD is a poor predictor of GFR in pregnancy. *Arch Dis Child Fetal Neonatal Ed*, 2011;**96**(Suppl 1), Fa99.

31. Davison JM, Lindheimer MD. Pregnancy and chronic renal disease. *Sem Nephrol* 2011;**31**:86–89.

32. Odukayo A, Hladunewich M. Obstetric nephrology: Renal hemodynamics and metabolic physiology in normal pregnancy. *Clin J Am Soc Nephrol* 2012;**7**:2073–2080.

33. Brosens I, Benagiano G (eds.). Obstetrics and gynaecology after organ transplantation. *Clinical Obstetrics and Gynaecology* 2014;**28**:1113–1277 and A1–A6.

34. Williams D (ed.). *Best practice and research clinical obstetrics and gynaecology* 2015;**29**:577–764.

35. Bramham, K, Hladunewich MA, Jim B, Maynard SE (eds.). Pregnancy and kidney disease. *NephSAP* 2016;**15**:109–229.

36. Cabbidu G, Castellino S, Gernone G, Santoro D, Moroni M, Giannattasio M. A best practice position statement on pregnancy in chronic kidney disease: The Italian Study Group on Kidney and Pregnancy. *J Nephrol* 2016;**29**:277–303.

37. Culshaw N, Pasupathy D, Kyle P. The value of obstetric surveillance systems within the National Health Service. *The Obstetrician and Gynaecologist* 2013;**15**:85–89.

38. Knight M. How will the new Confidential Enquiries into Maternal and Infant Death in the UK operate? The work of MBRRACE-UK. *The Obstetrician and Gynaecologist* 2013;**15**:65.

39. Nair M, Kurinczuk JJ, Brocklehurst P, Sellers S, Lewis G, Knight M. Factors associated with maternal death from direct pregnancy complications: A UK national case-control study. *BJOG* 2015;**122**:653–662.

40. Safer Maternity Care. The National Maternity Safety Strategy – Progress and Next Steps. November 28, 2017. www.gov.uk/dh.

Renal Physiology

Kate Bramham and Tracey Salter

Introduction

Remarkable and unique changes enable the kidneys to adjust to the increased metabolic demands of pregnancy. Renal adaption occurs following conception, is maximal prior to major increases in uteroplacental blood flow and is maintained until at least late gestation. Adjustment of systemic and renal homeostasis enables enhanced glomerular filtration, volume expansion, modified electrolyte and acid base balance and augmented erythropoietin and active vitamin D synthesis. These alterations are likely to contribute to successful pregnancy outcomes. Current understandings of underlying mechanisms of gestational transformations are outlined in what follows, and potential pathophysiological pathways of pregnancy-associated deterioration in renal function are discussed.

Gestational Changes in the Renal Tract

Increases in renal blood flow and interstitial space result in volume expansion of the kidneys up to 70 percent, equating to approximately 1 cm in length [1]. Dilatation of the renal tract (calyces, renal pelvis and ureter) is evident in 90 percent of women by the third trimester [1], and is more prominent on the right. This effect is proposed to be the consequence of the ureter passing over the right iliac artery. However, renal tract dilatation is also recognized in transplanted kidneys, implying that circulating factors are contributory. Urological complications are discussed in more detail in Chapter 15.

Renal Function in Pregnancy

Renal Blood Flow

Ovulation is followed by an increase in renal plasma flow, as measured by para-aminohippurate clearance. After conception, there are further increases in effective renal plasma flow, reaching rates 50–85 percent greater than nonpregnant values [2].

Longitudinal assessments of effective renal plasma flow in healthy women during pregnancy and postpartum consistently report augmented flow. There is discrepancy at later gestation, however, with some reports of up to 20 percent reduced flow toward term [3, 4], and others of sustained blood flow [5]. Positional changes in late pregnancy may influence renal hemodynamics [5], but this is not confirmed by all studies [3].

Glomerular Filtration

In parallel with changes in renal blood flow, prior to conception there is a 20 percent increase in glomerular filtration during the luteal phase of the menstrual cycle compared with the week of menstruation [6], and a 7 percent increase compared with the follicular phase [7].

Assessments of inulin and 24-hour creatinine clearance in healthy pregnant women report increases in glomerular filtration as early as four weeks post-conception [6], peaking at 40–65 percent postpartum values [3, 4] in the second trimester. In the last trimester, glomerular filtration, assessed by 24-hour creatinine clearance, appears to fall to nonpregnant values [8]. In a study of serial 24-hour creatinine clearance in early pregnancy, a 45 percent increase was present by nine weeks' gestation. Two women who subsequently had miscarriages had a less marked increase in creatinine clearance compared to women with uncomplicated pregnancies, evident three weeks prior to fetal loss, suggesting that adequate early renal adaptation appears to be important for successful pregnancy. Furthermore, in women with severe chronic kidney disease (CKD), a decline, rather than an improvement, in renal function with pregnancy is associated with lower birth weight [6].

Increments in glomerular filtration are less than renal plasma flow, suggesting that adjustments in regulation of glomerular filtration occur. Dextran sieving studies in healthy pregnant women, which enable assessment of relative filtration of different sizes of neutral molecules, suggest that there is a reduction in porosity to small molecules in early pregnancy that is more pronounced in later pregnancy [9]. Changes in breadth of glomerular pore size during pregnancy, as compared with postpartum, have also been reported, calculated by modeling from dextran clearances [10]. It is likely that there are dynamic changes throughout pregnancy in the magnitude of the filtration fraction and its constituents, with similar gestational changes in the glomerular filtration barrier permeability, but understanding remains limited.

Mechanisms of Gestational Change in Glomerular Filtration

The kidney has one of the largest pregnancy redistributions of blood flow compared with other nonreproductive organs. Yet, despite extensive recognition of this adaptation to pregnancy, there are few studies of pregnant women exploring potential mechanisms. In nonpregnant individuals, plasma volume expansion leads to increased glomerular filtration, and is likely in part to contribute to increased renal blood flow in pregnancy (see "Volume Regulation in Pregnancy" section later in this chapter). It is unlikely to exclusively mediate this, however, as maximal plasma volume expansion occurs at later gestation than the highest glomerular filtration rates.

Further augmentation of glomerular filtration can be achieved by protein loading, by amino acid infusion or by a high-protein meal. One study of 14 healthy pregnant women reported increments in glomerular filtration of 18, 10 and 12 percent following an amino acid infusion in early and late pregnancy and postpartum, respectively, compared with a control infusion of compound sodium lactate solution [11]. The authors propose this effect reflects recruitment of "dormant" nephrons, thus enabling assessment of "renal reserve." Rat studies of amino acid infusions in pregnant and nonpregnant animals confirm that there is a further increase in glomerular filtration in pregnant animals of the same magnitude as in the nonpregnant state, thus confirming that renal vasodilatory responses in pregnancy remain intact. Hence, mechanisms of autoregulation of glomerular filtration appear to remain intact and "renal

reserve" is maintained regardless of gestational adaptation.

Women with renal transplants also have renal adaptation during pregnancy comparable to healthy controls, despite preexisting compensatory renal hypertrophy, although the response is reduced. Interestingly, donor gender or age did not influence gestation-induced renal adaptation in a cohort of 20 renal transplant recipients [12].

Some authors propose that there is a reduction in threshold for autoregulation that may be protective against periods of hypoperfusion secondary to gestational hypotension, but this has not been formally assessed. Furthermore, the proportion of "renal reserve" recruitment in pregnancy is unclear. The contribution of limited reserve in women with CKD to renal function in pregnancy is explored in Chapters 2 and 5.

Glomerular Hemodynamic Studies

Single glomerular micropuncture studies measuring hydrostatic and oncotic pressure in Munich-Wistar rats have confirmed that there are no differences between pregnant and nonpregnant states despite an increased whole kidney glomerular filtration rate [13]. Although probable, the same mechanism for increased glomerular filtration in human pregnancy cannot be assumed as experimental changes in renal blood flow in rats appear to elicit a much wider response in glomerular filtration than is observed in humans. This is likely to be the consequence of filtration equilibrium occurring more proximally in the glomerular capillaries of rats than humans, and thus increments in plasma flow are able to continue to increase glomerular filtration. However, there is evidence from glomerular dynamic modeling studies in healthy pregnant women that changes in glomerular filtration are predominantly driven by augmented effective renal plasma flow [9], with some contribution from reduced plasma oncotic pressure [10]. Equal vasodilation of both afferent and efferent arterioles must be responsible, allowing increased renal plasma flow to augment ultrafiltration without increments in transglomerular hydrostatic pressure.

Hyperfiltration states (e.g. essential hypertension, type 1 diabetes) are considered to result in glomerular hypertension. The augmented filtration fraction necessary to maintain total glomerular filtration is associated with glomerular injury and secondary focal segmental glomerulosclerosis. Glomerular normotension is likely to explain why sequential pregnancies in women with normal kidney function are not associated with progressive renal injury, nor is there evidence of glomerular injury in multigravid rats.

Relaxin Studies

The presence of an intact corpus luteum plays an important, but not critical role in hemodynamic renal adaptation in pregnancy. The ovarian hormone relaxin rises minimally in the luteal phase then exponentially in early pregnancy, and has been demonstrated to mediate gestational changes. A study of nine women with pregnancies conceived by ovum donation, with undetectable serum relaxin, reported a reduction in plasma osmolality and an increase in creatinine clearance in the first trimester, but change from baseline was significantly less than in healthy controls with detectable relaxin [14].

Further mechanistic evidence is provided by rat models, which are summarized next [15]:

- Exogenous relaxin administration to chronically instrumented conscious nonpregnant, ovarectomized female and male rats results in renal hemodynamic changes comparable to those in pregnant animals.
- Anti-relaxin antibody administration to pregnant rats abrogates any gestational increase in renal blood flow or glomerular filtration.
- Relaxin infusion in nonpregnant rats reduces renal vasoconstrictor response to angiotensin II in vitro.

The relationship between relaxin concentration and renal adaption in humans is less clear. Healthy volunteers were administered intravenous human synthetic relaxin over six hours, but, despite a rapid rise in renal blood flow of up to 60 percent, there were no differences before and after treatment in glomerular filtration [16]. The absence of an association between relaxin administration and increased glomerular filtration may be temporal, as larger studies of chronic relaxin therapy over several weeks for heart failure and systemic sclerosis reported significant changes in creatinine clearance that were dose dependent. However, the influence of relaxin on the magnitude of gestational-associated change in filtration fraction is unknown.

The mechanism of relaxin-induced changes in renal blood flow has also been explored in rat models and appears to be mediated by the potent endothelial-derived vasodilator nitric oxide. Evidence is provided by the following studies [15]:

- Blockade of nitric oxide synthase with L-arginine analogs in chronically instrumented pregnant rats abrogated gestation-associated increases in renal blood flow and glomerular filtration, both with acute and chronic administration, and prevented renal adaptation if given in early pregnancy.
- L-arginine analogs blocked relaxin-induced increases in renal vasodilation and hyperfiltration and blunted myogenic reactivity in pregnant rats.
- Endothelial removal in rat renal arteries prevented relaxin-induced vasodilation.

The mechanism of induction of nitric oxide synthesis is unclear. There was no increase in endothelial nitric oxide synthase (eNOS) isoforms in mid-trimester pregnant rats compared with nonpregnant controls. One study reported reduced eNOS expression in pregnant animals, but higher renal inducible (iNOS) and neuronal (nNOS) expression than in nonpregnant animals, and increased protein abundance of the specific nNOS beta isoform in mid-trimester rats has been confirmed by others [15].

Endothelin B (ET_B) receptor activation appears to be contributory to gestation-associated renal adaptation. Evidence comes from the following studies [15]:

- ET_B receptor antagonists administered to pregnant rats prevented a gestational increase in renal vasodilation and hyperfiltration.
- ET_B receptor-deficient rats do not exhibit gestational renal adaptation.
- ET_B receptor antagonists abrogate renal adaptation in relaxin-treated nonpregnant rats.

It is unclear whether the renal effects of ET_B receptor activation are a consequence of increased expression, or another unknown mechanism. Similarly, the pathway by which relaxin elicits ET_B receptor activity has not been elucidated, as relaxin does not appear to stimulate ET_B receptor synthesis in vitro.

Matrix metalloproteinase-2 (MMP-2) has been proposed to be a potential downstream mediator of renal vasodilation in pregnancy by hydrolysis of big ET to ET_{1-32}, which interacts with ET_B receptors and is summarized in what follows [15]:

- MMP synthesis is increased in uterine fibroblasts in the presence of relaxin.
- MMP-2 is upregulated in small renal arteries of both midterm pregnant rats and nonpregnant rats with relaxin-induced renal vasodilation.

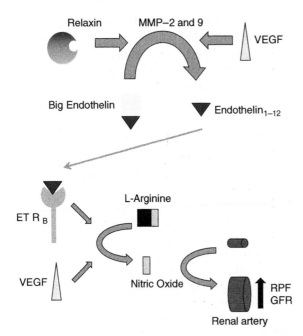

Figure 1.1 Mechanisms of glomerular hyperfiltration in pregnancy

- Inhibition of MMP-2 in pregnant rats or relaxin-treated rats reduced renal adaptation and enhanced renal artery myogenic reactivity.
- MMP-2 activity is increased in ET_B receptor-deficient rats, and therefore may act upstream of MMP-2 activation.

MMP-9 has been shown to be upregulated in small renal arteries isolated from short-term (four to six hours) relaxin-treated nonpregnant rats, but in this model MMP-2 expression was unchanged. Following administration of specific neutralizing antibodies MMP-9 was found to mediate relaxin-associated reduction in myogenic activity, but not MMP-2. However, if the rats were treated with relaxin for several days, MMP-2 activity was increased and the MMP-2 neutralizing antibody inhibited the blunting of myogenic activity. Thus length of exposure to relaxin in order to activate different mediator pathways is likely important.

McGuane and colleagues have recently reported the novel association between angiogenesis and relaxin-mediated vasodilation [17]. Nonpregnant rats were treated with a vascular endothelial growth factor (VEGR) receptor tyrosine kinase inhibitor (SU5416) before and during a five-day period of relaxin administration. Expected increases in renal plasma flow and GFR were abolished. *In vitro* studies support the role of angiogenic factors mediating relaxin-induced vasodilation. Pretreatment of small rat and mice renal arteries and human subcutaneous arteries with SU5416, placental growth factor (PlGF) or VEGF-neutralizing antibodies inhibited the vaso-dilator effects of relaxin, with evidence of upregulated MMP-2 activity [17].

Relaxin stimulates VEGF synthesis in endometrial cell lines and both VEGF and PlGF have been shown to upregulate MMP-9 in human aortic smooth muscle cells. Together these findings suggest that angiogenic factors may be important mediators of relaxin-induced vasodilation that have effects both upstream and downstream from vascular MMP activity.

A summary of the factors contributing to renal vasodilation and hyperfiltration with gestation is outlined in Figure 1.1.

Progesterone Studies

Evidence from pseudo-pregnancy in rats confirms that the feto-placental unit is not essential for renal adaptation to pregnancy. Furthermore, gestational increase in glomerular filtration occurs before maximal placental progesterone synthesis. However, removal of the placenta during mid-pregnancy abrogates changes in renal blood flow and glomerular filtration [18]. Progesterone, but not estrogen, administered to nonpregnant women results in up to 15 percent increase in inulin clearance and creatinine clearance, but only affected effective renal plasma flow, not glomerular filtration, when given acutely to men.

Other Glomerular Changes in Pregnancy

Glomerular Volume

A controversial study including renal biopsy specimens from 12 healthy pregnant women demonstrated increased glomerular volume. There was also evidence of glomerular endotheliosis despite the absence of proteinuria and hypertension, which had previously been proposed to be a hallmark of preeclampsia (although the severity of changes seen was less marked as compared to biopsies from women with preeclampsia) [19]. An autopsy series also confirmed that glomerular size is greater in in pregnancy compared with nonpregnant individuals, but that there were no differences in glomerular cellularity [20].

Glomerular Proteinuria

Total urinary protein excretion rises with gestation. The most widely recognized upper limit of "normal" is 300 mg/24 hours, derived from the upper 95 percent confidence interval (259.4 mg) from a study of 270 healthy pregnant women [21]. Older studies examined differences in protein filtration during pregnancy. Increased urine concentration of several plasma constituents is described (e.g. α-1 antitrypsin, transferrin, beta-lipoprotein, complement fractions β1-A-C, IgD and α-macroglobulin), whereas some urinary plasma proteins are reduced (e.g. thyroxine-binding prealbumin, IgG and IgA) and others are unchanged (e.g. hemopexin, haptoglobin and IgM) compared to nonpregnant women subjects, suggesting dynamic gestational changes in glomerular permeability.

There is a gestational increase in urinary albumin excretion with variable rates of resolution reported between 12 weeks and 12 months postpartum [9, 22, 23, 24]. Given the substantial increase in glomerular filtration and the molecular size of albumin, it might be anticipated that higher levels of albuminuria would be present. Tubular reuptake may reduce total urinary albumin concentrations, but gestation-associated increase in transferrin, a comparable-sized molecule to albumin, is considerably greater [25]. Selective tubular reuptake could be contributory, although it has been proposed that increased glomerular basement membrane negative charge could repel anionic plasma proteins, thus reducing their filtration and urinary excretion.

Vascular endothelial growth factor is responsible for the maintenance of podocyte and glomerular basement membrane integrity in nonpregnant individuals, and angiogenic balance is likely to play an important role in glomerular protein excretion during pregnancy, but direct relationships between glomerular structure and function and local or circulating angiogenic factors in healthy pregnancy are yet to be confirmed.

Tubular Changes in Pregnancy

Tubular Proteinuria

Renal tubules reabsorb most filtered proteins, but also catabolize proteins with excretion of constituent peptides and directly secrete proteins into urine. Filtered low-molecular proteins should be almost completely reabsorbed by the proximal tubule, but urinary levels of alpha-1 microglobulin, beta 2 microglobulin, retinol-binding protein and clara cell protein have been found to be increased in the second and third trimesters in healthy individuals in the absence of increased plasma concentrations [26]. This has led to the proposal that proximal tubular reabsorption capacity is either compromised during pregnancy or at capacity due to increased filtration.

Other changes in urinary protein composition with gestation include increased urinary excretion of tubular enzymes [25], which are of similar molecular weight to urinary lysosomal enzymes, suggesting further gestational changes in tubular function rather than increased filtration of circulating plasma enzymes.

Glycosuria

Glycosuria is more frequently recognized in pregnant than nonpregnant individuals despite no changes in serum glucose concentrations. Augmented glomerular filtration of glucose is likely to overwhelm proximal tubular reuptake [27], hence glucose is more readily detectable in the urine of pregnant women.

Uric Acid

Serum uric acid concentrations fall by approximately 25 percent in healthy pregnancy compared with nonpregnant controls, then increase toward term. Uric acid passes freely through the glomerulus, predominantly reabsorbed in the proximal tubule with reuptake of 90 percent of the filtered load along the nephron. Pregnancy is associated with altered handling of uric acid with lower plasma concentrations in early pregnancy associated with reduced tubular resorption [28]. Reuptake appears to be restored in later pregnancy, or increased plasma concentrations may be the consequence of a fall in glomerular filtration toward term.

Historically uric acid concentration was used as predictor of preeclampsia, as it was observed to rise before the onset of hypertension and proteinuria and was associated with reduced renal clearance. However, subsequently the ability of uric acid to differentiate between different hypertensive disorders has been disproven, and a meta-analysis of 41 studies including 3,913 women confirmed uric acid concentrations to be only a weak predictor of eclampsia and severe hypertension and not associated with intrauterine death [29]. Furthermore, discrimination between preeclampsia and preexisting renal disease is not possible. Assessment of uric acid concentration is no longer recommended to predict or diagnose hypertensive disorders of pregnancy.

Volume Regulation in Pregnancy

During pregnancy there is a net volume expansion of 6–8 liters, which includes 4–6 liters in the interstitium, and a 50 percent increase in plasma volume. There is a concomitant reduction in plasma osmolality of 10mOsm/kg, which is apparent in early pregnancy and persists until delivery. Postpartum there is substantial natriuresis to restore nonpregnant osmolality and extracellular volume [30]. Several reports suggest that inadequate volume expansion is associated with poor fetal growth, which is evident as early as weeks 5 and 10 [31].

Despite the reduction in osmolality, there is also progressive retention of approximately 900 mmol of sodium. Dynamic homeostatic mechanisms must be reset throughout gestation in order to accommodate changes in additional volume and reduced plasma osmolality. However, women given diuretics or salt restriction retain an appropriate neurohumoral antinatriuretic response [32].

It is unclear whether systemic vasodilatation leading to relative "underfill" is the primary stimulant for sodium and water retention or conversely if renal sodium reuptake is the initial event leading to plasma volume expansion. A study of women in the first trimester confirmed that both vasodilation and plasma volume expansion are already initiated by six weeks' gestation [33].

The following influences on volume and plasma osmolality have been described during pregnancy:

Vasodilation

Pregnancy-induced systemic vasodilation is predominantly mediated by nitric oxide and results in venous pooling, thus reducing effective circulating blood volume. "Underfill volume" sensing will be triggered, including renin-angiotensin-aldosterone system (RAAS) activity, atrial natriuretic peptide (ANP) suppression and antidiuretic hormone (ADH) release, leading to volume expansion throughout gestation.

Relaxin

Relaxin appears to play an important role in osmoregulatory gestational changes. Increments in circulating relaxin are temporally related to early plasma volume expansion [34]. A fall in plasma osmolality is blunted in women who conceived by ovum donation [14]. The presence of ovaries appeared to be critical to the development of plasma volume expansion and reduced plasma osmolality. Furthermore, relaxin-neutralizing antibodies infused in pregnant rats abolished gestational changes in plasma osmolality, and administration of exogenous relaxin to rats following ovarectomy was associated with a decrease in plasma osmolality [15].

Renin-Angiotensin-Aldosterone System (RAAS) Activation

In early pregnancy, plasma activity, total concentration and substrate or renin is enhanced in comparison with nonpregnant controls, resulting in increased plasma angiotensin II and aldosterone concentrations. Plasma aldosterone in pregnant women has been reported to be up to fourfold higher than in nonpregnant individuals [2]. RAAS activation occurs in spite of concurrent plasma volume expansion and increased renal blood flow. There is marked blunted vasopressor response to angiotensin II, while antinatriuretic activity is probably enhanced [35].

Although a resetting of activation of RAAS occurs, augmentation of activity is observed following usual triggers including sodium restriction, and reduced venous return due to supine or upright posture demonstrating highly sophisticated adaptation. Underlying mechanisms leading to enhanced renin synthesis are unclear. Increased circulating prostaglandins have been proposed to initiate vasodilation leading to relative volume depletion and stimulation of RAAS activity. In rat models, renin and aldosterone concentrations revert rapidly to prepregnant values after delivery, suggesting that nonpregnant sensing thresholds are quickly reestablished.

Atrial Natriuretic Peptide (ANP)

Atrial natriuretic peptide (ANP) concentrations are not increased in early pregnancy despite volume expansion. Elevated levels are found at later gestations corresponding to dilatation of the atrium. Resetting of plasma volume expansion stimulus for release must occur, and this is supported by meta-analysis [36]. ANP remains elevated postpartum with up to 148 percent increases in concentration compared with nonpregnant women [36], consistent with the period of natriuresis, and consistent with the finding of increased urinary cGMP postpartum, a mediator of ANP activity.

Some authors propose that there is a blunted response to ANP in pregnancy, which, although described in rats, has not been confirmed in humans. There is evidence of enhanced cGMP metabolism by phosphodiesterase-5 in the inner medullary collecting duct in gravid rat models, and inhibition of phosphodiesterase-5 abolished gestation associated refractoriness to ANP in pregnant rats. Whether this pathway is relevant in humans remains to be established.

Antidiuretic Hormone (ADH)/Vasopressin

In nonpregnant individuals, substantial ADH release would be elicited by a fall in plasma osmolality of 10mOsm/kg, inhibiting thirst and enhancing water excretion, but ADH does not appear to be triggered at the same threshold in pregnancy. Several human studies have demonstrated higher circulating ADH concentrations in pregnant women at the same plasma osmolality as nonpregnant controls, particularly in the first trimester, and these findings have been supported by rat models. One study of ADH concentrations reported no difference between pregnant and nonpregnant rats despite a reduction in plasma osmolality of 8mOsm/kg. Collecting duct aquaporin 2 expression was increased and appeared to be mediated by V2 vasopressin receptors [37].

Human chorionic gonadotrophin (hCG) may be contributory in early pregnancy adaptations in ADH. Six nonpregnant females were given hypertonic saline during the luteal phase of the menstrual cycle. Additional administration of hCG resulted in a reduction in plasma osmolality, ADH and thirst, which was not evident in control males [38].

ADH concentrations fall in later pregnancy compared with early pregnancy and ADH clearance increases three- to fourfold in the second and third trimesters. A placenta-derived vasopressinase has been identified, but its contribution to ADH mediated change is unclear.

Gestational volume expansion would also be expected to suppress ADH release, but does not occur in rat models This trigger may be "overridden" by systemic vasodilation leading to perceived under-filling of the vasculature, or due to resetting of the threshold for ADH release.

Tubuloglomerular Feedback

Tubuloglomerular feedback has been studied in chronically instrumented rats. In nonpregnant animals, plasma volume expansion is detected as increased tubular fluid volume delivery to the macular densa, leading to afferent arteriolar vasoconstriction and reduced glomerular filtration, thus regulating tubular fluid volume. In pregnant rats this response was not activated until higher rates of renal blood flow were present compared to nonpregnant controls [39], confirming a "resetting" of the threshold of volume expansion to suppress tubuloglomerular feedback. However, a response to increased renal plasma volumes was still observed, thus autoregulation is maintained in order to tolerate higher plasma volumes.

Electrolyte Homeostasis in Pregnancy

Volume expansion leads to net dilution of electrolytes during pregnancy. However, there is a net gain in total sodium, potassium and calcium achieved by the following mechanisms:

Sodium

Plasma sodium concentration falls by 4–5mmol/L during pregnancy. Filtered sodium load increases due to the elevated glomerular filtration rate, but reabsorption by the tubules is enhanced resulting in a net gain in sodium. Multiple contributory factors have been proposed and are outlined in Figure 1.2.

Aldosterone responsive epithelial Na channel (ENaC) activity in late pregnancy appears to be instrumental in sodium retention. ENaC channel mRNA expression in the renal collecting tubule has been demonstrated to increase in the presence of estrogen in vitro. Inhibition of renal ENaC in late pregnant rats blunted sodium retention and plasma volume expansion, and late gestation increase in blood pressure [40]. However, aldosterone responsive sodium chloride co-transporter (NCC) mRNA expression appears to be unchanged in pregnant rats compared to virgin controls [41] and an explanation for this discrepancy is unclear.

Potassium

There is a reduction in urinary potassium excretion during pregnancy leading to retention of approximately 350mmol of potassium despite elevated aldosterone concentrations and increased urinary bicarbonate excretion. Mineralocorticoids administered to healthy pregnant women in the third trimester had little effect on potassium excretion and the authors proposed this is due to the anti-

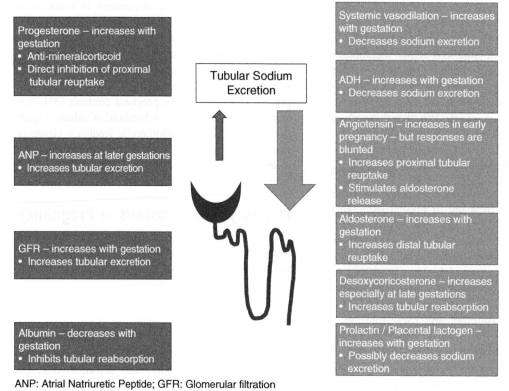

ANP: Atrial Natriuretic Peptide; GFR: Glomerular filtration

Figure 1.2 Influences on sodium excretion during pregnancy

mineralocorticoid effect of progesterone [42]. More recently, H+/K+ ATPase types 1 and 2 mRNA have been demonstrated to be increased in the cortex and medulla of late pregnant rats compared with virgin controls, which could explain the mechanism of potassium retention independent of aldosterone. [43] Precise gestational changes in potassium handing within the nephron are poorly understood.

Calcium

Calcium excretion increases during pregnancy by two- to threefold, and is proposed to be the consequence of increased glomerular filtration coupled with reduced reuptake in the thick ascending limb of the loop of Henle. Elevated plasma 1,25-dihydroxy-Vitamin D3 concentrations are observed in pregnancy, leading to increased intestinal absorption of calcium and suppression of parathyroid hormone (PTH) concentrations. PTH-induced tubular calcium reuptake is subsequently blunted. Calciuria is discussed in more detail in Chapter 18.

Acid-Base Homeostasis in Pregnancy

During pregnancy there is a net increase in hydrogen ion synthesis due to increased basal metabolic rate and calorific intake. Plasma pH is higher than healthy nonpregnant individuals during pregnancy, however, due to respiratory alkalemia driven by an elevated respiratory rate. A mild compensatory metabolic acidemia is also evident, with concentrations between 18 and 22mmol/l in healthy pregnant women. There is no evidence of gestational changes in renal bicarbonate reabsorption or hydrogen ion excretion in healthy pregnancy.

Assessment of Renal Function in Pregnancy

Creatinine production during pregnancy is unchanged during pregnancy, hence serum creatinine concentrations fall due to increased renal clearance. Gestation-specific reference ranges for creatinine concentration are not well defined. Accurate assessment

Table 1.1 Comparison for methods of assessment of glomerular filtration in pregnancy

Method of Assessment	Gold Standard Comparison	Overestimate/Underestimate
24-hour creatinine clearance	Inulin clearance	Significant correlation
Timed creatinine clearance	24-hour creatinine clearance	Significant correlation
	Inulin clearance	
Cockcroft Gault	Inulin clearance	Underestimates
	Creatinine clearance	Overestimates using current weight and underestimates using prepregnancy weight
Modified Diet in Renal Disease Formula	Inulin clearance	Underestimates
	24-hour creatinine clearance	
Chronic Kidney Disease – EPI	24-hour creatinine clearance	Underestimates
Cystatin-C	24-hour creatinine clearance	Underestimates

of glomerular filtration rate in pregnancy is challenging, and comparisons of estimates with formal infusion clearances are presented in Table 1.1.

Glomerular Filtration Rate (GFR) Estimation Formulae

Formulae to estimate glomerular filtration rate (GFR) have been studied during pregnancy. Comparing the modified diet and renal disease (MDRD) formula with inulin clearance [44] and the chronic kidney disease-EPI formula with creatinine clearance[45] both underestimate filtration by approximately 20 percent. These formulae should not be used during pregnancy. Similarly, formulae that include weight or body surface area underperform, as they are dynamic during pregnancy and do not reflect kidney size. For example, a study of the Cockcroft-Gault formula overestimated glomerular filtration by approximately 40mls/min compared with inulin clearance.[44]

Twenty-Four-Hour Creatinine Clearance

Twenty-four-hour creatinine clearance is the best assessment of glomerular filtration in clinical practice. Although there is the recognized limitation of variable proximal tubular creatinine secretion, independent changes in urinary creatinine excretion compared with serum creatinine concentration with gestation are not reported [6], thus alterations in tubular secretion are unlikely. However, pooling of urine in dilated ureters and incomplete bladder emptying may impair accurate timed collections resulting in falsely low clearance. Some authors propose that women should lie in the left lateral position prior to micturition for an hour in order to minimize this confounder, although this is unlikely to be practical for most women. Moreover, studies comparing 24-hour creatinine clearance with inulin clearance have not identified significant differences between measurements [4, 46].

Cystatin C

Cystatin is proposed to be a more accurate indicator of glomerular filtration at the higher end of the normal range than creatinine. Cystatin is freely filtered at the glomerulus, actively reabsorbed and catabolized by tubular cells. Several studies of cystatin in pregnancy identify limitations as a useful marker of glomerular filtration. Concentrations are shown to rise in the second trimester rather than the anticipated fall with increasing glomerular filtration. Cystatin is an anionic 13kDa molecule; thus it would be expected that increased filtration occurs as a consequence of the postulated reduced negative charge of the basement membrane with gestation. An explanation for this paradoxical finding is unclear.

Several reports support the role of cystatin as a diagnostic marker of preeclampsia with correlation reported between serum concentrations and 24-hour creatinine clearance [47]. Elevated concentrations are described in women with chronic hypertension, but the role of cystatin as a predictive or diagnostic marker of superimposed preeclampsia in women with CKD has not been explored.

Mechanisms of Pregnancy-Associated Progression in Renal Disease

The pathophysiology of pregnancy-associated progression of renal disease in women with more severe CKD is unclear. Micropuncture studies in healthy rats with five or more pregnancies confirmed no differences in glomerular or whole kidney hemodynamics compared with nonpregnant controls. In rat models of CKD due to anti-glomerular basement membrane glomerulonephritis, raised glomerular capillary pressure was observed in nonpregnant females, but pregnancy resulted in no further change in glomerular pressure [48]. There was a tendency for an increase in overall glomerular filtration, single nephron glomerular filtration and renal blood flow in pregnant rats with glomerulonephritis. However, in this model there were no differences in glomerular filtration between rats with experimental glomerulonephritis and controls, hence the severity of kidney disease may not be sufficient to be associated with an accelerated decline in function.

Baylis and Wilson assessed glomerular hyperfiltration in uninephrectomized rats with high dietary protein feeding following five repetitive pregnancies [49]. Again there was evidence of raised glomerular pressure and also elevated single nephron glomerular filtration and glomerular plasma flow rate in the nonpregnant operated animals compared with controls, but single nephron GFR and glomerular plasma flow rates were lower in repetitively pregnant rats compared with nonpregnant animals. There was still a significant but variable increase in single nephron glomerular filtration in response to amino acid infusion suggestive of preserved renal reserve.

Finally, pregnancy-associated glomerular hemodynamic changes were assessed in the spontaneously hypertensive rat. Despite marked glomerular hypertension compared with normotensive controls, there were no differences in glomerular pressure between mid-gestation pregnant and nonpregnant animals, nor any evidence of reduced glomerular filtration after repeated pregnancies [50]. Interestingly there was no increase at mid-gestation in renal vascular resistance, nor was there an increase in renal blood flow in response to an amino acid infusion in both moderately and severely hypertensive animals suggestive of a loss of renal vasodilatory response potentially due to structural adaptations.

Other proposed mechanisms of pregnancy-associated acceleration in renal disease include subacute thrombotic microangiopathy, podocyte loss, angiogenic imbalance and preexisting endothelial dysfunction; however, none has been studied in detail. A potential protective anti-fibrotic role of relaxin, described in nonpregnant patients with CKD, has not been explored in pregnancy.

Conclusion

Remarkable physiological adaptation to pregnancy occurs in the renal vasculature, glomerulus and tubules. Understanding the underlying mechanism of augmented glomerular filtration without hyperfiltration injury is evolving, and could be invaluable to inform development of therapeutic strategies for nonpregnant patients with CKD. However, pathophysiology of pregnancy-associated progression of renal impairment remains elusive, and requires further study in order to prevent this condition and the catastrophic consequences for new mothers, their infants and their families.

References

1. Brown MA. Urinary tract dilatation in pregnancy. *Am J Obstet Gynecol*. 1990;**164**:641–643.

2. Conrad KP GL, Lindheimer MD. The kidney in normal pregnancy and preeclampsia. In Lindheimer M, Roberts JM, Cunningham FG, ed. *Chesley's hypertensive disorders in pregnancy*. San Diego, CA: Elsevier Inc.; 2009:297–334.

3. Dunlop W. Investigations into the influence of posture on renal plasma flow and glomerular filtration rate during late pregnancy. *British journal of obstetrics and gynaecology*. 1976;**83**:17–23.

4. Sims EA, Krantz KE. Serial studies of renal function during pregnancy and the puerperium in normal women. *J Clin Invest*. 1958;**37**:1764–1774.

5. Assali NS, Dignam WJ, Dasgupta K. Renal function in human pregnancy: Effects of venous pooling on renal hemodynamics and water, electrolyte, and aldosterone excretion during gestation. *The journal of laboratory and clinical medicine*. 1959;**54**:394–408.

6. Davison JM, Noble MC. Serial changes in 24 hour creatinine clearance during normal menstrual cycles and the first trimester of pregnancy. *British journal of obstetrics and gynaecology*. 1981;**88**:10–17.

7. Paaby P, Brochner-Mortensen J, Fjeldborg P, Raffn K, Larsen CE, Moller-Petersen J. Endogenous overnight creatinine clearance compared with 51cr-edta clearance during the menstrual cycle. *Acta medica Scandinavica*. 1987;**222**:281–284.

8. Davison JM, Dunlop W, Ezimokhai M. 24-hour creatinine clearance during the third trimester of normal pregnancy. *British journal of obstetrics and gynaecology*. 1980;**87**:106–109.

9. Roberts M, Lindheimer MD, Davison JM. Altered glomerular permselectivity to neutral dextrans and heteroporous membrane modeling in human pregnancy. *Am J Physiol*. 1996;**270**:F338–343.

10. Milne JE, Lindheimer MD, Davison JM. Glomerular heteroporous membrane modeling in third trimester and postpartum before and during amino acid infusion. *Am J Physiol Renal Physiol*. 2002;**282**: F170–175.

11. Sturgiss SN, Wilkinson R, Davison JM. Renal reserve during human pregnancy. *Am J Physiol*. 1996;**271**: F16–20.

12. Smith MC, Ward MK, Sturgiss SN, Milne JE, Davison JM. Sex and the pregnant kidney: Does renal allograft gender influence gestational renal adaptation in renal transplant recipients? *Transplant Proc*. 2004;**36**:2639–2642.

13. Baylis C. The mechanism of the increase in glomerular filtration rate in the twelve-day pregnant rat. *J Physiol*. 1980;**305**:405–414.

14. Smith MC, Murdoch AP, Danielson LA, Conrad KP, Davison JM. Relaxin has a role in establishing a renal response in pregnancy. *Fertility and sterility*. 2006;**86**:253–255.

15. Conrad KP, Davison JM. The renal circulation in normal pregnancy and preeclampsia: Is there a place for relaxin? *Am J Physiol Renal Physiol*. 2014;**306**: F1121–1135.

16. Smith MC, Danielson LA, Conrad KP, Davison JM. Influence of recombinant human relaxin on renal hemodynamics in healthy volunteers. *J Am Soc Nephrol*. 2006;**17**:3192–3197.

17. McGuane JT, Danielson LA, Debrah JE, Rubin JP, Novak J, Conrad KP. Angiogenic growth factors are new and essential players in the sustained relaxin vasodilatory pathway in rodents and humans. *Hypertension*. 2011;**57**:1151–1160.

18. Matthews BF, Taylor DW. Effects of pregnancy on inulin and para-aminohippurate clearances in the anaesthetized rat. *J Physiol*. 1960;**151**:385–389.

19. Strevens H, Wide-Swensson D, Hansen A, Horn T, Ingemarsson I, Larsen S, Willner J, Olsen S. Glomerular endotheliosis in normal pregnancy and pre-eclampsia. *BJOG*. 2003;**110**:831–836.

20. Sheehan HL. Renal morphology in preeclampsia. *Kidney Int*. 1980;**18**:241–252.

21. Higby K, Suiter CR, Phelps JY, Siler-Khodr T, Langer O. Normal values of urinary albumin and total protein excretion during pregnancy. *Am J Obstet Gynecol*. 1994;**171**:984–989.

22. Taylor AA, Davison JM. Albumin excretion in normal pregnancy. *Am J Obstet Gynecol*. 1997;**177**:1559–1560.

23. Wright A, Steele P, Bennett JR, Watts G, Polak A. The urinary excretion of albumin in normal pregnancy. *British journal of obstetrics and gynaecology*. 1987;**94**:408–412.

24. Baweja S, Kent A, Masterson R, Roberts S, McMahon LP. Prediction of pre-eclampsia in early pregnancy by estimating the spot urinary albumin: Creatinine ratio using high-performance liquid chromatography. *BJOG*. 2011;**118**:1126–1132.

25. Cheung CK, Lao T, Swaminathan R. Urinary excretion of some proteins and enzymes during normal pregnancy. *Clinical chemistry*. 1989;**35**:1978–1980.

26. Kronborg C, Vittinghus E, Allen J, Knudsen UB. Excretion patterns of large and small proteins in pre-eclamptic pregnancies. *Acta Obstet Gynecol Scand*. 2011;**90**:897–902.

27. Davison JM, Hytten FE. The effect of pregnancy on the renal handling of glucose. *British journal of obstetrics and gynaecology*. 1975;**82**:374–381.

28. Dunlop W, Davison JM. The effect of normal pregnancy upon the renal handling of uric acid. *British journal of obstetrics and gynaecology*. 1977;**84**:13–21.

29. Thangaratinam S, Ismail KM, Sharp S, Coomarasamy A, Khan KS, Tests in prediction of pre-eclampsia severity review g: Accuracy of serum uric acid in predicting complications of pre-eclampsia: A systematic review. *BJOG*. 2006;**113**:369–378.

30. Lindheimer MD, Davison JM. Osmoregulation, the secretion of arginine vasopressin and its metabolism during pregnancy. *European journal of endocrinology / European Federation of Endocrine Societies*. 1995;**132**:133–143.

31. Duvekot JJ, Cheriex EC, Pieters FA, Menheere PP, Schouten HJ, Peeters LL. Maternal volume homeostasis in early pregnancy in relation to fetal growth restriction. *Obstet Gynecol*. 1995;**85**:361–367.

32. Lindheimer MD, Barron WM, Davison JM. Osmoregulation of thirst and vasopressin release in pregnancy. *Am J Physiol*. 1989;**257**:F159–169.

33. Chapman AB, Abraham WT, Zamudio S, Coffin C, Merouani A, Young D, Johnson A, Osorio F, Goldberg C, Moore LG, Dahms T, Schrier RW. Temporal relationships between hormonal and hemodynamic changes in early human pregnancy. *Kidney Int*. 1998;**54**:2056–2063.

34. Sherwood OD. Relaxin. In: Knobil E NJ, ed. *The physiology of pregnancy*. New York: Raven Press; 1994:861–1009.

35. Gant NF, Whalley PJ, Everett RB, Worley RJ, MacDonald PC. Control of vascular reactivity in pregnancy. *Am J Kidney Dis.* 1987;**9**:303–307.

36. Castro LC, Hobel CJ, Gornbein J. Plasma levels of atrial natriuretic peptide in normal and hypertensive pregnancies: A meta-analysis. *Am J Obstet Gynecol.* 1994;**171**:1642–1651.

37. Ohara M, Martin PY, Xu DL, St John J, Pattison TA, Kim JK, Schrier RW. Upregulation of aquaporin 2 water channel expression in pregnant rats. *J Clin Invest.* 1998;**101**:1076–1083.

38. Davison JM, Shiells EA, Philips PR, Lindheimer MD. Influence of humoral and volume factors on altered osmoregulation of normal human pregnancy. *Am J Physiol.* 1990;**258**:F900–907.

39. Barron WM, Durr JA, Schrier RW, Lindheimer MD. Role of hemodynamic factors in osmoregulatory alterations of rat pregnancy. *Am J Physiol.* 1989;**257**:R909–916.

40. West CA, Han W, Li N, Masilamani SM. Renal epithelial sodium channel is critical for blood pressure maintenance and sodium balance in the normal late pregnant rat. *Experimental physiology.* 2014;**99**:816–823.

41. West CA, McDonough AA, Masilamani SM, Verlander JW, Baylis C. The renal sodium chloride co-transporter, ncc, is unchanged in the mid pregnant rat and decreased in the late pregnant rat despite avid renal sodium retention. *Am J Physiol Renal Physiol.* 2015;ajprenal 00147 02015.

42. Ehrlich EN, Lindheimer MD. Effect of administered mineralocorticoids or acth in pregnant women: Attenuation of kaliuretic influence of mineralocorticoids during pregnancy. *J Clin Invest.* 1972;**51**:1301–1309.

43. West C, Qiu E, Baylis C, Gumz M. [312-pos]: Mechanisms of renal potassium retention during late pregnancy. *Pregnancy hypertension.* 2015;**5**:153.

44. Smith MC, Moran P, Ward MK, Davison JM. Assessment of glomerular filtration rate during pregnancy using the mdrd formula. *BJOG.* 2008;**115**:109–112.

45. Alper AB, Yi Y, Rahman M, Webber LS, Magee L, Von Dadelszen P, Pridjian G, Aina-Mumuney A, Saade G, Morgan J, Nuwayhid B, Belfort M, Puschett J. Performance of estimated glomerular filtration rate prediction equations in preeclamptic patients. *Am J Perinatol.* **28**:425–430.

46. Davison JM, Hytten FE. Glomerular filtration during and after pregnancy. *The Journal of obstetrics and gynaecology of the British Commonwealth.* 1974;**81**:588–595.

47. Moodley J, Gangaram R, Khanyile R, Ojwang PJ. Serum cystatin c for assessment of glomerular filtration rate in hypertensive disorders of pregnancy. *Hypertens Pregnancy.* 2004;**23**:309–317.

48. Baylis C. Renal disease in gravid animal models. *Am J Kidney Dis.* 1987;**9**:350–353.

49. Baylis C, Wilson CB. Sex and the single kidney. *Am J Kidney Dis.* 1989;**13**:290–298.

50. Baylis C. Immediate and long-term effects of pregnancy on glomerular function in the shr. *Am J Physiol.* 1989;**257**:F1140–1145.

Prepregnancy Counseling and Risk Assessment

Matt Hall and Liz Lightstone

Introduction

Fifty years ago, it was common for women with chronic kidney disease (CKD) to be advised against pregnancies, based on contemporary case series of very poor outcomes for mother and infant [1]. In recent times, pregnancy outcomes are far better, although women with CKD still represent a high-risk pregnancy group [2]. Increased risks are identified not only in women with advanced kidney disease but even in women with CKD stages 1 and 2 (baseline estimated glomerular filtration rate > 60 ml/min/1.73 m^2) [3]. Physicians in primary and secondary care need to be alert to advising women with renal disease prior to pregnancy that they might be at risk and inform them of the nature of those risks.

Aims of Prepregnancy Counseling

Prepregnancy counseling is an opportunity to:

- set expectations for likelihood of conception and pregnancy progress, and introduce patients to assisted conception, surrogacy or adoption options when appropriate;
- discuss potential risks to maternal health resulting from a pregnancy;
- discuss potential adverse fetal outcomes;
- adjust medications to minimize complication rates; and
- consider the optimal timing for a planned pregnancy.

Progressive improvements in maternal and fetal outcomes for women with CKD have meant that it is unusual to advise women with CKD against considering a pregnancy. Instead, the purpose of prepregnancy counseling should be to outline and attempt to quantify potential risks involved so that the patient and their partner can come to their decision on whether to, and when to, proceed with an attempted pregnancy. Observational surveys of patients' experiences reported that almost all women attending prepregnancy counseling found the process informative and useful in decision-making [4].

Who Should Have Prepregnancy Counseling?

Clinicians should consider whether a woman of childbearing age has a condition that might either directly influence the ability to complete a successful pregnancy, or require treatment that might adversely affect outcomes. This is particularly relevant for women with CKD where the treatment of even those with mild disease (for example, angiotensin-converting enzyme inhibitors for proteinuric glomerulopathies) could have a major effect on the fetus.

Identification of women with CKD has increased over the past decade, predominantly due to the widespread introduction of estimated glomerular filtration (eGFR) reporting by biochemistry laboratories. This calculated value accounts for some of the variability in relationship between serum creatinine and true GFR by factoring in the patient's age, gender and ethnicity. Most laboratories currently report estimated GFR derived from the CKD-EPI formula [5].

The incidence of adverse pregnancy outcomes is increased in women at all stages of CKD [3], so it can be argued that all women with CKD should be offered prepregnancy counseling, including those with normal excretory renal function. It is intuitive that women with more advanced renal disease, those receiving dialysis and those who have received a renal transplant are likely to be at higher risk of adverse outcomes than those with CKD stage 1 or 2, and this is reflected in case series. There is contradictory evidence from observational studies on whether women with early CKD, normal blood pressure and absence of albuminuria (for example, those with isolated microscopic hematuria) develop more adverse pregnancy outcomes than the general population. A prospective cohort study including 370 women with CKD stage 1 (baseline eGFR >

90ml/min/1.73 m^2) and 87 women with CKD stage 2 (baseline eGFR 60-89ml/min/1.73 m^2) reported higher rates of preterm delivery, lower birth weights, greater requirement for neonatal intensive care unit admission and higher rates of Caesarean section compared with healthy controls [3]. Conversely, a registry study of more than 5,000 pregnancies in Norway did not identify a difference in rates of adverse pregnancy outcomes between women with baseline eGFR 60–89ml/min/1.73 m^2 and those with eGFR $\geq$ 90ml/min/1.73 m^2 except in women also known to have hypertension [6]. Interpretation of both studies is partially limited by inadequate data on progression rates of CKD prior to pregnancy, confounding comorbidity status, degree of proteinuria or hypertension and longer-term follow-up. Whether to offer prepregnancy counseling to women with normal excretory renal function, normal blood pressure and absence of proteinuria will be determined in part by resource availability. Their risk of adverse pregnancy outcomes is likely to be similar to that of the general population, but, as yet, there is insufficient data to accurately identify those in need of enhanced monitoring.

Most published data identify baseline eGFR, blood pressure control and proteinuria as the key determinants to pregnancy outcomes, rather than the etiology of kidney disease. However, women with known, suspected or possible genetic components to their renal condition may benefit from genetic counseling and investigation in addition to standard prepregnancy counseling from the renal clinic, irrespective of their renal parameters. Rapid progress in renal genetics within the past 15 years has greatly enhanced the identification of genetic diagnoses for patients. Currently, about one in five patients developing kidney disease prior to 25 years of age have an identifiable monogenic cause, and this figure is likely to rise further as the linear annual increase in identified gene defects continues [7]. Therefore, women (or their partners) with a known family history of renal disease, onset of renal disease in childhood (particularly those with glomerular disease or multisystem syndromes) or phenotypes consistent with known monogenic diseases without family history (suggestive of *de novo* mutations causing, for example, autosomal dominant polycystic kidney disease) should be offered renal and genetic prepregnancy counseling. This can facilitate estimation of the risk of subsequent children inheriting the condition, and also allow consideration of preimplantation genetic diagnosis.

Irrespective of etiology of renal disease, baseline eGFR, blood pressure and proteinuria, women with renal disease and previous adverse pregnancy outcomes should be offered prepregnancy counseling within a multidisciplinary setting.

Every consultation should be individualized to the potential parents' circumstances. An example approach is given in Table 2.1.

Conception Advice

The optimum timing of pregnancy for women with CKD will be influenced by:

- ability to stabilize relapsing-remitting conditions, such as systemic lupus erythematosus (SLE), nephrotic syndromes or vasculitis;
- control of blood pressure;
- degree of renal dysfunction;
- rate of decline in renal function and potential for future renal transplantation;
- maternal age and fertility reserve;
- medication; and
- social and relationship factors.

Disease Remission and Control

Women with renal diseases associated with relapses should be advised to postpone pregnancy until their condition is stable and optimized. This is particularly true for SLE, as fully discussed in Chapter 14. Nephrotic syndrome in early pregnancy has been associated with particularly poor outcomes in reported series [8, 9]. It is intuitive that conditions amenable to treatment, such as minimal change disease or membranous nephropathy, should be in remission prior to a planned pregnancy on the minimum medication required, although interventional studies to support this approach are lacking. Similarly, women with small-vessel vasculitis should be in sustained remission and appropriate medication at minimized doses prior to pregnancy.

Blood Pressure Control

Chronic hypertension is a predictor of adverse pregnancy outcomes in the general population. Rates of preterm delivery (18 percent vs. 6 percent), small for gestational age (23 percent vs. 5 percent) and perinatal death (4.6 percent vs. 0.8 percent) are significantly

Table 2.1 Example structure for prepregnancy counseling discussion

Planning conception	• Confirmation of current pregnancy status prior to counseling
	• Identify risk factors for subfertility
	   . Age
	   . Severity of renal dysfunction
	   . Previous or current treatment with cytotoxic therapy and contraceptives
	• Evaluate optimum timing for planned pregnancy
	   . Disease/transplant function stability
	   . Likelihood/requirement for renal transplantation in near future
	   . Age and fertility
	• Medicine optimization
	   . Exchange teratogenic medication with pregnancy-safe alternatives (for example, mycophenolate derivatives for azathioprine)
	   . Minimize doses of corticosteroids while maintaining disease stability
	   . Omit nonessential medications when possible (for example, statins for cardiovascular disease primary prevention in CKD)
	• Discuss contraception if timing of pregnancy not currently optimal
	• Discuss assisted conception, preimplantation genetic diagnosis, surrogacy and adoption when appropriate

Assessing maternal and fetal risk	• Identify risk factors for adverse maternal and fetal outcomes
	   . Severity of renal dysfunction
	   . Blood pressure control
	   . Etiology of renal disease
	   . Proteinuria
	   . Past obstetric outcomes
	• Estimate adverse outcome risks
	   . Loss of maternal renal function
	   . Dialysis
	   . Preeclampsia
	   . Nephrotic syndrome and venous thromboembolism
	   . Urinary tract infection
	   . Renal transplant rejection/dysfunction
	   . Preterm delivery and sequelae
	   . Intrauterine growth restriction
	   . Stillbirth and neonatal death
	   . Neonatal intensive care unit admission

Set expectations	• Outline the recommended frequency of monitoring visits during a pregnancy • Discuss potential "worst case" scenarios to consider according to pregnancy risk profile • Reassure women that, following counseling, their decision to proceed with a planned pregnancy (or not) will be fully supported by the multidisciplinary team

higher for women with preexisting chronic hypertension but normal renal function [10].

A similar association has been identified in women with CKD; however, the data are less clear. Two retrospective studies identified hypertension at conception (mean arterial pressure > 105mmHg and diastolic blood pressure > 90mmHg, respectively) as an independent risk factor for subsequent fetal death with odds ratio of 10.5 and 20.5 [11, 12]. Other retrospective studies reported hypertension to be associated with poor fetal outcomes in univariate [13, 14] and multivariate [15] analyses.

A prospective study of 49 women with CKD stages 3 to 5 prior to pregnancy failed to identify hypertension as an independent predictor of fetal loss, small for gestational age or accelerated loss of maternal renal function, however [16]. Similarly, analysis of prospective data comparing controls with women with CKD stage 1 found that baseline hypertension was independently associated with preterm delivery and need for Caesarean section, but not small for gestational age or neonatal care unit admission [3]. It is plausible that the impact of chronic hypertension on pregnancy outcomes is overwhelmed by the impact of more advanced kidney disease to account for these findings, or that these studies are underpowered to estimate effect.

How to treat elevated blood pressure and *whether* to treat elevated blood pressure prior to pregnancy remains controversial. For women with hypertension during pregnancy but without CKD, the CHIPS trial offers support for the safety of targeting a diastolic blood pressure of 80–85mmHg versus 100–105mmHg), using labetalol predominantly, with no increase in reported adverse fetal events. The occurrence of severe maternal hypertension ($\geq$ 160/110mmHg) was lower in women treated to the lower target, but this did not result in any other benefits in terms of maternal morbidity [17]. For nonpregnant patients with CKD, progression of excretory dysfunction is reduced with tight blood pressure control [18, 19], but, during pregnancy, international guidelines fail to agree on target blood pressure [20], and there is no published evidence to support the benefit of blood pressure control prior to conception to improve pregnancy outcomes. Therefore, it is intuitive, but not evidence-based practice, to recommend that women with CKD are established on appropriate antihypertensive medication to achieve target blood pressure prior to conception in order to minimize their risk of CKD progression, rather than to prevent adverse maternal or fetal events during pregnancy.

Renal Dysfunction, Rate of GFR Decline and Fertility

Adverse maternal and fetal outcomes are more common with more severe renal dysfunction (see Risks to Maternal Health and Risks to Fetal Health). Although some outcomes for women with CKD stages 1 and 2 are not as good as for the general population [3], most pregnancies will result in delivery of a healthy infant with minimal, if any, long-term detriment to maternal health. Conversely, pregnancies for women with CKD stages 4 and 5 and those receiving dialysis are highly likely to result in early delivery, preeclampsia and maternal morbidity [21]. Finally, pregnancy outcomes for women with an established and well-functioning renal transplant are generally better than those for women with advanced CKD [22].

The timing of a planned pregnancy should be in the context of whether risks associated with the current level of renal function are acceptable to the mother or whether waiting until function has declined to the point of receiving a renal transplant would be preferential. This will, in turn, depend on the rate of decline of renal function, the patient's suitability for renal transplantation, the availability of donor organs and maternal fertility reserve. Following renal transplantation, published guidelines recommend that women wait for up to two years before attempting conception so that the risk of acute rejection is lower and medications are minimized (see Chapter 11). For example, a 25-year-old woman with progressive CKD 4, estimated GFR 18ml/min/1.73 m^2 and a sibling willing and able to donate a kidney might be best advised to await transplantation prior to attempted conception. Alternatively, a 38-year-old woman with stable CKD 4, estimated GFR 24ml/min/1.73 m^2 and multiple HLA antibodies might not have the possibility of or necessity for a renal transplant within the following five years, by which time fertility might be significantly impaired.

Fertility is also impaired by CKD. Conception rates have been reported as 60 per 1,000 women/year in the general UK population compared with 20–25 in renal transplant recipients and 5 in dialysis recipients [23–25]. Published conception rate data for women with pre-end-stage renal disease are unavailable; however, multiple pathophysiological alterations in CKD lead to impaired ovulation (hyperprolactinemia, decreased GnRH pulsatility) [26], decreased ovarian reserve [27] and reduced libido [28]. Options for assisted conception and associated risks are discussed in Chapter 4.

Risks to Maternal Health

Pregnancy-Induced Loss of Renal Function

Changes in systemic and renal physiology in pregnancy occur early (see Chapter 1). The ability of

Table 2.2 Risk of adverse maternal outcomes (14, 16, 21, 30) RRT, renal replacement therapy; SCr, serum creatinine; GFR, glomerular filtration rate

	Persistent loss of 25 percent kidney function following pregnancy	Need for RRT within one year of pregnancy	Preeclampsia
Baseline SCr < 140μmol/l, eGFR > 45 ml/min/1.73 m^2	0–6%	0–1%	15–25%
Baseline SCr 140-240μmol/l, eGFR 30-44 ml/min/1.73 m^2	33–55%	0–10%	20–60%
Baseline SCr > 240μmol/l, eGFR < 30ml/min/1.73 m^2	50–67%	10–35%	40–75%

renal parenchyma and vasculature to adapt to pregnancy reflects the magnitude of renal "reserve" as made available by vascular dilatation and mesangial relaxation. Most patients with mild renal disease – estimated GFR > 45 ml/min/1.73 m^2 – demonstrate a reduction in serum creatinine and blood pressure during mid-pregnancy, in common with women without renal disease, with parameters returning to baseline values shortly after pregnancy [29]. Those with more advanced renal disease may have a blunted physiological response to pregnancy, manifest as progressive hypertension and renal function decline.

Historic case series have defined baseline renal function as mild, moderate or severe based on serum urea [1], creatinine [14, 21] or estimated GFR [16, 30], making direct comparisons of results challenging. Nevertheless, irrespective of criteria used, the risk of losing renal function as a result of the physiological strain of pregnancy is dependent on baseline renal function. For women with normal or mildly impaired excretory renal function, it is unlikely that pregnancy will lead to loss of kidney function, and the risk of needing dialysis within a year of pregnancy is very low. Conversely, women with baseline creatinine > 180μmol/l or estimated GFR < 30 ml/min/1.73 m^2 are more likely than not to sustain a persistent loss of at least 25 percent of their kidney function after pregnancy and one in three will require dialysis within a year of pregnancy (Table 2.2) [2].

An independent, or confounding, effect of baseline blood pressure, proteinuria or etiology of renal disease on risk of pregnancy-induced loss of renal function has been less well defined. For women with CKD stage 1 (estimated GFR > 90 ml/min/1.73 m^2), multivariate regression analysis did not identify either hypertension or proteinuria as risk factors for CKD

progression [3]. Although maternal hypertension is linked to poor fetal outcomes [13–15], and is a known risk factor for progression of CKD outside of pregnancy, there is no evidence that its presence precipitates accelerated loss of renal function from pregnancy. For women with baseline estimated GFR < 40 ml/min/1.73 m^2, proteinuria > 1g/day was associated with accelerated loss of renal function postpartum as compared with lesser degrees of protein loss [16].

Loss of renal function following pregnancy is more common in renal transplant recipients than in other patients with CKD, particularly those with baseline serum creatinine > 150μmol/l. Twenty percent of patients had graft dysfunction during pregnancy, but a persistent increase in creatinine from baseline was not identified in those with baseline serum creatinine ≤ 150μmol/l. No difference in two-year graft survival was identified between renal transplant recipients who had completed a pregnancy and controls (93 percent vs. 94 percent, p = 0.7) [31] (see Chapter 11).

Prepregnancy counseling is an opportunity to forewarn patients of the potential impact of pregnancy on their renal disease. For most, it is a reassurance that long-term detrimental effects are unlikely and the risk of dialysis is very small. Women with advanced renal disease (estimated GFR < 30 ml/min/1.73 m^2) will need to be informed of the unpredictable but significant likelihood of needing dialysis during or shortly after pregnancy.

Preeclampsia

The incidence of preeclampsia in the general population is approximately 3–8 percent, depending on the criteria used (see also Chapter 18). The revised 2014

International Society for the Study of Hypertension in Pregnancy criteria define preeclampsia as:

- New-onset hypertension ($\geq$ 140mmHg systolic or $\geq$ 90mmHg diastolic) after 20 weeks' gestation; plus EITHER:
- Other maternal organ dysfunction:
  - Renal insufficiency (creatinine $\geq$ 90µmol/l), or
  - Liver involvement (elevated transaminases or upper abdominal pain), or
  - Neurological complications, or
  - Hematological complications, OR
- Fetal growth restriction, OR
- Proteinuria (24-hour urinary protein $\geq$ 300mg/day, or urine protein:creatinine ratio $\geq$ 30mg/mmol) [20].

Determining the incidence of preeclampsia in women with CKD is intrinsically complicated by the defining criteria used, since many women will have preexisting hypertension, proteinuria and/or renal insufficiency. No single parameter can reliably differentiate the development of preeclampsia from progressive or *de novo* renal disease, although the presence of extra-renal, extra-placental clinical features, such as hematological or liver abnormalities is strongly suggestive of the syndrome. There is increasing evidence to support the clinical utility of measuring angiogenic factors in serum to assist in diagnosing preeclampsia in this population [32], although this is not common practice at present.

It is, therefore, difficult to predict the risk of preeclampsia for individual women with CKD since the observational data available are not directly comparable. Nevertheless, it is accepted that CKD is a strong and independent risk factor for developing preeclampsia. Williams and Davison's review of published data between 1985 and 2007 reports the incidence of preeclampsia increased from 22 percent in women with baseline creatinine < 125µmol/l, to 40 percent with creatinine 125–180µmol/l, 60 percent with creatinine > 180µmol/l and 75 percent in women receiving dialysis [21]. Retrospective analysis of women with CKD who enrolled in the Vitamins in Preeclampsia trial found high rates of preeclampsia in women with CKD and baseline creatinine < 125µmol/l at 40 percent, with a third of these cases requiring delivery before 34 weeks' gestation [33].

Based on these and other results, the UK National Institute for Health and Clinical Excellence and the World Health Organization identify CKD as a risk factor for preeclampsia, and recommend that women with CKD are offered prophylactic treatment with low-dose aspirin during their pregnancy [34, 35]. There are no proven benefits from taking aspirin during attempted conception and recommendations suggest commencing aspirin 75mg daily between 12 and 20 weeks' gestation. Women should be advised that the beneficial effect of aspirin is significant but modest, with a risk reduction of approximately 25 percent [36]. With or without aspirin, enhanced monitoring for biophysical signs of impending preeclampsia is required for women with CKD.

Urinary Tract Infection

Episodes of bacteriuria are common in pregnancy due to physiological changes in renal anatomy. Increased renal blood flow, generalized smooth muscle relaxation and the compressive effects of a gravid uterus can lead to transient impairments of urine flow, stagnation and infection. Clinical practice guidelines report that, during pregnancy, asymptomatic bacteriuria is approximately four times more likely to progress to ascending pyelonephritis than in the non-gravid state, with a 21 percent risk of pyelonephritis if left untreated. Moreover, episodes of pyelonephritis may precipitate preterm labor and subsequent fetal morbidity. These data relate to three reports published between 1960 and 1969 [37]. A more recent randomized controlled trial of treatment for asymptomatic bacteriuria did not identify a decreased incidence of pyelonephritis or preterm delivery with treatment, and the absolute risk of adverse event was less than 3 percent with or without treatment [38].

Anatomical and functional abnormalities of the urinary tract leading to recurrent urinary tract infection (UTI) are the commonest causes of CKD in women attending renal-obstetric clinics in the United Kingdom [39]. Women with structural abnormalities of the renal tract and women receiving immunosuppression, with or without renal transplantation, are intuitively at increased risk of bacteriuria and UTI during pregnancy compared with the general population. Historical reports suggest that up to 40 percent of renal transplant recipients developed UTI in pregnancy [40]; however, there are no published data on the true incidence of infection rates in these populations in recent literature. Furthermore, it is common clinical practice to recommend that women in groups perceived to be at higher risk of ascending infection should have urine examined for the presence of bacteriuria, irrespective of symptoms, at least monthly during pregnancy [36], despite a lack of evidence to support this approach [41]. Conversely, studies do not report any evidence of harm in screening for, or treating, asymptomatic bacteriuria in pregnancy.

Despite the limited supportive evidence, it remains prudent to advise women with CKD and risk factors for UTI that (a) UTIs are more likely to occur during pregnancy; (b) screening for asymptomatic bacteriuria and subsequent treatment of positive results is recommended during pregnancy; and (c) prophylactic antibiotics are recommended during pregnancy for women already taking such treatment prior to conception, those with an episode of confirmed bacteriuria and taking immunosuppression and those with more than one episode of confirmed bacteriuria during pregnancy.

Caesarean Section

CKD is not an indication for instrumental or operative delivery per se and should only be performed for obstetric reasons. Nevertheless, women should be advised that the increased incidence of maternal and fetal morbidity found in pregnancies complicated by CKD results in an increased observed rate of Caesarean sections. For example, in an Italian cohort study, Caesarean section rates were 27.2 percent in the general population, 48 percent in women with CKD stage 1, 70 percent in women with CKD stage 2 and 78 percent in women with CKD stage 3 (p < 0.001) [3]. Similar incidences were described in an Indian cohort of 80 pregnancies with Caesarean section rates of 65 percent in women with CKD stages 1 and 2 and 71 percent in women with CKD stages 3 to 5. The commonest indications for Caesarean section were non-reassuring fetal heart rate (26 percent), severe preeclampsia (22 percent) and severe fetal growth restriction (19 percent) [42].

Proteinuria and Venous Thromboembolism

Pregnancy is a pro-thrombotic state – pregnant women have 4.3-fold higher risk of developing venous thromboembolism (VTE) compared to nonpregnant controls [43]. Proteinuria is also a pro-thrombotic state [44–46] as a result of hemoconcentration, venous stasis and imbalanced urinary losses of pro-thrombotic and anti-thrombotic factors [47], particularly in patients with a diagnosis of nephrotic syndrome due to membranous nephropathy and focal segmental glomerulosclerosis [48].

Women with established proteinuria outside pregnancy should be counseled that the physiological effects of pregnancy (and discontinuation of anti-proteinuric therapies) may convert asymptomatic proteinuria to overt nephrotic syndrome. There are no clinical studies to guide the necessity or effectiveness of thromboprophylaxis in pregnancy based on degrees of proteinuria and practice varies nationally and internationally. Consensus guidelines recommend that nephrotic syndrome in pregnancy is an indication for thromboprophylaxis in pregnancy and the puerperium, and lesser degrees of proteinuria may constitute a risk for thromboembolism that should inform the decision whether to use prophylaxis. Some centers commence thromboprophylaxis when proteinuria exceeds 1g per day. Others integrate degrees of proteinuria with serum albumin, edema and other VTE risk factors to determine thresholds for treatment.

Risks to Fetal Health

Prepregnancy counseling is an opportunity to set parental expectations for pregnancy outcomes. For most, a "successful pregnancy" is one resulting in a healthy infant coming home with the parents. Others might have specific pregnancy preferences, including location and method of delivery, that might not be safe in the context of their CKD.

Observational data have revealed that the incidence of adverse fetal outcomes is related to the severity of maternal renal dysfunction (Table 2.3), blood pressure control, etiology of maternal renal disease and, to a lesser extent, degree of proteinuria.

Miscarriage, Stillbirth and Neonatal Death

Recent studies have described a remarkable improvement in infant survival for women with CKD over the past 60 years. In the 1950s, infant survival was only 43 percent for women with baseline serum urea > 7mmol/l and 0% with urea > 21mmol/l [1]. Since the turn of the millennium, infant survival has been reported to be > 95% in women with CKD stages 3-5, and 86% in women receiving hemodialysis with an intensive schedule [3, 42, 49]. This progression – a combination of improved maternal medicine,

Table 2.3 Risk of adverse fetal outcomes [3, 21, 49, 55]. SGA, small for gestational age; LBW, low birth weight (< 2,500g); VLBW, very low birth weight (< 1,500g); NICU, neonatal intensive care unit admission; SCr, serum creatinine.

	Preterm delivery (< 34 weeks)	Preterm delivery (< 37 weeks)	SGA (< 10%) or LBW	SGA (< 5%) or VLBW	NICU	Failure to survive
Baseline SCr < 125μmol/l, eGFR > 60 ml/min/1.73 m^2	10%	30%	14–25%	5%	14%	1%
Baseline SCr 125-180μmol /l, eGFR 30-60 ml/min/1.73 m^2	38%	60–80%	19%	5%	44%	1%
Baseline SCr > 180μmol/l, eGFR < 30ml/min/1.73 m^2	44%	90%	50%	25%	70%	1%
Standard dialysis (17±5 hours/week)	80%	100%	44%	29%	NA	40–50%
Intensive dialysis (42±7 hours/week)	38%	50%	39%	6%	40%	13%

renal medicine and neonatal intensive care [2] – means that it should now be unusual to advise women with CKD that a pregnancy could not be considered.

Hypertension has been associated with increased rates of fetal loss. Some studies identify that controlling blood pressure prior to, or during, pregnancy increases survival [15] and (albeit in patients without CKD) reduces the risk of severe hypertension during superadded preeclampsia with a secondary effect on improved infant survival [17]. Other retrospective data suggest that, with or without antihypertensive treatment, hypertension is a strong risk factor for neonatal death with a hazard ratio of 21.9 (95 percent confidence interval 2.6–165) comparing women with baseline diastolic blood pressure (DBP) < 70mmHg with DBP > 90mmHg or receiving treatment [12].

The effect of maternal proteinuria on infant survival is less well defined. There are data to suggest that maternal nephrotic syndrome during pregnancy portends a very poor outlook for the pregnancy with 42 percent reported fetal mortality [9]; however, these findings are not matched by contemporary (albeit anecdotal) experience, which is far more favorable.

While stillbirth and neonatal death is now uncommon, doubt remains as to the true incidence of miscarriage in women with CKD. Irregular menstrual cycles are common, so early miscarriages may be mistaken for late and/or heavy periods, limiting the accuracy of available data.

Preterm Delivery and Impaired Fetal Growth

As compared with controls, the incidence of preterm delivery (< 37 weeks and < 34 weeks), low birth weight and, subsequently, neonatal intensive care unit (NICU) admission is higher in women with CKD. Of importance, this is true even for women with CKD stages 1 and 2, a cohort previously assumed to have minimal excess risk of adverse pregnancy events. In a prospective observational study of 91 pregnancies in women with CKD and 267 controls, rates of delivery before 37 weeks were eightfold in women with CKD stage 1–2 (40 percent vs. 4.9 percent), and admission to NICU sixteenfold (18 percent vs. 1.1 percent) [50]. The incidence of preterm delivery and impaired fetal growth increases with more advanced stages of renal dysfunction (Table 2.3) [3, 49, 50].

Further review reveals that preterm delivery is rarely due to spontaneous preterm labor. Of 91 pregnancies in women with CKD, 40 resulted in delivery before 37 weeks. Only three of these (7.5 percent) were due to spontaneous preterm labor, with the remainder iatrogenic due to maternal (65 percent), fetal (20 percent) or combined (7.5 percent) concerns [50].

The advice given to women at prepregnancy counseling, therefore, should be that pregnancies may not reach term, babies may be born smaller than normal and there is an increased chance that infants will require NICU support after delivery. Although enhanced monitoring during pregnancy to identify potential problems early will be required, it is not necessary to arrange early elective delivery if there is not an independent maternal or fetal indication to do so.

Disease-Specific Infant Complications

For most women, the etiology of their renal disease will not impact their infants above and beyond the degree of excretory dysfunction, hypertension or proteinuria with which it is associated. The predominant exceptions to this are women with CKD secondary to systemic conditions, including SLE (Chapter 11) and diabetes mellitus (Chapter 12), where effects of the primary disease confer risks independent of the renal disease.

Women with inheritable renal disease should receive counseling regarding the risk of transmitting their disease (or that of their partner) to their offspring. Commonly encountered monogenic causes of CKD in renal-obstetric clinics are autosomal dominant polycystic kidney disease (ADPKD), thin basement membrane nephropathy and Alport syndrome. Prepregnancy counseling should include discussion of the inheritance pattern and risk, and the option of preimplantation genetic diagnosis if feasible.

Congenital abnormalities of the kidneys and urological tract (CAKUT) encompasses a number of anatomical changes that predispose patients to urinary tract infection, obstruction and CKD (Chapter 10). The etiology of these conditions appears to be heterogeneous with variable degrees of genetic and environmental involvement that is poorly elucidated. Some patients appear to transmit their condition in an autosomal dominant manner, although this is infrequent. Advice regarding screening infants for inheritance varies from center to center; however, if no structural abnormality is identified on detailed intrauterine fetal scan and the infant does not exhibit signs suggestive of infections, screening the infant with postnatal ultrasound or micturating cystourethrogram is very unlikely to identify abnormalities and rarely recommended [51].

Teratogenicity and Medicines Management

An extensive medication history should be taken at prepregnancy counseling to identify previous and current prescribed medication, over-the-counter purchases of medications, illicit drugs and herbal or alternative remedies. Medicines management surrounding pregnancy is extensively discussed in Chapter 7.

Medications fall into one of four categories regarding potential pregnancies: 1) definitely harmful, 2) potentially harmful with insufficient safety data, 3) insufficient safety data but extensive experience of safe use in pregnancy and 4) proven safety data. These risks should be balanced against the treatments' benefits. Again, these can be categorized as: 1) essential, 2) preventative or 3) nonessential/symptomatic. Each treatment should be evaluated on its risks and benefits prior to pregnancy.

Advice should be given regarding the timing, safety and risks of changing prescribed treatments known to be harmful in preparation for a pregnancy. This is particularly pertinent for women (or their partners) receiving mycophenolate derivatives for renal transplantation or autoimmune conditions. They should be advised to exchange mycophenolate for an alternative agent (such as azathioprine) well in advance of pregnancy, following discussion with their primary renal physician, to allow elimination of the agent from the maternal system and to confirm disease stability on the new regime. This is likely to require three to six months.

Angiotensin-converting enzyme inhibitors (ACEi) and angiotensin receptor blockers (ARBs) are teratogenic in the second and third trimesters of pregnancy. Two conflicting studies cast doubt on whether they must be avoided prior to conception. In a comparison of 209 women exposed to ACEi in the first trimester against 202 women taking other antihypertensive treatments and 29,096 women with no antihypertensive treatment, ACEi exposure was associated with a risk ratio of 2.7 (95 percent confidence interval 1.7–4.3) of congenital malformation [52]. Subsequently, a larger registry study compared 400 pregnancies exposed to ACEi in the first trimester with 1,141 on other antihypertensive agents and 416,218 controls. The rate of major birth defects was higher in all patients receiving antihypertensive agents (adjusted odds ratio [aOR] 1.25 [95 percent CI 1.2–1.3]), but no different between those receiving ACEi and those on other agents (aOR 0.97 [0.67–1.41]) [53]. We advise women with a strong indication for an ACEi or ARB, such as heavy proteinuria, to continue taking therapy until they have a positive pregnancy test, then stop. We emphasize the need for regular pregnancy tests once they discontinue contraception in order to avoid second-trimester exposure.

Current recommendations suggest that HMG-CoA reductase inhibitors ("statins") should be stopped three months prior to pregnancy, although prospective cohort studies have not provided convincing evidence of an increased risk of adverse pregnancy outcomes or teratogenicity [54]. Their indication should be reviewed, but in most cases they should be stopped in advance. All prospective mothers should commence folic acid supplementation upon discontinuing contraception. For the majority of women with CKD, 400 micrograms is sufficient. Indications for high-dose folic acid (5mg per day) are predominantly related to patients' comorbidities, including diabetes, obesity or malabsorption disorders.

In the United Kingdom, further information regarding risks of medications in pregnancy can be obtained from the UK teratology information service (www.uktis.org) and the British National Formulary.

Conclusion

Prepregnancy counseling should be offered to all women with CKD contemplating pregnancy. A structured approach to the consultation should summarize assessment of fertility, optimal timing for a pregnancy, maternal and fetal risks of pregnancy and medicines management. It is unusual to recommend that women with CKD should not attempt a pregnancy, although for some, this should be postponed until reversible issues, such as disease stability, are addressed.

References

1. Mackay EV. Pregnancy and renal disease: A ten year survey. *Aust N Z J Obstet Gynecol* 1963;3:21.

2. Hall M. Pregnancy in women with CKD: A success story. *Am J Kidney Dis* 2016 Oct;68(4):633–639.

3. Piccoli GB, Cabiddu G, Attini R, Vigotti FN, Maxia S, Lepori N, et al. Risk of adverse pregnancy outcomes in women with CKD. *J Am Soc Nephrol* 2015 Aug;26(8):2011–2022.

4. Wiles KS, Bramham K, Vais A, Harding KR, Chowdhury P, Taylor CJ, et al. Pre-pregnancy counselling for women with chronic kidney disease: A retrospective analysis of nine years' experience. *BMC Nephrol* 2015 Mar 14;16: 28-015-0024-6.

5. Inker LA, Schmid CH, Tighiouart H, Eckfeldt JH, Feldman HI, Greene T, et al. Estimating glomerular filtration rate from serum creatinine and cystatin C. *N Engl J Med* 2012 Jul 5;367(1):20–29.

6. Munkhaugen J, Lydersen S, Romundstad PR, Wideroe TE, Vikse BE, Hallan S. Kidney function and future risk for adverse pregnancy outcomes: A population-based study from HUNT II, Norway. *Nephrol Dial Transplant* 2009 Dec;24(12):3744–3750.

7. Van Eerde AM, Krediet CT, Rookmaaker MB, Van Reekum FE, Knoers NV, Lely AT. Pre-pregnancy advice in chronic kidney disease: Do not forget genetic counseling. *Kidney Int* 2016 Oct;90(4):905–906.

8. McLigeyo SO, Otieno LS, Kinuthia DM, Mwongera FK, Wairagu SG. Outcome of pregnancy in nephrotic syndrome: A report on five cases. *East Afr Med J* 1991 Jun;68(6):477–483.

9. Yao T, Yao H, Wang H. Diagnosis and treatment of nephrotic syndrome during pregnancy. *Chin Med J (Engl)* 1996 Jun;109(6):471–473.

10. Sibai BM, Lindheimer M, Hauth J, Caritis S, Van Dorsten P, Klebanoff M, et al. Risk factors for preeclampsia, abruptio placentae, and adverse neonatal outcomes among women with chronic hypertension. National Institute of Child Health and Human Development Network of Maternal-Fetal Medicine Units. *N Engl J Med* 1998 Sep 3;339(10):667–671.

11. Jungers P, Chauveau D, Choukroun G, Moynot A, Skhiri H, Houillier P, et al. Pregnancy in women with impaired renal function. *Clin Nephrol* 1997 May;47(5):281–288.

12. Ferraro AJ, Somerset DA, Lipkin G, Al-Jayyousi RA, Carr S, Brunskill NJ, et al. Pregnancy in women with pre-existing renal disease: Maternal and fetal outcomes. *J Obstet Gynecol* 2005;25:S13.

13. Cunningham FG, Cox SM, Harstad TW, Mason RA, Pritchard JA. Chronic renal disease and pregnancy outcome. *Am J Obstet Gynecol* 1990 Aug;163(2):453–459.

14. Jones DC, Hayslett JP. Outcome of pregnancy in women with moderate or severe renal insufficiency. *N Engl J Med* 1996 Jul 25;335(4):226–232.

15. Bar J, Ben-Rafael Z, Padoa A, Orvieto R, Boner G, Hod M. Prediction of pregnancy outcome in subgroups of women with renal disease. *Clin Nephrol* 2000 Jun;53(6):437–444.

16. Imbasciati E, Gregorini G, Cabiddu G, Gammaro L, Ambroso G, Del Giudice A, et al. Pregnancy in CKD stages 3 to 5: Fetal and maternal outcomes. *Am J Kidney Dis* 2007 Jun;49(6):753–762.

17. Magee LA, Von Dadelszen P, Rey E, Ross S, Asztalos E, Murphy KE, et al. Less-tight versus tight control of hypertension in pregnancy. *N Engl J Med* 2015 Jan 29;372(5):407–417.

18. Tight blood pressure control and risk of macrovascular and microvascular complications in type 2 diabetes:

UKPDS 38. *UK Prospective Diabetes Study Group. BMJ* 1998 Sep 12;**317**(7160):703–713.

19. Hansson L, Zanchetti A, Carruthers SG, Dahlof B, Elmfeldt D, Julius S, et al. Effects of intensive blood-pressure lowering and low-dose aspirin in patients with hypertension: Principal results of the Hypertension Optimal Treatment (HOT) randomised trial. *HOT Study Group. Lancet* 1998 Jun 13;**351**(9118):1755–1762.

20. Tranquilli AL, Dekker G, Magee L, Roberts J, Sibai BM, Steyn W, et al. The classification, diagnosis and management of the hypertensive disorders of pregnancy: A revised statement from the ISSHP. *Pregnancy Hypertens* 2014 Apr;**4**(2):97–104.

21. Williams D, Davison J. Chronic kidney disease in pregnancy. *BMJ* 2008 Jan 26;**336**(7637):211–215.

22. Hou S. Pregnancy in renal transplant recipients. *Adv Chronic Kidney Dis* 2013 May;**20**(3):253–259.

23. Brown JH, Maxwell AP, McGeown MG. Outcome of pregnancy following renal transplantation. *Ir J Med Sci* 1991 Aug;**160**(8):255–256.

24. Okundaye I, Abrinko P, Hou S. Registry of pregnancy in dialysis patients. *Am J Kidney Dis* 1998 May;**31**(5):766–773.

25. Office for National Statistics (ONS). Vital Statistics: Population and Health Reference Tables. 2016; Available at: www.ons.gov.uk/peoplepopulationand community/populationandmigration/populationesti mates/datasets/vitalstatisticspopulationandhealthrefer encetables. Accessed February 6, 2017.

26. Holley JL. The hypothalamic-pituitary axis in men and women with chronic kidney disease. *Adv Chronic Kidney Dis* 2004 Oct;**11**(4):337–341.

27. Sikora-Grabka E, Adamczak M, Kuczera P, Szotowska M, Madej P, Wiecek A. Serum anti-Mullerian hormone concentration in young women with chronic kidney disease on hemodialysis, and after successful kidney transplantation. *Kidney Blood Press Res* 2016;**41**(5):552–560.

28. Palmer BF, Clegg DJ. Gonadal dysfunction in chronic kidney disease. *Rev Endocr Metab Disord* 2016 Sep 1.

29. Odutayo A, Hladunewich M. Obstetric nephrology: Renal hemodynamic and metabolic physiology in normal pregnancy. *Clin J Am Soc Nephrol* 2012 Dec;**7**(12):2073–2080.

30. Youssouf S, Hall M, Lightstone L, Brunskill NJ, Carr S. Pregnancy in a prospective cohort of women with CKD 3-5: Maternal outcomes. *J Am Soc Nephrol* 2011;**22**:16A.

31. Sibanda N, Briggs JD, Davison JM, Johnson RJ, Rudge CJ. Pregnancy after organ transplantation: A report from the UK Transplant pregnancy registry. *Transplantation* 2007 May 27;**83**(10):1301–1307.

32. Bramham K, Seed PT, Lightstone L, Nelson-Piercy C, Gill C, Webster P, et al. Diagnostic and predictive biomarkers for pre-eclampsia in patients with established hypertension and chronic kidney disease. *Kidney Int* 2016 Apr;**89**(4):874–885.

33. Bramham K, Briley AL, Seed PT, Poston L, Shennan AH, Chappell LC. Pregnancy outcome in women with chronic kidney disease: A prospective cohort study. *Reprod Sci* 2011 Jul;**18**(7):623–630.

34. Visintin C, Mugglestone MA, Almerie MQ, Nherera LM, James D, Walkinshaw S, et al. Management of hypertensive disorders during pregnancy: Summary of NICE guidance. *BMJ* 2010 Aug 25;**341**:c2207.

35. *WHO recommendations for prevention and treatment of pre-eclampsia and eclampsia.* Geneva: World Health Organization; 2011.

36. Duley L, Henderson-Smart DJ, Meher S, King JF. Antiplatelet agents for preventing pre-eclampsia and its complications. *Cochrane Database Syst Rev* 2007 Apr 18;(2)(2):CD004659.

37. Smaill F, Vazquez JC. Antibiotics for asymptomatic bacteriuria in pregnancy. *Cochrane Database Syst Rev* 2007 Apr 18;(2)(2):CD000490.

38. Kazemier BM, Koningstein FN, Schneeberger C, Ott A, Bossuyt PM, de Miranda E, et al. Maternal and neonatal consequences of treated and untreated asymptomatic bacteriuria in pregnancy: A prospective cohort study with an embedded randomised controlled trial. *Lancet Infect Dis* 2015 Nov;**15**(11):1324–1333.

39. Hall M, Brunskill N. Renal disease in pregnancy. *Obstetrics, Gynaecology, and Reproductive Medicine* 2016;**26**(2):46–52.

40. Davison JM, Milne JE. Pregnancy and renal transplantation. *Br J Urol* 1997 Jul;**80** Suppl 1:29–32.

41. Angelescu K, Nussbaumer-Streit B, Sieben W, Scheibler F, Gartlehner G. Benefits and harms of screening for and treatment of asymptomatic bacteriuria in pregnancy: A systematic review. *BMC Pregnancy Childbirth* 2016 Nov 2;**16**(1):336.

42. Bharti J, Vatsa R, Singhal S, Roy KK, Kumar S, Perumal V, et al. Pregnancy with chronic kidney disease: Maternal and fetal outcome. *Eur J Obstet Gynecol Reprod Biol* 2016 Sep;**204**:83–87.

43. Kayali F, Najjar R, Aswad F, Matta F, Stein PD. Venous thromboembolism in patients hospitalized with nephrotic syndrome. *Am J Med* 2008 Mar;**121**(3):226–230.

44. Kato S, Chernyavsky S, Tokita JE, Shimada YJ, Homel P, Rosen H, et al. Relationship between proteinuria and venous thromboembolism. *J Thromb Thrombolysis* 2010 Oct;**30**(3):281–285.

45. Go AS, Fang MC, Udaltsova N, Chang Y, Pomernacki NK, Borowsky L, et al. Impact of proteinuria and glomerular filtration rate on risk of thromboembolism in atrial fibrillation: The anticoagulation and risk factors in atrial fibrillation (ATRIA) study. *Circulation* 2009 Mar 17;**119**(10):1363–1369.

46. Kumar S, Chapagain A, Nitsch D, Yaqoob MM. Proteinuria and hypoalbuminemia are risk factors for thromboembolic events in patients with idiopathic membranous nephropathy: An observational study. *BMC Nephrol* 2012 Sep 10;**13**: 107–2369–13–107.

47. Mahmoodi BK, Ten Kate MK, Waanders F, Veeger NJ, Brouwer JL, Vogt L, et al. High absolute risks and predictors of venous and arterial thromboembolic events in patients with nephrotic syndrome: Results from a large retrospective cohort study. *Circulation* 2008 Jan 15;**117**(2):224–230.

48. Barbour SJ, Greenwald A, Djurdjev O, Levin A, Hladunewich MA, Nachman PH, et al. Disease-specific risk of venous thromboembolic events is increased in idiopathic glomerulonephritis. *Kidney Int* 2012 Jan;**81** (2):190–195.

49. Hladunewich MA, Hou S, Odutayo A, Cornelis T, Pierratos A, Goldstein M, et al. Intensive hemodialysis associates with improved pregnancy outcomes: A Canadian and United States cohort comparison. *J Am Soc Nephrol* 2014 May;**25**(5):1103–1109.

50. Piccoli GB, Attini R, Vasario E, Conijn A, Biolcati M, D'Amico F, et al. Pregnancy and chronic kidney disease: A challenge in all CKD stages. *Clin J Am Soc Nephrol* 2010 May;**5**(5):844–855.

51. Mallik M, Watson AR. Antenatally detected urinary tract abnormalities: More detection but less action. *Pediatr Nephrol* 2008 Jun;**23**(6):897–904.

52. Cooper WO, Hernandez-Diaz S, Arbogast PG, Dudley JA, Dyer S, Gideon PS, et al. Major congenital malformations after first-trimester exposure to ACE inhibitors. *N Engl J Med* 2006 Jun 8;**354** (23):2443–2451.

53. Li DK, Yang C, Andrade S, Tavares V, Ferber JR. Maternal exposure to angiotensin converting enzyme inhibitors in the first trimester and risk of malformations in offspring: A retrospective cohort study. *BMJ* 2011 Oct 18;**343**:d5931.

54. Karalis DG, Hill AN, Clifton S, Wild RA. The risks of statin use in pregnancy: A systematic review. *J Clin Lipidol* 2016 Sep–Oct;**10**(5):1081–1090.

55. Barua M, Hladunewich M, Keunen J, Pierratos A, McFarlane P, Sood M, et al. Successful pregnancies on nocturnal home hemodialysis. *Clin J Am Soc Nephrol* 2008 Mar;**3**(2):392–396.

Chapter 3

Contraception in Women with Renal Disease

Kate Wiles

Introduction

Advice regarding safe and effective contraception should be offered to all women of childbearing age with chronic kidney disease (CKD). This must include those women with advanced CKD and those receiving dialysis, women with active glomerulonephritis and women taking teratogenic medication. A wide range of contraceptive options is available for women with CKD. Women with CKD should be given advice about the efficacy, including "typical" as well as "perfect" use failure rates.

Safe and effective reversible forms of contraception, which can be used in all women with CKD, include the progesterone-only pill (desogestrel preparations), the contraceptive implant (Nexplanon®) and the intrauterine system (Mirena®). Emergency contraception can be safely prescribed. Combined contraceptives, which contain an estrogen component, carry an increased risk of hypertension, venous and arterial thrombosis and cervical cancer, which may be significant for women with CKD. Barrier methods, sterilization, fertility awareness, lactational amenorrhea and contraceptive drug interactions are discussed.

Contraception in Context

A key objective of global health policy is a reduction in the number of unplanned conceptions and one of the indicators of universal access to reproductive health is the extent to which the need for contraception is met. However, national survey data reveal that only 55 percent of pregnancies are planned in the United Kingdom [1]. Despite the free provision of contraception by the National Health Service (NHS), there were an estimated 225,600 unintended pregnancies in England in 2010, leading to 163,000 abortions and 53,900 unintended births at a cost of £193 m [2]. Unplanned pregnancy is associated with an increased risk of obstetric complications [3], even in the absence

of chronic health comorbidity. Consensus opinion is that contraceptive counseling improves patient choice and satisfaction and encourages a more sustained use of correct contraception [4]. However, it is essential that contraceptive counseling considers improper contraceptive use and reliability in order that contraceptive use has the capacity to limit the number of unintended pregnancies [2].

Contraceptive Reliability

When considering the likelihood of contraceptive failure, both "typical-use" and "perfect-use" pregnancy rates must be considered [5]. "Typical use" of a contraceptive method reflects how effective a contraceptive method is for the average person who may not always use the method consistently or correctly. The probability of a pregnancy with a year of use is a measure of contraceptive efficacy. Perfect-use and typical-use pregnancy rates for different contraceptive methods are outlined in Table 3.1. The difference between perfect and typical use gives an idea of how forgiving a contraceptive method is of imperfect use. For example, typical use of the male condom results in 18 percent of women experiencing an unintended pregnancy within a year, in contrast to a perfect-use failure rate of only 2 percent.

The Importance of Contraception in Women with CKD

CKD is estimated to affect 3 percent of women of childbearing age, and population trends of older primiparity and increasing obesity are predicted to increase prevalence in the future. The severity of pre-pregnancy CKD is the major determinant of adverse pregnancy outcome, including fetal growth restriction, preterm delivery, preeclampsia and perinatal death, as well as conferring a proportional risk of a postpartum decline in maternal renal function [6] (see Chapter 2). Mycophenolate mofetil and

Table 3.1 Contraceptive failure rates: Perfect and typical use. Adapted from [5].

Contraceptive Method		% women experiencing an unintended pregnancy within the first year	
		Perfect Use	Typical Use
No method		85	85
Combined contraceptives	Combined oral contraceptive (COC)	0.3	9
	Transdermal combined patch (Evra®)	0.3	9
	Vaginal ring (Nuvaring®)	0.3	9
Progesterone-only contraceptives	Progesterone-only pill (POP)	0.3	9
	Intramuscular depot (Depo-Provera®)	0.2	6
	Implant (Nexplanon®)	0.05	0.05
	Intrauterine system (Mirena®)	0.2	0.2
Copper IUD		0.6	0.8
Barrier Methods	Male condom	2	18
	Female condom	5	21
	Diaphragm	6	12
	Sponge	9–20	12–24
Sterilization		< 0.5	< 0.5
Fertility awareness methods		0.4–5	24

cyclophosphamide are known to be teratogenic, and angiotensin converting enzyme inhibitors and angiotensin receptor antagonists are fetotoxic after the first trimester. Therefore, it is essential that women of childbearing age be counseled regarding safe and effective contraception when these drugs are prescribed. However, a small UK study of women aged 20–47 with CKD revealed that only 48 percent had discussed contraception, 45 percent did not know the risks of pregnancy, 39 percent were unaware of potentially teratogenic medication and 29 percent had had an unplanned pregnancy [7].

Hormonal changes associated with end-stage renal disease include an absence of luteinizing hormone surge, low estradiol, low progesterone levels and a raised prolactin. Menstrual cycle irregularities occur as the glomerular filtration rate (GFR) falls below 15ml/minute and progress to amenorrhea with a GFR below 5ml/min [8]. As a result, end-stage renal failure and "uremia" are estimated to confer a fertility rate 10 times lower than that of the general population. However, conception and high-risk pregnancy can occur with 3.3 pregnancies per 1,000 patient years in recent cohorts [9]. In addition, rates of home hemodialysis are increasing in the United Kingdom, and isolated case reports suggest an increase in female

fertility in patients receiving intensified hemodialysis [8]. However, few nephrologists discuss fertility issues with their dialysis patients [10].

Following transplantation, fertility increases and ovulatory cycles can normalize within the first month. However, pregnancies in renal transplant recipients are associated with higher complication rates when compared to women with matched native renal function [11]. In addition, the teratogenicity of maintenance immunosuppression, specifically mycophenolate mofetil, needs to be considered. In the United Kingdom, 200–600 per million women aged 20–44 years have renal transplants, [12], and use of folate at conception in the United Kingdom suggests that more than one-third of patients with a renal transplant have an unintended pregnancy [13]. In the United States, 5–12 percent of renal transplants occur in women of childbearing age, of whom 50 percent have unintended pregnancies [14]. Such data are mirrored worldwide. In China, 15 percent of transplant patients report unplanned pregnancies, with 34 percent of these women having two or three. Of these, 56 percent were not using any method of contraception, largely due to a failure to realize that reproductive potential is restored after transplantation [15]. Less than 50 percent of a Brazilian transplant population was found to have received contraceptive advice following renal transplantation, and 92.9 percent of pregnancies in this group were unplanned [16]. In Iran, 92 percent of female transplant recipients in one cohort were using coitus interruptus as their only method of contraception, resulting in 29 percent of pregnancies being unintended [17].

Contraceptive Options in Women With Renal Disease

Evidence from "healthy" populations is used to determine the suitability of different contraceptive methods for women with CKD, as most studies of contraception will exclude participants with medical comorbidity. However, the UK Medical Eligibility Criteria for Contraceptive Use (UKMEC) offers evidence-based and expert consensus guidance for contraceptive use in the presence of different medical conditions [18]. Although renal disease is not considered as a separate entity within this guideline, advice applicable to women with hypertension, lupus, diabetes, venous thromboembolism and vascular risk is available.

In providing contraceptive counseling to renal patients, it must be remembered that the effectiveness of any contraceptive method is dependent upon the acceptability of the method to the patient and likely compliance. Although absolute contraindications to particular contraceptives may exist, the "safety" of a particular method is often not a discrete "yes-no" variable, but exists on a spectrum from recognized safety to a risk that potentially outweighs benefit. Acceptability must be considered in this context. In addition, contraceptive decision-making must consider the potentially significant risks of an unplanned pregnancy in CKD, particularly in women with unstable renal function and those taking tetratogenic medication.

Table 3.2 provides a summary of the advantages and disadvantages of different contraceptive methods, with specific reference to women with renal disease (see Table 3.2).

Combined Oral Contraceptives

The combined oral contraceptive contains an estrogen, most commonly ethinylestradiol, and a progestogen, to inhibit ovulation. The amount of estrogen in the combined pill has fallen over time due to the epidemiological link between estrogen and breast cancer and the association of estrogen with adverse thromboembolic, cerebrovascular and cardiovascular events. Today's combined pills contain approximately 30μg of estrogen compared to a historical 50μg. A further reduction in estrogen content to 20μg does not appear to have any advantage with no evidence of additional vascular risk reduction but an increase in menstrual bleeding disturbances [19].

When considering the combined pill for women with renal disease, the following recognized side effects must be considered:

1. Hemodynamic effects
2. Venous thromboembolism (VTE)
3. Arterial thrombosis
4. Cervical cancer risk

Hemodynamic Effects

Use of the combined pill is associated with a rise in blood pressure that is presumed due to dose-dependent hepatic activation of the renin-angiotensinogen-aldosterone axis by the estrogen component [20]. This is relevant to the renal population where rates of hypertension are much higher than in the general population. In a small prospective cohort of women with renal transplants taking combined hormonal contraceptive methods, 86 percent of patients were hypertensive at study entry and modifications in the type and doses of antihypertensives were required in 36 percent in order to maintain the same arterial pressure [21]. In contrast, small prospective studies have demonstrated that newer combined pills that contain estradiol as their estrogenic component do not affect 24-hour blood pressure readings, due to the fact that estradiol is a far less potent hepatic enzyme inducer than ethinylestradiol [20].

Combined pills have also been found to influence the kidney's hemodynamic response to salt. Salt-loading in women taking combined oral contraceptives produces an increased filtration fraction, which is hypothesized to be due to the effects of exogenous estrogen on nitric oxide and prostaglandins as well as the renin-angiotensin system [22]. Although these data come from women without concomitant renal disease, it has been hypothesized that an equivalent hyperfiltration response to the combined pill in those with preexisting renal impairment has the potential to accelerate glomerular sclerosis and exacerbate proteinuria.

Table 3.2 Summary of the advantages and disadvantages of contraceptive methods for women with renal disease. Adapted from [48].

Contraceptive Method		Advantages	Disadvantages
Combined contraceptives	Combined oral contraceptive (COC)	Reduced ovarian and endometrial cancer risk	Increased VTE risk (~x2 background) Blood pressure rise Increased arterial thrombosis risk Increased cervical cancer risk
	Transdermal combined patch (Evra®)	Not affected by vomiting or malabsorption	Higher risk of VTE than COC pill Blood pressure rise Increased arterial thrombosis risk Increased cervical cancer risk
	Vaginal ring (NuvaRing®)		
Progesterone-only contraceptives	Progesterone-only pill (POP)	Safe for those for whom estrogens are contraindicated, including VTE, hypertension and lupus	Small compliance window (not desogestrel eg Cerelle®/Cerazette®)
	Intramuscular depot (Depo-Provera®)	Not affected by vomiting or malabsorption Effective for 12 weeks	Increased breakthrough menstrual bleeding Adverse lipid profile (increased LDL, reduced HDL) Reversible decrease in bone-mineral density
	Implant (Nexplanon®)	Not affected by vomiting or malabsorption Effective for three years	Increased breakthrough menstrual bleeding
	Intra-uterine system (Mirena®)	Reduced menstrual bleeding Not affected by vomiting or malabsorption Effective for five years	Irregular light bleeding in first six months after insertion, overall reduction in menstrual bleeding Possible increase in breast cancer risk
Copper IUD		Not affected by vomiting or malabsorption Can be used as emergency contraception Effective for 10 years	Increased breakthrough menstrual bleeding
Barrier Methods	Male condom Female condom Cervical cap Diaphragm Sponge	Convenient Protection against sexually-transmitted disease (condoms) Not affected by vomiting or malabsorption	Failure rate with typical use Increased UTIs (diaphragm) Genital ulceration and HIV risk with spermicide use

Table 3.2 (cont.)

Contraceptive Method	Advantages	Disadvantages
Sterilization	Effective	Irreversible Operative risk
Fertility awareness methods		High failure rate Signs and symptoms affected by medication
Lactational amenorrhoea	Benefits of breast-feeding for infant	Difficult to "diagnose" postpartum amenorrhea Finite time span

Venous Thromboembolism (VTE)

Use of the combined oral contraceptive pill approximately doubles the risk of VTE from an incidence of 3.01 per 10,000 women years in never or former users to 6.29 per 10,000 women years in current users [23]. A higher estrogen content and the use of the progestogens desogestrel, gestodene and drospirenone are associated with increased risk. An increased VTE risk is evident even when women taking medication for diabetes, heart disease, hypertension and hyperlipidemia are excluded from study data. Such an increase in VTE risk is unacceptable for patients with a history of VTE and for patients with lupus and either positive, or unknown, antiphospholipid antibodies. Nephrotic syndrome is not considered as a discrete entity in either UK or international contraceptive guidelines, presumably due to its rarity in the young female population. However, nephrosis leads to urinary losses of anticoagulants with a concomitant increase in hepatic synthesis of procoagulants and a shift in the hemostatic balance toward thrombosis. The additional thrombotic risk of the combined pill in the context of either sustained or remitting proteinuric disease needs to be considered and alternative contraceptive methods should be prescribed.

Arterial Thrombosis

Meta-analysis data from the general population show that current use of combined pills containing < 50µg of ethinylestradiol confer a twofold risk of vascular disease, including myocardial infarction and ischemic stroke [24]. The vascular risk of combined pills means they are contraindicated in established vascular disease. In addition, the risks of estrogen-containing contraceptives outweigh any advantage in obesity (BMI > 35 kg/m^2), cigarette smoking, diabetes with microvascular complications and patients with hypertension, even when controlled on treatment. In CKD, a reduced glomerular filtration and proteinuria are both independent vascular risk factors and the excessive cardiovascular mortality associated with end-stage renal disease is well described. Of specific relevance to the female population is a large prospective cohort study that demonstrates an increased risk of cardiovascular death in women with CKD stage 3 or above, even in the absence of baseline cardiovascular disease [25]. The vascular risk of estrogen-containing contraceptives means that they cannot be recommended for use in women with stage 3–5 CKD.

Cervical Cancer Risk

Although population data show that use of the combined pill is protective against both ovarian and endometrial cancer [4], an increased risk of cancer of the cervix is recognized [26]. Cancer risk is relevant to the transplant population who are exposed to an increased lifetime risk of cancer as a product of long-term immunosuppression. This includes an estimated fivefold risk of cervical cancer, and there is concern that this risk may be further increased by the concomitant use of an estrogen-containing contraceptive. In addition, an increased cancer burden is described in the dialysis population, including an increased risk of all human papilloma virus (HPV)-associated cancers [27]. The role of the HPV vaccine in reducing the risk of cervical cancer in women with CKD is unknown.

Non-oral Combined Hormonal Contraceptives

The transdermal combined patch (Evra®) and the vaginal ring (NuvaRing®) utilize a combination of estrogen and progestogen to inhibit ovulation in the same way as the combined oral contraceptive. In addition, these non-oral methods suppress endometrial growth and increase cervical mucous viscosity, thereby inhibiting migration of the sperm to the uterus. The combined patch adheres to the skin and is changed weekly. The ring is placed into the vagina with hormonal transport across the vaginal wall into the bloodstream. The vaginal ring is worn for three weeks followed by a one-week break. Both of these contraceptive methods can be considered equivalent to the combined pill in terms of efficacy, but have the added advantage of being unaffected by nausea, vomiting or gastrointestinal malabsorption. The use of the vaginal ring has been described in renal patients following transplantation without affecting body mass index, blood pressure, biochemical parameters or immunosuppressive drug levels [28].

Data on the adverse effects of these non-oral methods are more limited than for the combined pill. However, cohort data suggest an even higher risk of venous thromboembolism with the combined patch and vaginal ring than with the combined pill [29]. Myocardial infarction and ischemic stroke data are limited by the small number of users of these methods and the rarity of these events in the population. In addition, long-term data, including cancer association, are not yet available. However, in the absence of these data, the clinical considerations, cautions and contraindications to the use of non-oral combined contraceptives should be considered the same as the estrogen-containing pill.

Progesterone-Only Methods

Progesterone-only methods of contraception include oral, parenteral and intrauterine progesterone delivery. The advantage of progesterone-only preparations is their safety profile in patients for whom estrogens are contraindicated. In the renal population, they can be used in patients with venous thromboembolism and thrombophilia, and in the context of hypertension, smoking and obesity.

Progesterone-Only Pill

Oral methods include a variety of formulations of the progesterone-only pill. Most progesterone-only pills provide contraception by thickening the cervical mucous to prevent entry of sperm into the female genital tract and making the endometrium less suitable for implantation. Ovulation is not always inhibited. Such preparations therefore depend upon

compliance within a three-hour window every day, and therefore "typical-use" efficacy may be less than with an estrogen-containing pill. Additional contraceptive protection is needed if the woman is more than three hours late taking her daily tablet as mucous impermeability is considered lost 27 hours after tablet intake. The exception to this is the desogestrel pill (Feanolla®, Cerelle®, Cerazette®, Aizea®, Nacrez®), which provides more consistent inhibition of ovulation even with a 12-hour delay in tablet re-dosing.

In relation to renal disease, a cohort study of two progesterone-only oral contraceptive agents in 187 patients with systemic lupus including 23 percent with renal disease, 9 percent with nephrotic syndrome and 29 percent with detectable antiphospholipid antibodies showed that the use of the progesterone-only pill did not increase the incidence of lupus nephritis, and found the progesterone-only pill to be an effective, well-tolerated contraceptive method [30].

Parenteral Progesterone Methods

Parenteral methods of progesterone delivery include:

- Depo-Provera®: an intramuscular injection of a long-acting progestogen repeated at 12 weekly intervals
- Nexplanon®: a surgically placed implant inserted under local anesthetic effective for three years
- Mirena®/Intrauterine system (IUS): Intrauterine progesterone delivery via a slow-releasing reservoir of levornorgestrel causing reversible atrophy of the endometrium, effective for five years (see also Intrauterine Devices).

Efficacy varies between these progesterone-only methods. Injectable and intrauterine progesterone-only contraceptives do not rely on daily compliance and therefore have lower failure rates than both combined and progesterone-only pills, even when "typical use" is considered (see Table 3.1). Depo-Provera® requires re-dosing every 12 weeks, but Nexplanon® and Mirena® are longer-acting and have lower failure rates than sterilization. Use of the levornorgestrel intrauterine system carries an unintended pregnancy rate of 0.2 percent in the first year of use, and the progestogen-based implant 0.05 percent [5]. In the United States, it is estimated that if 10 percent of women switched from oral contraception to these long-acting reversible methods, then medical costs due to contraceptive user error would be reduced by $288 m/year [31].

Adverse Effects of Progesterone-Only Methods

Progesterone-only preparations can lead to altered menstrual bleeding patterns. The Mirena® IUS is beneficial in reducing bleeding and is used in the management of menorrhagia. In contrast, the progesterone-only pill and the Nexplanon® implant can both exacerbate breakthrough menstrual bleeding. For women with CKD, this spectrum of effects needs to be considered in the context of anticoagulation, lupus thrombocytopenia and uremic bleeding. Desogestrel is an inactive prodrug that is converted to active etonogestrel for its contraceptive effect. This is the same progestogen as in Nexplanon®. Desogestrel pills (Cerazette®, Cerelle®, Aizea®, Nacrez®) can therefore be trialed to assess bleeding effect before insertion of Nexplanon® if desired.

There are no absolute contraindications to the use of progesterone-only methods of contraception. However, depot medroxyprogesterone (Depo-Provera®) has been shown to be associated with a decrease in bone mineral density, which is reversible with discontinuation of treatment. Although the quality of evidence is insufficient to determine whether this translates into an increased fracture risk [32], this may be a consideration for renal patients taking high-dose or long-term steroid therapy. There are also conflicting and inconsistent data linking synthetic progestogen use to an adverse lipid profile. This includes a transient increase in low-density lipoprotein (LDL) cholesterol [33]. The use of depot formulations in vascular disease and complicated diabetes is therefore not recommended in UK guidance [18]. However, to date, this finding remains a surrogate end point and there is an absence of evidence that this translates into a significant clinical effect.

Recent prospective data demonstrates an increase in the relative risk of breast cancer with both oestrogen and progesterone-only contraceptive formulations [34]. The absolute risk is higher for women over the age of 40 for whom non-hormonal based contraception (eg copper IUD) should be considered.

Intrauterine Devices (IUD)

Intrauterine devices (IUD) include both the progestogen-releasing intrauterine system (IUS or Mirena®) (see Progesterone-Only Methods) and the copper IUD. The copper IUD works due to immobilization of sperm and inhibition of fertilization. It is effective for 10 years and is a very cost-effective contraception.

The copper IUD can also be used as an effective emergency contraceptive device up to five days following unprotected intercourse to prevent implantation [4].

In contrast to the Mirena®, which reduces menstrual bleeding, the main side effect of the copper coil is that it can increase menstrual flow by 30 percent and cause dysmenorrhea [4]. For women with CKD, this may be important for those with lupus thrombocytopenia, those who require therapeutic anticoagulation and those who are at risk of uremic bleeding. In addition, a Cochrane review has recommended the use of non-steroidal anti-inflammatory drugs as the best management of IUD-associated menorrhagia and dysmenorrhea [35], which are contraindicated for most women with CKD.

There are no reports of intrauterine contraceptive failure in renal transplant recipients in contemporary literature. Although no studies have been performed to specifically examine the efficacy of IUD in the renal population, there is no clinical evidence to suggest an excess of intrauterine contraceptive failure in women with renal transplants [36]. This contrasts with an historical report of IUD failure in two renal transplant recipients more than 30 years ago [37]. The theoretical concern presented at that time was that intrauterine contraception was less effective in a patient maintained on immunosuppressive therapy due to an attenuation of the uterine inflammatory response that forms part of the contraceptive mechanism. Such concern is now considered unfounded. It is recognized that macrophages play the most important role in the uterine milieu and that calcineurin inhibitors, antimetabolites and biological agents, including basiliximab and daclizumab, which act primarily via T-cell inhibition, are unlikely to affect this process. In addition, steroid therapy is recognized to increase macrophage activity via activation of macrophage migration inhibiting factor. In addition, the Mirena® IUS does not have an immunological basis for its action but utilizes endometrial inhibition and cervical mucosal thickening. IUDs remain one of the most effective contraceptive methods available and they should not be denied to renal transplant recipients on the basis of hypothesised, but unsubstantiated, biological theory [38].

A second theoretical concern regarding the use of intrauterine methods in the transplant population is one of infection. However, small, retrospective studies of renal transplant patients using the Mirena® IUS have failed to show any cases of either pelvic infection or unplanned pregnancy [39]. Large-scale studies have not been carried out in solid organ transplant recipients, but data from patients who are immunosuppressed due to human immunodeficiency virus (HIV) show no correlation between infectious complications of IUDs and immune competence as measured by CD-4 count [40]. Observational evidence indicates that IUDs do not increase the risk of pelvic inflammatory disease unless they are inserted in women with preexisting, untreated infection [4]. Although universal screening for gonorrhea and chlamydia is not recommended prior to IUD insertion, screening can be considered for women taking immunosuppressive medication [38].

The use of IUDs in the peritoneal dialysis population remains understudied. Current advice is poorly informed by historical, isolated case reports of peritonitis in association with copper IUD use in patients undergoing peritoneal dialysis [41]. Such anecdotal data should be appropriately balanced with an understanding of both the relative contraindications and typical use failure rates of alternative contraceptive methods, and the known risks of an unintended pregnancy.

Barrier Methods

Barrier methods of contraception include condoms, cervical caps, diaphragms and sponges. They offer convenience and avoid the possibility of drug interaction. In addition, condoms prevent the transmission of HIV and sexually transmitted infections. Their effectiveness depends upon consistent and correct use by the patient or her partner. Therefore, failure rates are variable and it is important to consider their "typical-use" effectiveness (see Table 3.1).

Both male and female condoms are available with "typical-use" failure rates of 18 percent and 21 percent, respectively [5]. For this reason, for women for whom an unintended pregnancy would be unacceptable either on health or personal grounds, sole use of a barrier method is not an appropriate contraceptive choice. Male and female condom use should not be combined due to an increased chance of slippage of both devices [38].

Diaphragms are thin, dome-shaped devices that lie between the posterior fornix and pubic bone. Cervical caps are smaller and fit directly over the cervix. Both caps and diaphragms need to be sized appropriately for the individual patient. They stay in place for six hours after intercourse. Use of caps and diaphragms should be combined with a spermicide in order to achieve acceptable levels of efficacy [38]. The contraceptive

sponge covers the cervix in a similar manner to the cap, but can be used without prior pelvic examination and individual fitting. It is impregnated with a spermicide that is activated when water is applied before use. Efficacy of these female barrier methods, even with "perfect use," varies between 80–94 percent with increased parity being a negatively contributing factor. "Typical use" is even less effective, with 12–24 percent of women experiencing an unintended pregnancy in the first year of use [5].

An increased frequency of urinary tract infection (UTI) has been associated with both diaphragm use and the use of spermicide-coated condoms. This may have relevance for women with CKD who experience recurrent UTIs, especially following transplantation. In addition, spermicides in the United Kingdom contain nonoxinol-9 (N-9), which is associated with epithelial disruption in the vagina and rectum with repeated and high-dose use and may increase transmission of blood-borne viruses. There is no evidence that condoms lubricated with a spermicide provide a greater level of contraception than those lubricated with a non-spermicidal agent, and so the use of N-9–lubricated condoms cannot be recommended [42].

Sterilization

Voluntary sterilization can be offered to all women who understand the nature of the procedure, including its low failure rate and effective irreversibility, in combination with a certainty that they do not want any more children. This may not be easy for either the patient or consulting clinician to determine. The probability of regret following sterilization has been found to be higher for women sterilized before the age of 30 compared to those older than 30 [43]. However, life events can also become sources of regret in family-planning decisions [4]. Such life events can be prevalent in the complex disease journey of the renal patient who transitions from disease stability to disease decline, renal replacement and, potentially, in and out of transplantation.

Laparoscopic female sterilization can be associated with increased risk for women with CKD, largely dependent on the severity of their underlying disease. The requirement for an operative procedure means that hypertension, diabetic control, bleeding time, fluid balance and vascular risk are important considerations in being able to provide an appropriate level of perioperative and anesthetic care.

Hysteroscopic sterilization is a less invasive alternative to standard operative sterilization and can be performed as an outpatient procedure without the need for anesthesia. A hysteroscope is used to place micro inserts into the fallopian tubes, which induce ingrowth, fibrosis and eventual blockage. Patients must continue to use alternative, effective contraception for three months following the procedure and wait until correct placement of the micro inserts is confirmed by pelvic x-ray, transvaginal ultrasound or hysterosalpingogram imaging. It is estimated that 10 percent of women will be unable to undergo the procedure due to tubal spasm, occlusion or anatomical variation.

Based on the number of kits distributed worldwide, pregnancy rates following hysteroscopic sterilization are estimated to be 0.15 percent. When compliance and misinterpretation of follow-up imaging are factored out, pregnancy rates fall to two pregnancies for every one million kits [44]. Hysteroscopic sterilization avoids the need for an operative procedure in women with CKD. If confirmation of tubal occlusion requires hysterosalpingography, then contrast volume will be small with almost immediate drainage from the uterus upon conclusion of the radiographic procedure [45]. Although concurrent immune suppression is not an absolute contraindication to hysteroscopic sterilization, manufacturers of the different available micro inserts generally caution against its use due to a theoretical concern that the tissue response that leads to tubal occlusion will be inhibited by immunosuppressive therapy. However, isolated case reports of successful hysteroscopic sterilization exist in women with renal transplants [46].

Fertility Awareness Methods

Fertility awareness–based methods of contraception require identification of the fertile days of the menstrual cycle through monitoring of cycle days, cervical secretions or basal body temperature. This is then combined with either abstinence or barrier methods within the fertile window. Studies of these methods are not methodologically robust and are poorly reported [47], but fertility awareness is estimated to result in 24 percent of women experiencing an unintended pregnancy within a year [5]. Drugs that affect cycle regularity, cycle hormones and fertility signs and symptoms will further reduce the contraceptive efficacy of these methods. For the renal patient, relevant drugs include steroids, cytotoxic medications, antidepressants and lithium. Couples using fertility awareness–based methods should be counseled that there is little evidence that these methods are effective and that the typical use failure rate is high. Other contraception options should be offered.

Lactational Amenorrhea

Lactational amenorrhea utilizes a physiological birth spacing tool. Breastfeeding an infant inhibits gonadotrophin release and suppresses ovulation. In order to ensure a sufficient contraceptive effect, the baby must be exclusively breastfed and the mother should be amenorrheic, both within six months of childbirth. When applied correctly, this is estimated to be 98 percent effective as a contraceptive method [4]. However, this contraceptive approach is largely promoted only when other forms of contraception are unavailable. As a form of contraception, it is limited both by the inherent difficulties in "diagnosing" amenorrhea in the postpartum period, particularly in those with advanced CKD and by its finite timespan. A Cochrane review of lactational amenorrhea for family planning concluded that a wiser approach to the postpartum period would be to encourage breastfeeding and, in addition, to motivate the mother to use an alternative form of contraception if contraception is required [48].

Emergency Contraception

The most widely used emergency contraceptive contains levonorgestrel at either a single high dose of 1,500µg, or two doses of 750µg taken 12 hours apart, within a 72-hour window of unprotected sexual intercourse. As a progesterone-only preparation there are no contraindications to use in renal disease, hypertension, coagulopathy and lupus. In addition, there is no evidence of an associated increase in cardiovascular risk [18].

The copper IUD can also be used as an emergency contraceptive device and is effective up to five days post-coitus (see Intrauterine Devices) [4].

Drug Interactions

Patients with renal disease can be prescribed a variety of different long-term and short-term medications. The interaction between these drugs and patients' contraceptive choice needs to be appreciated by all prescribing clinicians. Reassuringly, drugs that are commonly prescribed to women with CKD are considered to have a clinically insignificant effect on

Table 3.3 Interactions between renal drugs and contraception. Adapted from [49,50].

Class of Drug	Effect/Interaction	Effect on Contraceptive Efficacy	Recommendations
Antihypertensives	May be antagonized by combined contraceptives	None expected	Monitor BP
Diuretics	1. Estrogens may antagonize diuretic effect 2. Theoretical risk of hyperkalemia when potassium sparing diuretics are used with drospirenone	None expected	Monitor serum potassium and fluid balance
Statins		Minor to moderate increase in ethinylestradiol. Clinical significance unknown. Effect likely to be small.	None
Antidiabetic drugs	Estrogens and progestogens antagonize hypoglycemic effect		Monitor blood glucose
Immunosuppressants	1. Plasma levels of tacrolimus possibly increased by ethinylestradiol, gestodene and norethisterone 2. Ciclosporin levels possibly increased by estrogens and progestogens – unconfirmed and uncertain clinical significance	Tacrolimus theoretically inhibits metabolism of estrogens and progestogens. Clinical significance unknown. Effect likely to be small.	Monitor tacrolimus and ciclosporin levels.
Proton-pump inhibitors and H2 receptor blockers	Increased gastric pH theoretically reduces absorption of ulipristal acetate	Reduced efficacy of ulipristal acetate	Use alternative emergency contraception

contraceptive efficacy. The inverse effect whereby contraception affects other drugs prescribed to women with CKD is already encompassed in the routine clinical surveillance, namely monitoring of blood pressure, potassium, fluid state and calcineurin inhibitor levels. Drug interactions of particular relevance to the nephrologist are outlined in Table 3.3.

Conclusion

Contraceptive counseling is important for all women in their childbearing years, including women with CKD, yet there is a paucity of evidence that contraceptive counseling is being routinely and comprehensively provided for women with CKD. Unintended pregnancies occur in women with CKD despite the recognized risk of adverse pregnant outcomes. Safe and effective contraceptive advice should be offered to all women of childbearing age with CKD. This must include those women with the highest risk of adverse outcome in the event of an unintended pregnancy such as women with advanced or progressive CKD, women on dialysis, women with active glomerulonephritis and women taking teratogenic medication including ACE-inhibitors, angiotensin antagonists, mycophenolate mofetil and cyclophosphamide.

A wide range of contraceptive options is available for women with CKD. Women with CKD should be given advice about the efficacy of each method including "typical use" failure rates, which may be very different and less acceptable to women than the failure rates associated with "perfect use."

Safe and effective reversible forms of contraception that can be used in all women with CKD include the progesterone-only pill with an extended re-dosing window (Cerazette®, Cerelle®, Aizea®, Nacrez®), the contraceptive implant (Nexplanon®) and the intrauterine system (Mirena®). Emergency contraception can also be safely prescribed. For other methods, potential side effects, "typical-use" failure rates, anticipated length of use and acceptability should be considered on an individual basis. Non-hormonal methods should be considered for women over the age of 40 years.

References

1. Wellings K, Jones KG, Mercer CH, et al. The prevalence of unplanned pregnancy and associated factors in Britain: Findings from the third national survey of sexual attitudes and lifestyles (natsal-3). *Lancet* 2013, 382: 1807–1816.

2. Montouchet C, Trussell J. Unintended pregnancies in England in 2010: Costs to the National Health Service (NHS). *Contraception* 2013, 87: 149–153.

3. Shah PS, Balkhair T, Ohlsson A, et al. Intention to become pregnant and low birth weight and preterm birth: A systematic review. *Matern Child Health J* 2011, 15: 205–216.

4. Amy JJ, Tripathi V. Contraception for women: An evidence based overview. *BMJ* 2009; 339: b2895.

5. Trussell J. Contraceptive failure in the United States. *Contraception* 2011, 83: 397–404.

6. Williams D, Davison J. Chronic kidney disease in pregnancy. *BMJ* 2008, 336(7637): 211.

7. Baines LA, Smith MC, Davison JM, et al. Estimating the need for prepregnancy care in women with chronic kidney disease (CKD). *Archives of Disease in Childhood – Fetal and Neonatal Edition* 2011, 96(S1): Fa107.

8. Hladunewich M, Hercz AE, Keunen J, et al. Pregnancy in end stage renal disease. *Semin Dial* 2011, 24: 634–639.

9. Shahir AK, Briggs N, Katsoulis J, et al. An observational outcomes study from 1966–2008, examining pregnancy and neonatal outcomes from dialysed women using data from the ANZDATA registry. *Nephrology (Carlton)* 2013, 18: 276–284.

10. Kimmel PL, Patel SS. Psychosocial issues in women with renal disease. *Adv Ren Replace Ther* 2003, 10: 61–70.

11. Stratta P, Canavese C, Quaglia M. Pregnancy in patients with kidney disease. *J Nephrol* 2006; 19(2): 135–143.

12. The Renal Association. *UK renal registry: The 17th annual report*. The Renal Registry, Bristol, Dec 2014.

13. Bramham K, Nelson-Piercy C, Gao H, et al. Pregnancy in renal transplant recipients: A UK national cohort study. *Clin J Am Soc Nephrol* 2013, 8: 290–298.

14. Yildirim Y, Uslu A. Pregnancy in patients with previous successful renal transplantation. *Int J Gynaecol Obstet* 2005, 90: 198–202.

15. Xu L, Yang Y, Shi JG, et al. Unwanted pregnancy among Chinese renal transplant recipients. *Eur J Contracep Reprod Health Care* 2011, 16(4): 270–276.

16. Guazzelli CA, Torloni MR, Sanches TF, et al. Contraceptive counseling and use among 197 female kidney transplant recipients. *Transplantation* 2008, 86 (5): 669–672.

17. Ghazizadeh S, Lessan-Pezeshki M, Khatami M, et al. Unwanted pregnancy among kidney transplant recipients in Iran. *Transplant Proc* 2005, 37(7): 3085–3086.

18. Faculty of Sexual and Reproductive Healthcare. *UK medical eligibility criteria for contraceptive use*. Royal College of Obstetricians and Gynaecologists, England, 2009.

19. Gallo MF, Nanda K, Grimes DA, et al. 20 μg versus > 20 μg estrogen combined oral contraceptives for contraception. *Cochrane Database Syst Rev* 2013, 8: CD003989.

20. Grandi G, Xholli A, Napolitano A, et al. Prospective measurement of blood pressure and heart rate over 24 h in women using combined oral contraceptives with estradiol. *Contraception* 2014, 90(5): 529–534.

21. Pietrzak B, Bobrowska K, Jabiry-Zieniewicz Z, et al. Oral and transdermal hormonal contraception in women after kidney transplantation. *Transplant Proc* 2007, 39(9): 2759–2762.

22. Pechère-Bertschi A, Maillard M, Stalder H, et al. Renal hemodynamic and tubular responses to salt in women using oral contraceptives. *Kidney Int* 2003, 64(4): 1374–1380.

23. Lidegaard O, Lokkegaard E, Svendsen AL. Hormonal contraception and risk of venous thromboembolism: National follow up study. *BMJ* 2009, 339: b2890.

24. Baillargeon JP, McClish DK, Essah PA, et al. Association between the current use of low-dose oral contraceptives and cardiovascular arterial disease: A meta-analysis. *J Clin Endocrinol Metab* 2005, 90(7): 3863–3870.

25. Kurth T, de Jong PE, Cook NR, et al. Kidney function and risk of cardiovascular disease and mortality in women: A prospective cohort study. *BMJ* 2009, 338: b2392.

26. Appleby P, Beral V, Berrington de González A, et al. Cervical cancer and hormonal contraceptives: Collaborative reanalysis of individual data for 16,573 women with cervical cancer and 35,509 women without cervical cancer from 24 epidemiological studies. *Lancet* 2007, 370 (9599):1609–1621.

27. Skov Dalgaard L, Fassel U, Østergaard LJ, et al. Risk of human papillomavirus-related cancers among kidney transplant recipients and patients receiving chronic dialysis – an observational cohort study. *BMC Nephrol* 2013, 14: 137.

28. Paternoster DM, Riboni F, Bertolino M, et al. The contraceptive vaginal ring in women with renal and liver transplantation: Analysis of preliminary results. *Transplant Proc* 2010, 42(4): 1162–5.

29. Lidegaard O, Nielsen LH, Skovlund CW, Løkkegaard E. Venous thrombosis in users of non-oral hormonal contraception: Follow-up study, Denmark 2001–10. *BMJ* 2012, 344: e2990.

30. Chabbert-Buffet N, Amoura Z, Scarabin PY, et al. Pregnane progestin contraception in systemic lupus erythematosus: A longitudinal study of 187 patients. *Contraception* 2011, 83(3): 229–237.

31. Trussell J, Henry N, Hassan F, et al. Burden of unintended pregnancy in the United States: Potential savings with increased use of long-acting reversible contraception. *Contraception* 2013, 87(2): 154–161.

32. Lopez LM, Grimes DA, Schulz KF, et al. Steroidal contraceptives: Effect on bone fractures in women. *Cochrane Database Syst Rev* 2014, 6: CD006033.

33. Berenson AB, Rahman M, Wilkinson G. Effect of injectable and oral contraceptives on serum lipids. *Obstet Gynecol* 2009, 114(4): 786.

34. Morch LS, Skovlund CW, Hannaford PC et al. Contemporary hormonal contraception and the risk of breast cancer. NEJM 2017, 377:2228–2239.

35. Grimes DA, Hubacher D, Lopez LM, et al. Non-steroidal anti-inflammatory drugs for heavy bleeding or pain associated with intrauterine-device use. *Cochrane Database Syst Rev* 2006(4): CD006034.

36. Krajewski CM, Geetha D, Gomez-Lobo V. Contraceptive options for women with a history of solid-organ transplantation. *Transplantation* 2013, 95 (10): 1183–1186.

37. Zerner J, Doil KL, Drewry J, et al. Intrauterine contraceptive device failures in renal transplant patients. *J Reprod Med* 1981, 26(2): 99–102.

38. Estes CM, Westhoff C. Contraception for the transplant patient. *Semin Perinatol* 2007, 31(6): 372–377.

39. Ramhendar T, Byrne P. Use of the levonorgestrel-releasing intrauterine system in renal transplant recipients: A retrospective case review. *Contraception* 2012, 86(3): 288–289.

40. Morrison CS, Sekadde-Kigondu C, Sinei SK, et al. Is the intrauterine device appropriate contraception for HIV-1-infected women? *BJOG* 2001, 108(8): 784–790.

41. Plaza MM. Intrauterine device-related peritonitis in a patient on CAPD. *Perit Dial Int* 2002, 22: 538.

42. Faculty of Sexual and Reproductive Healthcare. *Barrier methods for contraception and STI prevention.* Royal College of Obstetricians and Gynaecologists, England, Aug 2012.

43. Hillis SD, Marchbanks PA, Tylor LR, et al. Poststerilization regret: Findings from the United States collaborative review of sterilization. *Obstet Gynecol* 1999, 93(6): 889–895.

44. Munro MG, Nichols JE, Levy B, et al. Hysteroscopic sterilization: 10-year retrospective analysis of worldwide pregnancy reports. *J Minim Invasive Gynecol* 2014, 21(2): 245–251.

45. Widmark JM. Imaging-related medications: A class overview. *Proc (Bayl Univ Med Cent)* 2007, 20(4): 408–17.

46. Speir VJ, Razmara A, Saberi NS. Hysteroscopic sterilization in an immunosuppressed patient. *J Minim Invasive Gynecol* 2012, 19(3): 391–392.

47. Grimes DA, Gallo MF, Grigorieva V, et al. Fertility awareness-based methods for contraception. *Cochrane Database Syst Rev* 2004(4): CD004860.

48. Van der Wijden C, Kleijnen J, Van den Berk T. Lactational amenorrhea for family planning. *Cochrane Database Syst Rev* 2003(4): CD001329.

49. Turner, Goldsmith, Himmelfarb, Lameire, Remuzzi, Winearls eds. *Oxford textbook of nephrology.* 4th edn. Oxford University Press, Oxford, 2015 [in press].

50. Faculty of Sexual and Reproductive Healthcare. *Drug interactions with hormonal contraception.* Royal College of Obstetricians and Gynaecologists, England, Jan 2012.

Assisted Reproduction in Women with Renal Disease

Jason Waugh and Ian Aird

Introduction

Nearly 40 years ago when Louise Brown was born, history was made as the first child conceived through *in vitro* fertilization was delivered [1]. It is perhaps just as important to note that in 2018 it will be 60 years since the first child was born to a woman who had received a renal transplant [2]. There can be no doubt that advances in medical care have dramatically improved the quality of life and life expectancy of women with chronic kidney disease (CKD). With these changes have come improvements in fertility and as such it is now necessary to consider prepregnancy counseling for all women with CKD of reproductive age. For most women, this counseling will center on a risk assessment for pregnancy, a discussion about the likely outcomes of a pregnancy based on this risk assessment and then a consideration as to the timing of pregnancy, with advice being given regarding contraception, prepregnancy optimization of both renal function and general prepregnancy dietary supplementation, and other factors such as smoking cessation (see Chapters 2 and 3).

At the same time as advances have been seen in the medical management of CKD, women will be aware of improvement in the management of subfertility, with many of these services being available through publicly funded healthcare systems or being affordable to many women through the private medical system.

It is therefore relevant to bring together in this chapter some of the issues that relate to the management of subfertility in women with renal disease. There will also be a small number who will seek advice on subfertility where there are other factors such as tubal occlusion or male factor infertility where, in the presence of mild or mild/moderate renal impairment, prepregnancy counseling may be similar to that for those couples who are planning for spontaneous conception.

Additional advice will be necessary regarding complications of assisted reproduction treatments (ART). Recent developments within the field of ART have led to strategies to reduce the risk of complications associated with these treatments – namely multiple pregnancy and ovarian hyperstimulation syndrome – the consequences of which will be very much more significant in women with impaired renal function.

Sexual Dysfunction in CKD

In 1999, 41,056 women commenced therapy for end-stage renal disease (ESRD) in the United States, and this is just the tip of the iceberg compared with the estimated 6 million people in the United States with reduced renal function who are often unaware of this as they remain completely asymptomatic [3, 4]. Of the ESRD population, approximately 30 percent have a functioning renal transplant, and this group may well have seen their renal function improve significantly [5].

Sexual dysfunction has been found to be significantly more common in women (and men) with CKD than in the general population [6]. Fifty-five percent of female dialysis patients report difficulty with sexual arousal [7]. Dysmenorrhea, delayed sexual development, impaired vaginal lubrication, dyspareunia and difficulties reaching orgasm are also frequently observed [8, 9].

Disturbances in the Hormonal Milieu

The detailed abnormalities that occur within the hypothalamic-pituitary-ovarian axis in women with CKD are not fully understood. There is evidence for abnormalities at both the hypothalamic and pituitary levels. Inappropriate cyclical release of gonadotrophin-releasing hormone (GnRH) from the hypothalamus leads to loss of normal pulsatile luteinizing hormone (LH) release by the pituitary, which, in turn, leads to impaired ovulation. The exact cause of the abnormal cyclical release of GnRH is unclear. Possible etiologies include raised levels of prolactin and endorphins or reduced clearance of GnRH and LH by the kidney leading to abnormally high levels [10].

Little is understood about the hormonal milieu in men and women with ESRD. Changes to dialysis regimens as well as the concomitant use of erythropoietin (EPO) have added to the variation seen in studies in this area over the past 30 years. Early reports suggested that fewer than 10 percent of premenopausal women on dialysis have regular menstruation [11] (and probably ovulation), but later surveys have suggested menstruation rates of up to 42 percent [12]. There are no recent studies on ovulatory patterns in women on dialysis. Early studies reported anovulatory patterns in general and the presumed mechanism for this is a loss of the cyclic components of gonadotrophin secretion that are a feature of women with normal renal function. The low levels of estradiol and the loss of the pre-ovulatory peak in LH and estradiol are similar to patterns seen in anovulatory women without ESRD. While a disturbance in the positive feedback pathway of estradiol is almost certain, as supplementing exogenous estrogen fails to invoke an LH surge, an acquired hypothalamic defect in women with ESRD has been suggested and is supported by the loss of the LH surge and persistently low progesterone levels [11].

Of interest, clomifene, a competitor for estrogen at the hypothalamus, increases LH and FSH, suggesting that the hypothalamus can respond to LH-releasing hormone in women with CKD. This would support the view that a defect at the hypothalamic level exists with an intact negative feedback of gonadotrophin release by low-dose estradiol contributing to the anovulatory mechanisms in these women [13].

Elevated levels of endogenous endorphins secondary to reduced renal clearance in ESRD have also been implicated as they are also known to inhibit gonadotrophin release [14].

The view that the negative feedback loop is intact is further supported by the observation that in postmenopausal women on dialysis, FSH and LH levels are "normal" (the same as postmenopausal women without ESRD). What is unknown is why the menopause tends to occur earlier in women with ESRD [15].

Elevated prolactin concentrations are commonly observed in patients with ESRD and this appears to be autonomous as it is resistant to interventions designed to inhibit or stimulate its release. This may contribute to hypothalamic-pituitary dysfunction as similar presentations are seen in women with elevated prolactin levels who do not have ESRD. The difference for women with ESRD is that when treated with bromocriptine, they may normalize their prolactin levels, but they will rarely resume normal menses and may continue to have galactorrhea [16].

More detailed studies in this area are required to explore these pathways and to elucidate the mechanisms for anovulation and menstrual disorders in ESRD as therapeutic interventions might significantly improve quality of life for dialysis patents.

Psychosocial Issues

Treatment of ESRD can result in stresses from many sources. For a woman, the illness may limit functional capacity, which means she may be prevented from fulfilling the role she both desires and believes she is capable of. This will include impaired libido and sexual and reproductive function, but does go further to include dietary restrictions and the physical limitations and time constraints of long-term dialysis treatment. While many women adapt to these challenges and lead successful and happy lives, marital discord and family dysfunction can result [17].

Depression and Psychiatric Morbidity

While large epidemiological studies are lacking, depression is widely recognized as the most common psychiatric morbidity in ESRD. It affects women more than men and reported rates of hospitalization are as high as 10 percent for psychiatric disease [18].

Marital and Family Issues

Marital disruption is relatively common in couples where one individual has ESRD, especially if on hemodialysis. This has been reported in up to 50 percent of cases [19] and would appear to be unrelated to levels of renal impairment or associated depressive symptoms. However, it is common (in up to 25 percent) to find associated depressive symptoms in the spouse of a patient with ESRD (see later in this chapter) [20]. It has also been reported by Berkman, Katz and Weissman [21] that, for women having home dialysis, the finding of high rates of sexual dysfunction do not correlate well with marital problems and many couples were comparable with the general population in terms of marital and social adaptation.

A Word on Men

While the issues of pregnancy will be restricted to women, much of the psychological morbidity associated with ESRD and its management is not. Men may be involved in this process in three ways.

- They may be the principal carer for a woman with ESRD. This role has been associated with a high rate of psychological morbidity and depressive symptoms are common. The additional burden of the risks associated with assisted conception might precipitate more problems with the result being either marital or family breakdown. Husbands of women with CKD have been reported as showing greater levels of stress and anxiety than the women themselves [22].

- It is possible that the consultation regarding pregnancy and assisted conception will be with a woman who is well but whose partner has ESRD. While it is recognized that depressive symptoms in a female carer are fewer than in a male carer, it should be remembered that the marital and family setting will be complex and very different from the clinician's perception of the norm [23]. There may be many issues present for this woman that will need exploration ahead of embarking on a long course of investigation and treatment.

- It is possible that both partners in the relationship might have some degree of renal impairment or even ESRD: the social contact associated with regular dialysis has on occasion led to relationships being established.

Sexual dysfunction in men is extremely common in ESRD. In brief, erectile dysfunction has been reported in up to 70 percent [24]. Reduced libido and difficulty reaching orgasm are also frequently reported in men with CKD [25].

ESRD is also associated with impaired spermatogenesis and testicular damage resulting in oligospermia with low motility or azoospermia. There is also impaired endocrine function in the testis with low total and free testosterone [26]. Add to this abnormal prolactin metabolism with elevated levels and gynecomastia in 30 percent of men [27], and the psychological morbidity common to ESRD and the problem can be very complex, especially if both partners have the disease.

The Ethics of Pregnancy in ESRD

In the past 50 years thousands of women around the world with ESRD who have received a transplant have had successful pregnancies [28]. As well as the kidney transplant population, there are well-documented series of pregnancies following other organ transplants, and while these numbers can only be expected to grow, the issue of subfertility in women with primary organ failure will sometimes not wait until transplantation "cures" their infertility and they can conceive spontaneously. Fifty percent of reported pregnancies in transplanted populations are unplanned. When counseling women with ESRD regarding pregnancy, three questions should be considered: "What effect will pregnancy or fertility treatment have on my disease?"; "What effect will my disease have on my pregnancy or fertility treatment?"; and "What issues particularly relate to the child who might be born after my pregnancy?" There is now a wealth of data that can be drawn upon to discuss risk for this group of women, and some of these issues are worthy of expansion, especially when taken to the extreme of a woman who is considering fertility treatment despite the associated risks to and from her underlying disease.

What Effect Will Pregnancy or Fertility Treatment Have on My Disease?

The outcome from pregnancy in women with CKD of varying degrees of severity is covered in Chapters 2 and 5. Suffice it to summarize that worsening renal function is associated with worsening outcomes for both mother and fetus, with permanent loss of residual renal function being likely and in proportion to the degree of impairment at conception. As suggested, and as has been confirmed in the literature, successful transplantation often restores both normal function and fertility, and this is discussed as a treatment modality for subfertility later in this chapter.

What Effect Will My Disease Have on My Pregnancy or Fertility Treatment?

There is approximately a 70 percent live birth rate for pregnancies spontaneously conceived in women who have received a transplant. The figure is less for those on hemodialysis (HD) or peritoneal dialysis (PD), and exact figures for specific renal conditions vary. In proportion to the degree of impairment, increasing rates of pregnancy loss (12 percent), preterm delivery (45–60 percent), hypertension, preeclampsia (up to 30 percent) and intrauterine growth restriction (20–30 percent) are seen [28]. At the extreme end of the spectrum of renal disease are women on dialysis where pregnancy complications are almost universal when pregnancy does occur [29].

What Issues Particularly Relate to the Child Who Might Be Born after My Pregnancy?

This is a complex ethical area. First, there are pharmacological considerations from fetal exposure to immunosuppressive agents in mothers who have been transplanted. While birth defects in women on established immunosuppressants would appear to be similar to background rates, concerns remain with newer agents such as mycophenolate mofetil [30]. The potential from intrauterine exposure for problems in childhood or adult life such as autoimmune disease, cancer or infertility is yet to be fully evaluated.

Babies born preterm have significant risk of long-term disability and the additional effect of being born to a transplanted mother is not known [31]. This knowledge has to be evaluated against a background of a potentially shorter life expectancy for the mother dependent upon her primary disease. This raises a number of additional questions.

Is Pregnancy Ethically Wrong?

From the child's perspective, the answer is "probably not," as there is no guarantee that any parent will remain healthy while a child grows to adulthood. However, clinicians do have an obligation to raise such concerns so that women can consider issues such as who would help rear a child with developmental problems and who could take over as a primary carer in the event of the mother's death. According to the Human Fertilisation and Embryology Authority (HFEA) code of practice, it is essential that, prior to commencing fertility treatment, the treating clinic take into account the welfare of any child who may be born as a result of that treatment (including the need of that child for supportive parenting) [32].

Who Is the Patient?

Pregnant women can refuse treatment if they so choose, but most will often choose to take additional risks for the sake of the fetus. Complicated risk–benefit evaluations of different treatment regimens need to be considered and discussed with women, but no woman can be compelled to act in the best interest of her fetus even by the courts.

Should Women Receive a Further Transplant if Their Primary Transplant Deteriorates as a Result of Pregnancy?

Ethicists have discussed this issue and continue to do so. Some argue that it should not be possible to receive a second organ while others have not received a first; some argue that it is unethical to receive a second organ if you have lost the first owing to "voluntary risk taking," and some would include pregnancy with deteriorating renal function in this group [33]. This particular argument fails morally as organ failure is multifactorial and pregnancy has only a part to play in this process. Veatch [34] suggests treatment based on present need, urgency and need over a lifetime, thus prioritizing younger women who would have fewer quality-adjusted life years (QALYs) without transplantation than an elderly patient awaiting a first transplant.

What Treatments Should Be Offered for Infertility?

As discussed, the transition from ESRD on dialysis to post-transplant stability could be viewed as treatment of infertility, as fecundity rates improve to such a degree post transplantation that urgent contraceptive advice is required following transplantation to prevent unwanted/unplanned pregnancy. However, advice on infertility will still be sought by some women for whom this remains an issue. Their options include assisted conception, adoption or a decision not to have a family. Does a woman have a right to become a parent? Lainie Ross [35] explores this question of rights in today's society. The right not to become a parent (a negative right) is clear through the right to contraception and abortion, but the positive right to become a parent is less clear. Article 16 (1) of the Human Rights Act states, "men and women of full age, without any limitation due to race, nationality or religion, have the right to marry and to found a family." The right to conceive applies only to spontaneous conception, and assisted reproduction programs retain the right to restrict access if the best interests of the resulting child would be compromised [32]. Whether they choose to enforce this is variable and often regulations are dependent upon the host nation state.

Pharmacology of Assisted Conception

Clomifene Citrate

As described earlier, clomifene citrate may be prescribed in women with infertility and associated renal disease.

The indications are likely to be coincident conditions causing subfertility through anovulation, the most common cause of which is polycystic ovarian syndrome (PCOS).

Clomifene acts by inducing gonadotrophin release by antagonizing estrogens in the hypothalamus and disrupting feedback mechanisms. Chorionic gonadotrophin has been used as an adjunctive therapy. Women with ESRD on dialysis are unlikely to benefit from clomifene despite hypothalamic sensitivity (see earlier in this chapter).

Clomifene is mainly excreted via the fecal route with only 8 percent being excreted via the kidney; as such, there are no reported contraindications in relation to renal disease.

Adverse effects include ovarian hyperstimulation syndrome (OHSS). A review of more than 8,000 cycles of clomifene therapy reported that OHSS occurred in 13.5 of cycles with only sporadic reports of moderate and severe forms of the condition [36]. OHSS is discussed further in what follows.

Multiple pregnancy, the importance of which cannot be overemphasized, occurs in approximately 10 percent of cycles and the majority of these are twin pregnancies. For this reason, the recently updated National Institute of Health and Clinical Excellence (NICE) guideline for the management of fertility recommends the offer of ultrasound monitoring during at least the first cycle of treatment to reduce the risk of multiple pregnancy [37]. In patients with CKD, we would argue that it is mandatory for every cycle of treatment to be monitored and cycles where there is more than one mature follicle should be abandoned. Less severe but more common problems of clomifene therapy include breast tenderness, nausea, vomiting and headaches.

According to NICE, the options for women who are resistant to clomifene include laparoscopic ovarian drilling, combined treatment with clomifene and metformin or treatment with gonadotrophins. Metformin may be contraindicated in women with CKD due to the risk of lactic acidosis; the British National Formulary (BNF) recommends avoidance of metformin if eGFR is less than 30 ml/min/1.73 m^2 to the risk.

Aromatase inhibitors have recently been proposed as an alternative for anovulatory women resistant to clomifene. Aromatase inhibitors induce ovulation by blocking estrogen biosynthesis, thereby reducing negative estrogenic feedback at the pituitary. The most studied aromatase inhibitor for ovulation induction is letrozole. It should be emphasized that aromatase inhibitors are not currently licensed for use in ovulation induction. However, they have certain potential advantages over clomifene, particularly for women with CKD; these include: a higher rate of monofollicular development, which should theoretically reduce the risk of multiple pregnancy, no direct anti-estrogenic effects on the endometrium or cervical mucus, due to an absence of peripheral estrogen blockade and a shorter half-life, which would predict a lower risk of teratogenicity.

Gonadotrophins

Follicle-Stimulating Hormones and Luteinizing Hormone

These are available as purified extracts from human postmenopausal urine (Menotrophins e.g. Merional or Menopur [75 units FSH, 75 units LH] or Follitropin e.g. Fostimon [75 units FSH]) or as recombinant preparations (Gonal-F, Puregon [FSH], Luveris [LH]).

The indications for gonadotrophin therapy include the treatment of women with proven hypogonadotropic hypogonadism, hypopituitarism, those who do not respond to clomifene citrate and for controlled ovarian stimulation in assisted reproduction treatments (ART). The most significant adverse effects are OHSS (discussed later in this chapter) and multiple pregnancy from the resultant ART cycle.

Again, women are often troubled by nausea and vomiting and venous thromboembolic events have been described. There are no data related to the use of these drugs in women with significant renal impairment, although it is likely that women with a reduced glomerular filtration rate (GFR) and/or creatinine clearance or women with nephrotic syndrome would be more susceptible to complications. Approximately 10 percent of these hormones are excreted through the kidney unchanged and so plasma levels may be elevated if renal function is compromised.

Human Chorionic Gonadotrophin

Human chorionic gonadotrophin (hCG) is given in superovulatory cycles for intrauterine insemination (IUI) to mimic the LH surge and promote ovulation.

In *in vitro* fertilization (IVF) cycles, it is given as a precursor to egg collection to induce final oocyte maturation. It is also given to support the luteal phase after embryo transfer. HCG is available as Choragon and Pregnyl, which are purified urinary-derived products, and Ovitrelle, which is a recombinant preparation. Exposure to hCG appears to be a critical "trigger" in the development of OHSS in women who have been previously exposed to gonadotrophins. Choragon and Pregnyl carry a warning against their use in renal impairment.

Gonadotrophin-Releasing Hormone Agonists

The gonadotrophin-releasing hormone agonists buserelin goserelin, nafarelin and leuproelin are used to downregulate the gonadotrophin-releasing hormone receptors, thus switching off endogenous FSH and LH and both preventing premature ovulation and promoting multiple follicle development. Removal of endogenous LH and FSH activity also allows for easier cycle planning, which facilitates management of the IVF laboratory workload.

Adverse Effects

The most significant adverse effects are hypertension, edema, altered blood lipids, bone demineralization and fluid retention. These drugs carry a warning against their use in women with renal impairment. Downregulation of the pituitary gland prior to ovarian stimulation also leads to a larger cohort of follicles being stimulated to develop, which in turn increases the risk of ovarian hyperstimulation syndrome.

Gonadotrophin-Releasing Hormone Antagonists

Gonadotrophin-releasing hormone antagonists, including ganirelix and cetrorelix, are a relatively new introduction to IVF treatments. They have an advantage over GnRH agonists in that they do not need to be given before ovarian stimulation and they therefore reduce exposure to drugs and lessen the treatment burden. They also have the advantage over GnRH agonists in that the final oocyte maturation prior to oocyte collection may be achieved by use of a GnRH agonist trigger. If this protocol is combined with cryopreservation of all embryos with subsequent transfer in frozen thawed embryo transfer cycles, it may abolish almost completely the risk of OHSS [38]. Unfortunately for women with CKD, current BNF recommendations are that GnRH antagonists should be avoided in moderate or severe renal impairment.

It should be remembered that all these drugs would be given simultaneously with other medication for renal disease. The issues related to hypertensive medication and immunosuppression will be dealt with elsewhere, but there are no data regarding the coadministration of these drugs in terms of maternal toxicity or fetal teratogenicity. With the altered pharmacodynamics related to changes in volume of distribution with the hemodynamic changes of ovarian induction/hyperstimulation (see later in this chapter), the fetus might be exposed to significantly higher doses of these agents than has previously been described.

Complications of Assisted Conception

The complications of ART are not to be underestimated for women whose renal function is impaired. OHSS is discussed in what follows as it can result in renal failure even when renal function is normal at the time treatment commences.

Ectopic Pregnancy

Current rates of ectopic pregnancy following assisted conception are between 2 percent and 5 percent, although rates in some older series were as high as 10 percent. Such a complication, even if detected early in a subclinical phase, would prove a significant challenge to a woman with ESRD. Issues would include the possibility of general anesthesia for either laparoscopic or open surgical management, hemorrhage either before or after surgery and the difficulties of treating conservatively with methotrexate. Women should be made aware of this complication and the risks involved. Avoidance of multi-embryo transfer during IVF treatment will help to reduce the incidence of ectopic pregnancy and the even harder-to-diagnose condition of heterotopic pregnancy, which is more common after IVF when more than one embryo is transferred.

First-Trimester Miscarriage

Once conception is confirmed, the miscarriage rate in the general population is approximately 25 percent, and this is higher in older women and those with other risk factors. Again, the risks of associated hemorrhage, anesthesia and surgery need to be highlighted to any woman planning this course of treatment [39].

Multiple Pregnancy

The impact of assisted conception on multiple pregnancy rates is substantial. A multiple pregnancy for a woman with significant CKD could be catastrophic. The hemodynamic and renal response to pregnancy will be amplified, with total blood volume increasing by an extra 500 ml in a twin gestation compared with a singleton gestation and there is a greater drop in total peripheral resistance and diastolic blood pressure. This coupled with an exaggeration in the nausea and vomiting of early pregnancy and a higher prevalence of hyperemesis gravidarum may be sufficient to precipitate overt renal failure. Anemia is more common, the nutritional burden is greater and the fetuses more difficult to assess. All antenatal obstetric complications are increased and include higher prematurity rates, more preeclampsia and a higher perinatal mortality. Add to this the complications specific to monochorionic twins, the increase in rates of surgical delivery and postpartum hemorrhage for all twins, and the picture is still far from complete.

From a fetal and neonatal perspective, the biggest risk factor for twins is prematurity and low birth weight. Compared with singletons, twins are four times more likely to die in pregnancy and seven times more likely to die shortly after birth, and they have six times the risk of cerebral palsy [40].

In light of the aforementioned increase in neonatal and maternal risks, in 2007 the HFEA introduced its multiple birth reduction strategy. The central aim of this policy was to reduce the rates of multiple births following IVF from nearly 25 percent in 2006 to 10 percent over a number of years. IVF treatment centers would be required to devise their multiple births minimization strategy involving greater use of single embryo transfer (SET) [41].

Minimizing the risk of multiple pregnancy by adopting a policy of SET needs to be balanced against the risk of jeopardizing the live birth rate. For younger women producing good-quality embryos, any reduction in live birth rate caused by the transfer of a single embryo disappears if one compares the cumulative live birth rate of repeated SET (either two cycles of fresh SET or one cycle of fresh SET followed by one frozen SET in a natural or hormonal stimulated cycle) [42]. For women with CKD, it should be borne in mind that SET policies may increase the number of treatment cycles required to achieve a pregnancy with associated treatment-related risks, but this would surely be more than offset by reducing the potentially life-threatening risks associated with multiple pregnancy. In order to maximize the effectiveness of SET, it is important to select the embryo for transfer that has the highest implantation potential and transfer this embryo to a uterine/endometrial environment that is as receptive as possible.

More recent developments within the IVF laboratory have led to prolonging embryo culture to the blastocyst stage (usually day 5 post fertilization). It is known that blastocyst embryos have a higher implantation potential than cleavage stage embryos (day 2 or 3 post fertilization).

A significant cause of implantation failure is genetic abnormality within the transferred embryo. Preimplantation genetic screening is a technique whereby the developing embryo is biopsied to remove a cell or cells and these cells undergo genetic tests such as fluorescent in situ hybridization (FISH) or comparative genomic hybridization (CGH) to identify genetically competent embryos that are more likely to implant, less likely to miscarry [43].

Embryo biopsy is, however, an invasive procedure resulting in damage and potential loss of the embryo. The genetic tests to screen the embryo are also expensive and not currently widely available. Recently a noninvasive technique of imaging developing embryos using time lapse monitoring (TLM) has shown promise in identifying embryos with higher and lower implantation potential – though currently there is a need to perform properly designed prospective randomized controlled trials to confirm the value of this technique before it is incorporated into routine practice [44].

For women with CKD, where multiple pregnancy could have catastrophic consequences, these new techniques should be adopted to enable selection of a single blastocyst embryo with the highest potential to maximize the chance of implantation leading to a healthy singleton birth and reducing the chance of a dangerous multiple pregnancy.

It should, however, be remembered that prolonging embryo culture to the blastocyst stage in a nonphysiological environment and manipulation of the embryo during procedures such as embryo biopsy is associated with a higher incidence of monozygotic twinning [45]. These issues covered throughout this section should be fully discussed before a woman embarks on fertility treatment [46].

Ovarian Hyperstimulation Syndrome

All women who respond to ovarian stimulation have a degree of hyperstimulation usually recognized as ovarian enlargement, nausea and vomiting. Clinical OHSS is best defined as the presence of ascites, which probably results from increased vascular permeability and hemoconcentration as a result of this fluid loss [47]. OHSS is usually termed severe when there are also thromboembolic events or respiratory or renal failure. Little is known regarding the progression of this condition, but studies have started to map the changes as OHSS develops and then resolves. Evbuomwan, Davison and Murdoch [48] have studied healthy women longitudinally and shown that during superovulation cycles following hCG administration, first there is a 20 percent reduction in blood volume between day 2 and day 4 and then a sustained rise in blood volume (30 percent) between days 8 and 12 in women who develop OHSS. None of these changes were seen in women who did not develop clinical OHSS. Also reported was a sharp drop in serum osmolality between day 0 and day 2 in those who do not develop OHSS, which recovered to normal by day 2. In those who did develop OHSS, osmolality increased by 6 mOsm/kg between day 2 and day 0 followed by a decrease of 8 mOsm/kg by day 2 sustained to day 12. Despite this hypo-osmolar state, women with OHSS had a concentrated and then dilute urine output. Further studies by this group have suggested that the osmotic threshold for arginine vasopressin secretion and thirst are reset to lower plasma osmolality during superovulation and this is maintained until at least day 10 after hCG in OHSS.

The fluid shifts associated with this condition are considerable and, when abdominal distension precipitates clinical intervention with paracentesis, up to 7 l of ascites can be removed. Renal failure in healthy women is thought to result from poor renal perfusion secondary to hemoconcentration and the fluid shifts are so considerable that these changes would be sufficient to compromise any residual function in a diseased kidney or to jeopardize the survival of a grafted kidney. There are no data on OHSS or superovulation in women with preexisting CKD, and it is unlikely that any will exist outside isolated case reports.

Assisted Reproduction in CKD

There are no data from which recommendations can be made with regard to safety or outcome for either mother or baby in women with preexisting renal disease who might request assisted conception treatment. A strategy of as little disturbance as possible should be considered. Whether an approach is taken where donor ova are used to reduce the risks of ovarian stimulation or conventional IVF cycles are used, considerable risks remain, particularly those related to preeclampsia.

In women with renal disease who are not dialysis dependent, both obstetric and nephrological complications will be dependent upon their renal function prior to treatment. For those with only mild impairment and possibly moderate impairment, such treatment might be deemed reasonable after careful and extensive counseling regarding the risks and complications outlined earlier.

For those women who are dialysis dependent, it would seem difficult to justify assisted conception using the "best interest of the child" argument (Welfare of the Child HFEA). However, transplantation in this group could be seen not only as treatment of their renal disease, but also the most promising way forward in their quest for parenthood.

Likewise, for those women who have had a successful renal transplant and who have normal or near-normal renal function and a stable graft, it would seem reasonable to consider requests for assisted conception favorably where all other criteria were met.

The situation is most complicated for those women who have severe renal impairment but are not yet on dialysis and those with an unstable graft post transplantation where any pregnancy could jeopardize any renal reserve. Under these circumstances, it would seem difficult to justify assisted conception when most clinicians would be advocating contraception to preserve renal reserve. However, the window of opportunity for pregnancy might be getting smaller as these women are not yet "sick" enough to be placed on the transplant waiting list.

Conclusion

Both nephrologists and obstetricians are likely to meet with requests from women/couples for advice regarding assisted conception. Few data exist nor are likely to exist in the future.

The ethical dilemmas in this area have been explored and a woman's right to choose will mean such requests are forthcoming, but the majority of decisions can be made on clinical grounds based on data extrapolated from spontaneously conceived pregnancies that have been well described in ESRD.

The additional risks associated with superovulation mean that assisted conception should be reserved for women with the best and most stable renal function. Obstetricians and nephrologists may still be left caring for women where assisted conception has been sought against the best medical advice. Despite assisted conception, termination of pregnancy may be the only way to preserve renal function or to prolong the mother's life expectancy. As in any such difficult situation, it is important that the mother's autonomy is respected and that she is supported in any decision she takes.

References

1. Steptoe PC, Edwards RG. Birth after the reimplantation of a human embryo. *Lancet* 1978;2:336.

2. Murray JE, Reid DE, Harrison JH, Merrill J. Successful pregnancies after human renal transplantation. *N Engl J Med* 1963;269:341–343.

3. US Renal Data System. *USRDS 2001 annual report.* Bethesda, MD: National Institutes of Health, National Institute of Diabetes and Digestive and Kidney Diseases; 2001.

4. Jones CA, McQuillan GM, Kusek JW, Eberhardt MS, Herman WH, Coresh J, et al. Serum creatinine levels in the US population: Third national health and nutrition examination survey. *Am J Kidney Dis* 1998;32:992–999.

5. Patel SS, Kimmel PI, Singh A. The new clinical practice guidelines for chronic renal disease: A framework for K/DOQI. *Semin Nephrol* 2002;22:449–458.

6. Laumann EO, Paik A, Rosen RC. Sexual dysfunction in the United States: Prevalence and predictors. *JAMA* 1999;28(6).

7. Finkelstein F, Shirani S, Wuerth D, Finkelstein SH. Therapy insight: Sexual dysfunction in patients with chronic kidney disease. *Nat Clin Pract Nephrol* 2007;3:200–207.

8. Bellinghieri G, Santoro D, Mallamace A, Savica V. Sexual dysfunction in chronic renal failure. *J Nephrol* 2008;21:s113–s117.

9. Peng YS, Chiang CK, Kao TW, Hung KY, Lu CS, Chiang SS, Yang CS, Huang YC, Wu KD, Wu MS, Lien YR, Yang CC, Tsai DM, Chen PY, Liao CS, Tsai TJ, Chen WY.: Sexual dysfunction in female haemodialysis patients: A multicenter study. *Kidney Int* 2005;68:760–765.

10. Holley JL. The hypothalamic-pituitary axis in men and women with chronic kidney disease. *Adv Chronic Kidney Dis.* 2004;11:337–341.

11. Lim VS, Henriquez C, Sievertsen G, Frohman LA. Ovarian function in chronic renal failure: Evidence suggesting hypothalamic anovulation. *Ann Intern Med* 1980;93:21–27.

12. Lim VS. Reproductive function in patients with renal insufficiency. *Am J Kidney Dis* 1987;9:363–7.

13. Holley JL, Schmidt RJ, Bender FH, Dumler F, Schiff M. Gynecologic and reproductive issues in women on dialysis. *Am J Kidney Dis* 1997;29:685–690.

14. Ginsberg ES, Owen WF, Jr. Reproductive endocrinology and pregnancy in women on hemodialysis. *Nephron* 1984;37:195–199.

15. Schmidt RJ, Holley JL. Fertility and contraception in end stage renal disease. *Adv Ren Replace Ther* 1998;5:38–44.

16. Zingraff J, Jungers P, Pelissier C, Nahoul K, Feinstein MC, Scholler R. Pituitary and ovarian dysfunctions in women on haemodialysis. *Nephron* 1982;30:149–153.

17. Sacks CR, Peterson RA, Kimmel PL. Perception of illness and depressions in chronic renal disease. *Am J Kidney Dis* 1990;15:31–39.

18. Kimmel PL, Thamer M, Richard CM, Ray NF. Psychiatric illness in patients with end stage renal disease. *Am J Med* 1982;105:214–221.

19. Finkelstein FO, Finkelstein SH, Steele TE. Assessment of marital relationships of hemodialysis patients. *Am J Med Sci* 1976;271:21–28.

20. Wicks MN, Milstead EJ, Hathaway DK, Cetingok M. Subjective burden and quality of life in family caregivers of patients with end stage renal disease. *ANNA J* 1997;24: 527–528, 531–538.

21. Berkman AH, Katz LA, Weissman R. Sexuality and life style of home dialysis patients. *Arch Phys Med Rehabil* 1982;63:272–275.

22. Binik YM, Mah K. Sexuality and end stage renal disease: Research and clinical recommendations. *Adv Renal Replace Ther* 1994;1:198–209.

23. Deneker B, Kimmel PL, Renich TP, Peterson RA. Depression and marital dissatisfaction in patients with ESRD and their spouses. *Am J Kidney Dis* 2001;38:839–846.

24. Rosas SE, Joffe M, Franklin E, Strom BL, Kotzker W, Brensinger C, et al. Prevalence and determinants of erectile dysfunction in hemodialysis patients. *Kidney Int* 2001;12:2654–2663.

25. Finkelstein F, Shirani S, Wuerth D, Finkelstein SH. Therapy insight: Sexual dysfunction in patients with chronic kidney disease. *Nat Clin Pract Nephrol* 2007;3:200–207.

26. Procci WR, Goldstein DA, Adelstein J, Massry SG. Sexual dysfunction in the male patient with uremia: A reappraisal. *Kidney Int* 1981;**19**:317–323.

27. Gómez F, de la Cueva R, Wauters JP, Lemarchand-Béraud T. Endocrine abnormalities in patients undergoing long term hemodialysis. The role of prolactin. *Am J Med* 1980;**68**:522–530.

28. Armenti VT, Radomski JS, Moritz MJ, et al. Report from the National Transplant Registry (NTPR): Outcomes of pregnancy after transplantation. In *Clinical transplants 2002*. Los Angeles, CA: UCLA Tissue Typing laboratory, 2002, pp. 121–130.

29. Davison JM. Dialysis, transplantation and pregnancy. *Am J Kidney Dis* 1991;**17**:127–132.

30. Tendron A, Gouton J-B, Decramer S. *In utero* exposure to immunosuppressive drugs: Experimental and clinical studies. *Paediatr Nephrol* 2002;**17**:121–130.

31. Bhutta AT, Cleves MA, Casey PH, Cradock MM, Anand KJ. Cognitive and behavioural outcomes of school age children who were born premature: A meta-analysis. *JAMA* 2002;**288**:728–737.

32. HFEA Code of Practice (8th edition) www.hfea.gov.uk/code.html.

33. Ubel PA, Arnold RM, Caplan AL. Rationing failure: The ethical lessons of the retransplantation of scarce vital organs. *JAMA* 1993;**270**:2469–2474.

34. Veatch RM. *Transplantation ethics*. Washington, DC: Georgetown University Press, 2000.

35. Friedman Ross L. Ethical considerations related to pregnancy in transplant recipients. *N Engl J Med* 2006;**354**:1313–1316.

36. Schenker JG and Weinstein D. Ovarian hyperstimulation syndrome: A current survey. *Fertil. Steril.*, 1978;**30**, 255±268.

37. NICE Clinical Guideline 156 (2013) Fertility: Assessment and treatment for people with fertility problems.

38. Youssef MA, Van der Veen F, Al-Inany HG, Mochtar MH, Griesinger G, Nagi Mohesen M, Aboulfoutouh I, Van Wely M. Gonadotropin-releasing hormone agonist versus HCG for oocyte triggering in antagonist-assisted reproductive technology. *Cochrane Database Syst Rev*. 2014 Oct 31;**10**:CD008046. doi: 10.1002/14651858.CD008046

39. McFaul PB, Patel N, Mills J. An audit of the obstetric outcome of 148 consecutive pregnancies from assisted conception: Implications for neonatal services. *BJOG* 1993;**100**:820–825.

40. Braude P. One child at a time – Reducing multiple births after IVF. Report of the Expert Group on Multiple Births after IVF. October 2006. www.hfea.gov.uk/docs/MBSET_report.pdf.

41 Multiple births and single embryo transfer review. www.hfea.gov.uk/Multiple-births-after-IVF.html.

42. Pandian Z, Marjoribanks J, Ozturk O, Serour G, Bhattacharya S. Number of embryos for transfer following in vitro fertilisation or intracytoplasmic sperm injection. *Cochrane Database Syst Rev* Jul 2013;**29**(7):CD003416. doi: 10.1002/14651858

43. Keltz MD, Vega M, Sirota I, Lederman M, Moshier EL, Gonzales E, Stein D. Preimplantation genetic screening (PGS) with Comparative genomic hybridization (CGH) following day 3 single cell blastomere biopsy markedly improves IVF outcomes while lowering multiple pregnancies and miscarriages. *J Assist Reprod Genet*. 2013 Oct;**30**(10):1333–9. doi: 10.1007/s10815-013-0070-6. Epub 2013 Aug 16.

44. Kaser DJ, Racowsky C. Clinical outcomes following selection of human preimplantation embryos with time-lapse monitoring: a systematic review. *Hum Reprod Update*. 2014 Sep-Oct;**20**(5):617–31. doi: 10.1093/humupd/dmu023. Epub 2014 Jun 2.

45. Knopman JM, Krey LC, Oh C, Lee J, McCaffrey C, Noyes N. What makes them split? Identifying risk factors that lead to monozygotic twins after in vitro fertilization. *Fertil Steril*. 2014 Jul;**102**(1):82–9. doi: 10.1016/j.fertnstert.2014.03.039. Epub 2014 Apr 29.

46. MRC Working Party. Births in Great Britain resulting from assisted conception, 1978–87. MRC working party on children conceived by *in vitro* fertilisation. *BMJ* 1990;**300**:1229–33.

47. Balasch J, Fabreques F, Arroyo V. Peripheral arterial vasodilatation hypothesis: a new insight into the pathogenesis of ovarian hyperstimulation syndrome. *Hum Reprod* 1999;**13**:2718–30.

48. Evbuomwan IO, Davison JM, Murdoch AP. Coexistent hemoconcentration and hypoosmolality during superovulation and in severe ovarian hyperstimulation syndrome: a volume homeostasis paradox. *Fertil Steril* 2000;**74**:67–72.

CKD and Pregnancy

Patterns of Care and General Principles of Management

Lucy Mackillop and Mark Brown

Introduction

There have been two significant changes in the approach to management of women with CKD in pregnancy over the past few years. First, although women with preserved GFR generally have good pregnancy outcomes [1], it is now recognized that women with even mild CKD (e.g. stage 2) may have an increased risk of adverse pregnancy outcomes [2–4]. Second, there is now a greater emphasis on the possibility of successful pregnancy outcome with dialysis, following the observation that long and frequent dialysis, with almost normalization of blood biochemistry, leads to a high likelihood of a successful pregnancy [5]. A further issue that requires greater study is that outside of pregnancy, even mild CKD and non-nephrotic range proteinuria appear to be associated with increased risk of thromboembolism [6], a problem that could be further exacerbated in pregnancy.

Basic Principles of Antenatal Care

Management of the pregnant woman with chronic kidney disease (CKD) ideally begins prior to pregnancy to allow time for appropriate counseling regarding the potential risks and likely outcomes not only of the pregnancy (see Chapter 2) but also for the woman postpartum (see Chapter 9). Attitudes have changed over the past 20–30 years and CKD is no longer seen as an automatic contraindication to pregnancy [7]. Nevertheless, the data used to counsel women today are generally those derived from a few key studies published more than 10 years ago [8–16], summarized clearly in a systematic review [17].

Controversy remains as to whether the primary underlying renal disorder affects the pregnancy outcome or, more likely, the outcome is dependent upon the baseline level of renal function, with the exception of systemic lupus erythematosus (SLE). In either case, maternal hypertension and the presence of preconception proteinuria are significant independent adverse risk factors [16, 18]; live births now occur in 64–98 percent of pregnancies depending upon the degree of renal impairment and the presence or absence of hypertension and/or proteinuria.

On occasion, women with CKD have an accelerated course toward dialysis, either during pregnancy or postpartum [18]. In women with advanced renal failure, this possibility should be discussed before conception in the context of possible preemptive transplantation or early and frequent dialysis, which is usually associated with a better chance of having a successful pregnancy (see Chapter 2). Very occasionally, unplanned pregnancies occur in women with poorly controlled disease or very low GFR and in this instance discussion of termination of pregnancy should be considered as one of the options along with aggressive hemodialysis, which also can be associated with good pregnancy outcomes [5].

The key principles of antenatal care in women with chronic renal disease are:

1. measurement, interpretation and management of hypertension;
2. measurement, interpretation and management of changes in glomerular filtration rate (GFR);
3. measurement, interpretation and management of proteinuria, including nephrotic syndrome;
4. consideration of the primary underlying renal disease and its specific problems;
5. identification of abnormalities of renal tubular function;
6. identification and management of urinary tract infection;
7. clinical assessment and maintenance of volume homoeostasis;
8. consideration of appropriate "renal" and antihypertensive medications throughout pregnancy;

9. management of the medical consequences of CKD in pregnancy, including anemia and bone health;
10. identification of superimposed preeclampsia; and
11. assessment of fetal well-being.

Hypertension

Blood pressure normally falls by the end of the first trimester of pregnancy as part of a vasodilator response, accompanied by an increase in cardiac output and stimulation of the renin–angiotensin system [19]. Most women with impaired GFR will not exhibit this fall in blood pressure, and many will undergo an increase in blood pressure as the pregnancy progresses. Factors mediating this progression are unclear, given that in normal pregnancy, the majority of vascular factors favor dilatation of blood vessels; although circulating renin and aldosterone concentrations are increased, there is typically some refractoriness to the vascular effects of pressor substances. Whether this refractoriness is lost in women with underlying CKD is unknown. Pregnancy is accompanied by significant volume expansion, which under normal circumstances does not induce hypertension [19]. However, in the context of chronic renal impairment outside of pregnancy, there is often an inability to excrete a sodium load with accompanying hypertension, and it is likely that this mechanism is partly involved in the development of hypertension in these women during pregnancy. Regardless of the cause, persistence of hypertension is an adverse factor in pregnancy outcome [20], and it is therefore imperative that considerable attention is paid to the blood pressure of women with CKD during their antenatal care.

Measurement of blood pressure has traditionally used mercury sphygmomanometry, but this has slowly been replaced by a range of automated blood pressure recorders. It is probable that most of the automated blood pressure recorders used in routine clinical practice have not been validated for use in pregnancy. Even those that have been tested and have received appropriate grading from the British Hypertension Society (BHS) [21] or the Association for the Advancement of Medical Instrumentation (AAMI) [22] are not necessarily accurate in an individual pregnant woman. Where possible, blood pressure should still be recorded using mercury sphygmomanometry, recording the phase 5 sound as the true diastolic pressure [23]. An accurate alternative is the liquid crystal display sphygmomanometer [24]. Hypertension is generally defined as a blood pressure above 140/90 mmHg and in pregnancy, treatment is generally reserved for blood pressures above this level. For a time it was recommended that the target blood pressure for most women with CKD outside pregnancy be below 130/80 mmHg and so arose the question whether a period of 40 weeks or so of blood pressures above this level could lead to progressive renal impairment after the pregnancy. More recent analysis of the data suggests that in patients with CKD and low levels of proteinuria a target BP below 140/90 mmHg is sufficient.

Most women with CKD, particularly those with proteinuria above 1 g/day, will be receiving angiotensin-converting enzyme inhibitors (ACEi) or angiotensin II receptor blockers (ARBs) before pregnancy. These should be discontinued, preferably before pregnancy and certainly once pregnancy is diagnosed, owing to increased risks of fetal growth restriction, oligohydramnios, neonatal renal failure and possibly cardiac and neurological development abnormalities [25–27]. The concerns about ACE inhibitors in pregnancy have been modified somewhat, but it is our belief that in the absence of a very compelling indication such as cardiac failure, it is still best to avoid these agents during pregnancy. Likewise, chlorothiazides should also be discontinued. Suitable antihypertensives are summarized in Table 5.1 and in Chapter 8. Fear of using antihypertensives in pregnancy can be associated with poorer pregnancy outcomes, at least in women with renal transplants [28]. Target blood pressures should probably be in the region of 110–140/80–90 mmHg, seeking to preserve maternal renal function while not lowering the blood pressure so far as to reduce uteroplacental perfusion, although recent data suggest that in women with chronic hypertension without CKD aiming for a diastolic of 85 mmHg is not associated with a significant decrease in birth weight [29]. It is also important to appreciate that blood pressure will often rise significantly soon after delivery; therefore, blood pressure measurement must be just as diligent in the early postpartum period as during pregnancy.

Glomerular Filtration Rate

The GFR should rise by about 40 percent during normal pregnancy, typically apparent by the end of the first trimester. This arises from many factors, a key one being the production and effects of relaxin. One

Table 5.1 Antihypertensives in pregnancy. Adapted from NICE Hypertension in Pregnancy Guideline [76].

Drug	Route	Safety Data
Centrally Acting		
Methyldopa	oral	Mild hypotension in babies in the first two days of life
		No obvious association with congenital malformations
Beta-blockers		
Labetalol	oral/IV	No obvious association with congenital malformations
		Rare mild hypotension in babies in the first 24 hrs. of life
		Very rare neonatal hypoglycemia
Atenolol	oral	No obvious association with congenital malformations
		Possible association with fetal growth restriction [59]
Metoprolol	oral/IV	No obvious association with congenital malformations
Oxprenolol	oral	No obvious association with congenital malformations
Pindolol	oral	No obvious association with congenital malformations
Alpha blockers		
Prazosin	oral	No obvious association with congenital malformations
Calcium channel blockers		
Nifedipine	oral	No obvious association with congenital malformations
Amlodipine	oral	No reports
Verapamil	oral	No obvious association with congenital malformations
Diuretics		
Bendroflumethizide	oral	No adverse fetal effects
		Maternal hypovolemia
Frusemide	Oral/IV	No obvious adverse effects; may cause maternal hypovolemia
Vasodilators		
Hydralazine	IV	No obvious association with congenital malformations

study has suggested that failure to increase GFR is associated with miscarriage [30] (see Chapter 1).

Under experimental conditions, ensuring both adequate hydration and urine output, GFR is measured as either creatinine clearance or inulin clearance. From a practical point of view, clinicians rely on serum creatinine as the main measurement of GFR during pregnancy. Measurement of creatinine clearance requires 24-hour urine collection, which is cumbersome and even when conducted diligently may be inaccurate because of ureteric dilatation, which results in pooling of urine and an incomplete collection. Cystatin C has been used to measure GFR during pregnancy [31] together with beta-2 microglobulin. Cystatin C correlated weakly with 24-hour creatinine clearance but less well than serum creatinine in one study [32], and beta-2 microglobulin correlated weakly with serum creatinine in another [33].

However, there are problems with both measurements and serum creatinine remains the main tool for assessing GFR during pregnancy.

The CKD-Epi and Modification of Diet in Renal Disease (MDRD) formulae are now used widely outside of pregnancy [34], but are not accurate during pregnancy [35] and have never been recommended for this purpose. Similarly, the Cockcroft–Gault formula [36] has also not been validated; this formula depends on body weight as a reflection of muscle mass and body weight changes considerably during pregnancy, not because of changes in body mass but largely as a result of volume expansion, maternal fat and the fetus. Some have suggested that eGFR might be suitable to measure GFR in pregnancy [37], but others have not [38], and for now we recommend to continue to use serum creatinine as the best marker of GFR in pregnancy.

BOX 5.1 Stages of Chronic Kidney Disease Based upon Estimated GFR [77]

Stage	Description	Estimated GFR ml/min/1.73 m^2
1	Kidney damage with normal or raised GFR	≥ 90
2	Kidney damage with mildly low GFR	60–89
3a	Moderately low GFR	45–59
3b		30–44
4	Severely low GFR	15–29
5	Kidney failure	< 15 or dialysis

For practical purposes, a serum creatinine above 90 µmol/l is considered abnormal for pregnancy, reflecting impaired GFR. A serum creatinine above 130 µmol/l means that the pregnant woman carries substantial fetal and maternal hypertensive and renal impairment risks throughout her pregnancy. However, even in women with CKD stage 1 (see Box 5.1), there is an increased risk, at least in one population, above that of women with no renal disease for Caesarean section, preterm delivery and NICU admission [3, 4].

Proteinuria

In the nonpregnant woman, protein excretion is generally less than 150 mg/day, consisting of up to 20 mg/day albumin with the remainder being other proteins, often of tubular origin [39]. Albumin excretion during normal pregnancy appears to be unchanged, but total protein excretion is increased across all trimesters with an upper limit of excretion around 300 mg/day. The mechanisms of this increased excretion are unclear, but appear to relate to increased glomerular porosity [40] rather than to substantial changes in glomerular hemodynamics.

There has been a shift in nephrology practice outside of pregnancy to measure urinary protein excretion as the spot urine protein/creatinine ratio (PCR) instead of 24-hour urinary protein excretion. However, examination of source studies leading to this conclusion reveals often poor agreement between a single PCR and 24-hour urinary protein excretion. Lane and colleagues [41] showed that while there was statistically significant correlation between the spot PCR and 24-hour urinary protein excretion, agreement between predicted and actual 24-hour urinary protein excretion was poor for protein excretion above 1 g/day. On the other hand, spot PCR provided good threshold values that discriminated between protein excretions above or below excretion rates of 300 mg/day, 500 mg/day, 1 g/day and greater than 3 g/day.

Urinalysis alone is a poor predictor of protein excretion in pregnancy [42, 43]. Use of spot PCR in pregnancy has become a popular and reasonably reliable method of determining whether protein excretion is abnormal, i.e. above 300 mg/day [44], and is most often needed to diagnose the presence of proteinuric preeclampsia. There have been no studies to date testing whether serial spot PCR during pregnancy in a woman with CKD is a reliable method of predicting changes in 24-hour urinary protein excretion in that individual. While it is likely that this would be the case, 24-hour urine protein excretion remains the gold standard for assessing true changes in protein excretion during pregnancy within an individual woman. A practical approach is to consider measuring 24-hour urinary protein and creatinine excretion at the initial visit and determine the PCR from that collection, as a way of "validating" the PCR in that woman. Subsequent PCR will provide a guide to changes in her protein excretion, although it needs to be acknowledged that this is a guide only.

Even where there is a true change in protein excretion during pregnancy in women with underlying renal disease, very few therapeutic options are available apart from ensuring blood pressure control. ACE inhibitors and ARBs or aldosterone antagonists should not be used for this purpose during pregnancy, although diltiazem can be used and may have a small benefit [45]. There is thus no great imperative to keep measuring 24-hour urinary protein excretion in these women, other than to detect nephrotic syndrome. Some advocate increasing protein excretion as a marker of superimposed preeclampsia in women with underlying renal disease, although no studies have been able to confirm this, and protein excretion may increase in these women owing to appropriate increases in glomerular filtration or progression of the underlying primary renal disease or suboptimal blood pressure control. In other words, an increase in urinary protein excretion should highlight the need for the clinician to look for features of preeclampsia but by itself is not sufficient to make a diagnosis of super-imposed preeclampsia. Moreover, proteinuria is not felt to be an independent predictor of adverse pregnancy outcome in preeclampsia and should not be used by itself as an indicator for delivery [46].

Benign proteinuria is sometimes observed during pregnancy, so-called gestational proteinuria [47], where an otherwise healthy pregnant woman is found to have increased protein excretion, usually detected first by urinalysis and subsequently by a spot PCR, in the absence of any other feature of preeclampsia or hypertension and with a normal serum creatinine, i.e. normal GFR. In some cases this may represent *de novo* orthostatic proteinuria while others appear to be just a benign increase in protein excretion during normal pregnancy that generally returns to normal after pregnancy. For some, however, this is the first sign of preeclampsia, before a blood pressure rise [48], and we recommend increased surveillance for preeclampsia in such women. It is unknown if such women have any later propensity to significant renal disease. The main management issue is that urinalysis is reassessed three to six months postpartum in these women and appropriate nephrological assessment undertaken if this is persistent (see Chapter 9). New evidence suggests that normal protein excretion may be greater in twin pregnancies and this too should be taken into account when assessing kidney disease in pregnancy [49].

Nephrotic Syndrome

The term "nephrotic syndrome" refers to a distinct constellation of clinical and laboratory features of renal disease. It is specifically defined by the presence of heavy proteinuria (protein excretion greater than 3.5 g/24 hours), hypoalbuminemia (less than 30 g/L) and peripheral edema. Hyperlipidemia and thrombotic disease are also frequently observed. The most common cause of nephrotic syndrome during pregnancy is preeclampsia; however, nephrotic syndrome during pregnancy is also a problem for women with underlying primary glomerular disease. Serum albumin normally falls during pregnancy, partly owing to volume expansion, but values below 30 g/l should raise suspicion of the development of nephrotic syndrome. A spot urine PCR above 230 mg/mmol signifies a strong likelihood that protein excretion is above 3 g/day [41]. These women will generally have edema, although this is a poor diagnostic sign during pregnancy as it accompanies two-thirds of normal pregnancies. There is little diagnostic benefit from measuring serum cholesterol, usually a component of the nephrotic syndrome, as this is increased during normal pregnancy.

Women with nephrotic syndrome are at risk of losing vitamin D-binding protein, transferrin, immunoglobulins, antithrombin III (also accompanied by increased hepatic synthesis of clotting factors) and have a propensity for intravascular volume contraction in severe cases. The net result of these changes and management options are tabulated in Table 5.2. Low molecular weight heparin (LMWH) is suitable in nonpregnant patients if GFR is above 30 ml/min/1.73 m [2], but unfractionated heparin should be used in those with lower GFR, but in the absence of formal estimates of GFR in pregnancy choice of heparin requires clinical judgment. Follow-up of proteinuria after pregnancy is important not only in women with known CKD but also in women who have had preeclampsia. Bar and colleagues [42] found that 42 percent had albuminuria three to five years after delivery, signifying either underlying renal disease before the pregnancy or renal damage consequent upon preeclampsia. Most would not find such a high figure in usual clinical practice, but the clear message is that women with early onset or severe preeclampsia should be assessed several months postpartum to ensure underlying renal disease is excluded.

The Primary Underlying Renal Disease and Its Specific Problems

Management of specific renal diseases is addressed in other chapters in this book. However, it is integral to proper antenatal care of women with underlying renal disease to consider the nuances of the underlying primary disorder. The most common renal diseases predating pregnancy in this age group are presented in Table 5.3 along with the basic principles of care. Pregnancy in women with IgA nephropathy and mild renal impairment did not alter disease progression in a multicenter cohort study of 223 women [1]. Long-term follow-up of childhood IgA nephropathy showed that later pregnancy was complicated by hypertension in half the cases and preterm birth in

Table 5.2 Nephrotic syndrome

Diagnosis	Risks	Management Options
• heavy proteinuria (protein excretion greater than 3.5 g/ 24 hours)	• calcium deficiency • iron deficiency	• calcium and vitamin D3 supplementation • iron supplementation
• hypoalbuminemia (less than 30 g/L)	• increased likelihood of infection • venous thromboembolism	• LMWH • regular fetal growth and amniotic fluid estimation
• peripheral edema, hyperlipidemia and thrombotic disease are also frequently observed	• reduced uteroplacental blood flow with fetal growth restriction • renal function decline	• regular serum creatinine • (rarely) intravenous albumin

Table 5.3 Common renal disease and principles of management

Common renal diseases predating pregnancy	Basic principles of care

• primary glomerulonephritis
  . IgA nephropathy
  . focal and segmental glomerulosclerosis (FSGS)
  . minimal change
  . membranous
• reflux nephropathy
• diabetic nephropathy
• autosomal dominant polycystic kidney disease
• lupus nephritis
	• detection of deterioration in GFR and its extent
	• detection and treatment of anemia with iron and erythropoietin if indicated
	• assessment of bone health and treatment with calcium and vitamin D3 as indicated
	• prescription of low-dose aspirin for preeclampsia prophylaxis by 12 weeks' gestation
	• midstream urine culture at the beginning of pregnancy, then on two or three other occasions even in the absence of symptoms to assess for underlying urinary tract infection (particularly in those with reflux nephropathy)
	• good control of blood sugar and blood pressure to offset the disadvantage of not being able to use ACE inhibitors or ARBs in diabetic nephropathy
	• optimization of intravascular volume
	• use of appropriate immunosuppression when required in lupus nephritis, as well as determining whether the woman has anticardiolipin antibodies or lupus anticoagulant or has the anti-SSA/B antibodies with a propensity for fetal atrioventricular (AV) node disorders
	• counseling regarding inherited renal disorders and timing of screening of offspring

one-third [50], but these outcomes are not specific to this form of nephropathy. While lupus nephritis is not a common cause of end-stage renal failure overall, it is a disorder with a large preponderance toward young women and, as such, is another renal disease commonly seen by obstetric medicine physicians. In general, women with SLE should have quiescent disease pre-pregnancy to offer the best chance of a successful pregnancy outcome [51].

Inherited renal disorders are likely to have been diagnosed prior to the pregnancy and the specific implications of this for the offspring will have been discussed. The most common such renal disorder is autosomal dominant polycystic kidney disease (ADPKD); IgA nephropathy and reflux nephropathy are not inherited by specific Mendelian traits but tend to co-segregate within families, and the pregnant woman and her partner need to be aware of this.

While still uncommon, inherited disorders such as Alport's syndrome and familial hyperuricemic nephropathy [52] occur in this age group and appropriate counseling needs be provided before and during pregnancy.

Assessment of Renal Tubular Function

There are substantial changes in renal physiology during pregnancy that are largely centered on changes in renal blood flow and GFR. There are subtle changes in renal tubular function that include decreased proximal tubular glucose reabsorption, probably mediated through a volume expansion effect, leading to glycosuria in many women without reflecting diabetes. Normal pregnant women have a mixed respiratory alkalosis and metabolic acidosis with an increased urinary pH. Studies have shown the anion gap in pregnancy to be slightly lower than that postpartum [53] (see Chapter 1).

Tubular catabolism of albumin is probably normal as the fractional excretion of albumin is unchanged in pregnant compared with nonpregnant women [54]. The very large increase in filtered sodium is offset by increased tubular reabsorption, largely through resistance to atrial natriuretic peptide and increased renin and aldosterone production causing distal nephron sodium retention with accompanying potassium secretion and a tendency for low normal serum potassium levels [55]. While there is a resetting of plasma osmolality to about 10 mosm/kg below normal, renal concentrating and diluting abilities are intact [56].

The clinical implications for women with primary renal disease are as follows. Those with glomerular disorders such as primary glomerulonephritis or lupus nephritis are unlikely to have significant changes in renal tubular function but are more likely to have exaggerated sodium retention if GFR is reduced. Those with disorders affecting the tubulo-interstitial system such as reflux nephropathy, medullary cystic disease and ADPKD may have a propensity to sodium loss and thus experience volume contraction and fetal growth restriction, or occasionally impaired urinary concentrating ability, which exaggerates the predisposition to volume contraction.

However, from a practical point of view, changes in renal tubular function in women with underlying primary renal disorders are rare with only a few case reports in the literature [57, 58]. Measurement of serum sodium, potassium and bicarbonate together with creatinine is generally sufficient to ensure significant tubular dysfunction has not been missed in women with underlying CKD during pregnancy.

Plasma uric acid is commonly measured as a potential marker of preeclampsia, although its utility in preeclampsia is largely to heighten suspicions of fetal growth restriction. In renal transplant patients in particular, where urate excretion is influenced by both tubular function and drugs such as calcineurin inhibitors there is no point in measuring uric acid during such pregnancies. Uric acid undergoes reabsorption in the proximal tubule then secretion followed by post-secretory reabsorption and its excretion therefore can be influenced at several points along the nephron. Elevated plasma urate has been suggested as being pathogenic [59] or else a marker of renal vasoconstriction. In one small study, preeclamptic women receiving probenecid had lower serum uric acid and creatinine (but no difference in creatinine clearance) and higher platelet counts than women in a control group, but pregnancy outcomes were similar [60]. Consequently, a baseline uric acid level is only useful so that an elevated level is not interpreted by others later in pregnancy as indicating preeclampsia; serial measurement of uric acid in women with CKD is not of much value in clinical management.

Urinary Tract Infection

It is generally accepted that urine culture at the commencement of pregnancy is a cost-effective means of detecting asymptomatic bacteriuria, which should be treated in all pregnant women. This is of greater importance in women with underlying renal disease as they appear to have a predisposition to urine infection [61, 62], and this includes women who have had successful surgical correction of vesicoureteric reflux in childhood [63]. Ascending urine infection, or infection that leads to bacteremia, may precipitate a decline in renal function with subsequent fetal risks of impaired growth or preterm birth, as well as increased risk of preterm rupture of membranes.

A reasonable approach is to ensure that all women with underlying renal disease have a routine urine culture at the commencement of pregnancy. Women with a history of prior urine infections or surgical correction of a urinary tract anomaly, those taking immunosuppressive drugs, including renal transplant recipients, and those with impaired GFR should have further routine cultures done at around 24, 28 and

32–34 weeks of gestation. Assuming an initial uninfected sample, the remainder of women should have repeat urine cultures performed only if they develop symptoms of urinary tract infection or if routine urinalysis demonstrates new onset pyuria or nitrites, noting that pyuria is common in normal pregnancy.

Organisms responsible for urinary tract infection during pregnancy are generally the same as in nonpregnant women, with *Escherichia coli* being the predominant organism. Renal ultrasound is generally not indicated unless for some reason renal imaging has never been undertaken or if the infection fails to respond to initial antibiotic treatment. Normal ureteric and renal pelvic dilatation will be seen (see Chapter 1), and the temptation to decompress the urinary tract with nephrostomy should be resisted unless there is generalized sepsis and/or deteriorating GFR failing to respond to intravenous antibiotics.

There are no controlled trials to determine the optimum management of urinary tract infection in women with underlying renal disease during pregnancy. Conventional practice is to treat the initial infection for approximately one week and thereafter maintain a low dose of antibiotics, e.g. cephalexin or nitrofurantoin. This may be continued until shortly after delivery to avoid episodes of pyelonephritis with its fetal and maternal risks.

Clinical Assessment and Management of Volume Homoeostasis

Adequate intravascular volume is essential for preservation of GFR thereby optimizing pregnancy outcome for mother and baby regardless of the underlying renal disorder. However, it is particularly difficult to assess maternal volume homoeostasis clinically during pregnancy. Typical clinical signs used in nonpregnant women, such as edema, are of little value in assessing volume homoeostasis during pregnancy. For this reason, the hematocrit should be measured in women with underlying CKD as part of the full blood count at the initial first-trimester visit, together with serum albumin. Both measures should fall slightly as pregnancy progresses. A rise in either value strongly suggests intravascular volume contraction, although there is no discriminant value above which it is certain that volume depletion is definite [64]. Conversely, a significant fall in either value does not necessarily mean excessive volume expansion because the hematocrit depends on other factors,

such as the ability to maintain adequate red cell production, and serum albumin may fall in patients with nephrotic syndrome who in turn may have reduced intravascular volume. In practice, even if volume excess has occurred, provided that there is no respiratory compromise and that blood pressure can be controlled, this is a more favorable situation to preserve maternal renal function and fetal growth than if there is volume depletion. Therefore, when there is concern about fetal growth or deteriorating GFR in women with CKD, it is prudent to check the change in hematocrit and albumin from baseline. If these suggest reduced intravascular volume, then a trial of intravenous normal saline of no more than 1 liter per day under observation in hospital is a reasonable clinical approach, based on first principles alone.

Appropriate Use of Medications for Treatment of Renal Disease in Pregnancy

Specific medications for specific renal diseases and hypertension management are considered in Chapters 7 and 8. However, this is an important aspect of antenatal care and as discussed earlier, control of blood pressure is imperative to successful pregnancy outcome in women with underlying renal disease. Some commonly used drugs in CKD patients and considerations in pregnancy are summarized in Table 5.4.

Management of the Medical Consequences of CKD in Pregnancy

Chronic kidney disease has far-reaching effects on other organ systems and is certainly not limited to the kidney. In addition to the association with increased risk of cardiovascular disease (with or without hypertension) women with CKD are at risk of renal bone disease and anemia. Pregnancy is a time of changes in bone metabolism, favoring demineralization, and increased iron requirements and therefore particular attention needs to be paid to the increased chance of significant anemia, osteopenia and active vitamin D deficiency in pregnant women with CKD.

Iron deficiency anemia is very common in pregnancy and also in women with CKD. It is therefore suggested that all women with CKD should have a serum ferritin check at their first antenatal visit and iron deficiency treated proactively. In addition, consideration must be given to starting erythropoietin in pregnancy in women with CKD and refractory

Table 5.4 Commonly used drugs in CKD patients and considerations in pregnancy

Drugs	Considerations in pregnancy
Antibiotics	
Cephalosporins	Considered safe in pregnancy and breastfeeding
Amoxicillin	Considered safe in pregnancy and breastfeeding
Coamoxiclav	Associated with an increased risk of necrotizing enterocolitis in the newborn if given near preterm delivery
Nitrofurantoin	Associated with hemolytic anemia in the newborn if administered near delivery
Trimethoprim	Partial folate antagonist therefore avoid in first trimester
	Rarely can be associated with maternal hyperkalemia
Quinolones	Usually avoided but can be used if strongly indicated
Aminoglycosides	Use with caution, risk of auditory and vestibular nerve damage in the neonate when used in the second and third trimesters; use only when compelling indication
Immunosuppressants	
Prednisolone	Safe in pregnancy and breastfeeding, but may be associated with IUGR with prolonged high-dose use in pregnancy
Azathioprine	Considered safe in pregnancy and breastfeeding
Ciclosporine	Considered safe in pregnancy; less evidence for safety in breastfeeding
Hydroxychloroquine	Considered safe in pregnancy and breastfeeding
Tacrolimus	Considered safe [4]
	Rarely can be associated with neonatal hyperkalemia [62]
Mycophenolate mofetil and myfortic acid	Associated with increased risk of congenital malformations; do not use in pregnancy
Cyclophosphamide	Associated with increased risk of congenital malformations
mTOR inhibitors (sirolimus and everolimus)	Contraindicated in pregnancy and breastfeeding
Other drugs	
Low-dose (< 150mg od) aspirin	Used for preeclampsia prophylaxis. Considered safe in women with CKD.
Recombinant erythropoeitin	No association with adverse fetal effects
	May be associated with maternal hypertension, therefore increased surveillance for this is warranted
Intravenous iron	Considered safe in pregnancy and breastfeeding

mTOR: Mechanistic Target of Rapamycin

anemia despite adequate iron replacement. It is, however, important to remember that in some women erythropoiesis-stimulating agents may worsen blood pressure control [65] and more frequent blood pressure measurement is needed.

Like iron deficiency, vitamin D deficiency is common in the general obstetric population and, given the requirement for vitamin D to be converted to its active metabolite in the kidney, it is unsurprising that vitamin D deficiency is common in pregnant women with CKD. It is suggested therefore that women with CKD should be screened for a low calcium diet and vitamin D deficiency and treated as necessary. Alphacalcidol (1-alpha-hydroxycholecalciferol) or calcitriol (1–25 dihydroxycholecalciferol) should be used instead of cholecalciferol preparations in women with eGFR < 30ml/min.

The Paris collaborative trial has confirmed that aspirin is of benefit in preventing preeclampsia, although approximately 56 women require treatment to prevent one case [66]. Few studies have examined the prophylactic benefit of aspirin in women with underlying renal disease. However, these studies suggest that aspirin reduces the likelihood of developing preeclampsia in women with underlying CKD, with the number needed to treat being 9–57 to prevent preeclampsia and 42–357 to prevent perinatal death [67].

The effects of low doses of aspirin (up to 150 mg/day) on renal function are minimal, and, in general, this is a safe approach, particularly for women who have had previous early-onset severe preeclampsia and/or fetal loss. Therefore, women with CKD, including transplant recipients, should receive low-dose aspirin beginning in the first trimester to help optimize maternal and fetal outcomes.

Identification of Superimposed Preeclampsia

Preeclampsia is a placental disorder of unknown etiology discussed in detail in Chapter 17. It is apparent that the development of superimposed preeclampsia in a woman with CKD will lead to a worsening of renal function, exaggerated hypertension and proteinuria with risks of nephrotic syndrome, short-term and long-term risks to maternal renal function as well as increased risks for fetal growth restriction, preterm birth and perinatal mortality. However, it is very difficult to diagnose superimposed preeclampsia in a woman who begins her pregnancy with hypertension, renal impairment and/or proteinuria. An increase in blood pressure, rise in creatinine or increasing protein excretion can all be due to progression of the underlying renal disorder rather than superimposed preeclampsia. As yet, there is no validated diagnostic test to distinguish between these two scenarios, although work examining the use of serum biomarkers such as sFlt-1[68] to differentiate between preeclampsia and progression of underlying renal disease is promising [69]. In any case, when these features are accompanied by neurological signs such as hyper-reflexia and clonus or by abnormal liver transaminases or new-onset thrombocytopenia (except in SLE, where this may be an autoimmune phenomenon), then it is likely that superimposed preeclampsia has developed.

In many ways this is an academic distinction as clinicians caring for women with underlying renal disease should be vigilant for these changes in all cases, leading to increased surveillance not only of the mother but also of fetal well-being (see later in this chapter). The indications for delivery in women with superimposed preeclampsia are broadly the same as those in women with progressive underlying renal disease, i.e. inability to control blood pressure, deteriorating GFR with no reversible component, neurological abnormalities, progressively deteriorating thrombocytopenia, increasing liver transaminases or failure of fetal growth. Therefore, clinicians should not worry too much about distinguishing superimposed preeclampsia from progressive underlying renal disease, but rather focus on being vigilant throughout pregnancy for any of the aforementioned situations that would necessitate delivery.

Assessment of Fetal Well-Being

Traditional assessment of fetal well-being has depended upon a fetal morphology scan at around 20 weeks of gestation followed by regular ultrasound scans to assess fetal growth and amniotic fluid index, as well as Doppler studies of umbilical artery blood flow. The introduction of routine blood tests at 12 weeks of gestation, such as human chorionic gonadotrophin, alpha-fetoprotein and pregnancy-associated plasma protein A (PAPP-A), in combination with measurement of placental length and uterine artery pulsatility index at 20–23 weeks' gestation, has provided a good negative predictive test for adverse fetal outcome in women with high-risk pregnancies [70, 71]. In the 1990s it was noted that women with renal transplants undergoing serum screening for Down syndrome had a high false positive rate [72]. This was due to high hCG levels seen in women with renal disease. Mechanisms for high hCG are reduced renal clearance and possibly that the associated vasculopathy leads to reduced perfusion in the intervillous circulation of the placenta, with subsequent hypoxia and increased hCG production. For a serum creatinine of greater than 125micromol/l the false positive rate (FPR) is 48 percent vs. 12 percent for controls. Where total hCG rather than free hCG is used in the assay the FPR falls to 25 percent versus 15 percent for controls [73]. False positives are also seen in dialysis patients [74]. HCG is a large molecule and is not readily filtered out during dialysis causing levels to remain high; AFP and estriol fall post dialysis [75].

Consideration should, therefore, be given to whether screening in women with CKD should focus on maternal age and nuchal screening. There is no

Table 5.5 A suggested schedule of visits and management plan for pregnant women with CKD

Proposed Schedule	Appropriate Tests/Management Plan
Initial visit – first trimester	• Blood tests: full blood count, serum creatinine and electrolytes, uric acid, liver function, ferritin, calcium, vitamin D • Midstream urine culture • 24-hour urinary protein proteinuria is apparent on dipstick testing. (The PCR can be calculated from the 24-hour urine collection and used as a baseline.) • Organize serum screening and nuchal translucency scan • Start low-dose aspirin • Start calcium and vitamin D as indicated • Review current medications and ensure they are optimized for pregnancy • Consider LMWH if indicated
From 12 weeks to 28 weeks of gestation, alternate visits to the obstetrician and to the nephrologist should occur such that the pregnant woman is seen fortnightly if abnormal GFR and monthly if normal GFR	• Full blood count, creatinine and electrolytes, liver function and spot urinary PCR should be performed four weekly for women with abnormal GFR and eight weekly for women with normal GFR at initial visit. • MSU should be performed four weekly or more frequently if high risk of documented recurrent UTIs • A detailed anomaly scan should be offered between 18 and 22 weeks • Uterine artery Doppler assessment at 23–24 weeks may be offered
Thereafter until delivery, visits to the obstetrician and nephrologist should be fortnightly, alternating so that the pregnant woman is seen weekly	• Full blood count, creatinine and electrolytes, liver function and spot urinary PCR should be performed two weekly for women with abnormal GFR and four weekly for women with normal GFR at initial visit • MSU should be performed four weekly or more frequently if high risk of documented recurrent UTIs • For women with impaired GFR, monthly growth scan, umbilical Dopplers and amniotic fluid measurement is suggested
Following delivery, routine obstetric review at six weeks postpartum is required, but nephrology review should occur within the first four weeks as impairment of renal function may occur even after delivery in women with underlying renal disease	

literature currently on the impact of renal disease on free fetal DNA concentrations. If these are unaffected by CKD, then noninvasive prenatal diagnosis may be appropriate in these women to avoid unnecessary invasive testing.

Models of Antenatal Care

Women with underlying renal disease in pregnancy are best managed jointly by an obstetrician and renal or obstetric medicine physician in conjunction with a specialist midwife. It is imperative that the obstetrician has an understanding of maternal CKD in pregnancy and that the physician has an understanding of the possible fetal issues that may occur. Ideally, these women's pregnancies are managed through a high-risk pregnancy clinic or a day assessment unit. A suggested schedule of visits and management plan for these "at-risk" pregnancies is presented in Table 5.5.

Conclusion

Clinicians and pregnant women are limited by the paucity of published guidelines dedicated to the management of renal disease in pregnant women. While these pregnancies are certainly high risk compared with that in a normal pregnant woman, it is important for clinicians to remember that, provided a diligent approach such as that recommended in this chapter is taken, the final pregnancy outcome in most cases is successful for both mother and baby. For this reason, it is appropriate that clinicians managing a pregnant woman with CKD take a positive approach to the pregnancy, at all times emphasizing the need for diligence and assessment for potential complications, but highlighting that the end result in most cases will be good, which will in turn help to relieve some of the stress that accompanies pregnancy for these women.

References

1. Limardo M, Imbasciati E, Ravani P, Surian M, Torres D, Gregorini G, et al. Pregnancy and progression of IgA nephropathy: Results of an Italian multicenter study. *American Journal of Kidney Diseases* 2010;**56** (3):506–512.

2. Alsuwaida A, Mousa D, Al-Harbi A, Alghonaim M, Ghareeb S, Alrukhaimi MN. Impact of early chronic kidney disease on maternal and fetal outcomes of pregnancy. *Journal of Maternal-Fetal and Neonatal Medicine* 2011;**24**(12):1432–1436.

3. Piccoli GB, Attini R, Vasario E, Conijn A, Biolcati M, D'Amico F, et al. Pregnancy and chronic kidney disease: A challenge in all CKD stages. *Clinical Journal of the American Society of Nephrology* 2010;**5**(5):844–855.

4. Piccoli GB, Fassio F, Attini R, Parisi S, Biolcati M, Ferraresi M, et al. Pregnancy in CKD: Whom should we follow and why? *Nephrology Dialysis Transplantation* 2012;**27**(suppl 3):iii111–iii8.

5. Hladunewich MA, Hou S, Odutayo A, Cornelis T, Pierratos A, Goldstein M, et al. Intensive hemodialysis associates with improved pregnancy outcomes: A Canadian and United States cohort comparison. *Journal of the American Society of Nephrology* 2014.

6. Mahmoodi BK, Gansevoort RT, Næss IA, Lutsey PL, Brækkan SK, Veeger NJGM, et al. Association of mild to moderate chronic kidney disease with venous thromboembolism: Pooled analysis of five prospective general population cohorts. *Circulation* 2012;**126** (16):1964–1971.

7. Lindheimer MD, Davison JM, Katz AI. The kidney and hypertension in pregnancy: Twenty exciting years. *Semin Nephrol* 2001;**21**:173–189.

8. Jungers P, Chauveau D. Pregnancy in renal disease. *Kidney Int* 1997;**52**:871–885.

9. Jones DC. Pregnancy complicated by chronic renal disease. *Clin Perinatol* 1997;**24**:483–496.

10. Hou S. Pregnancy in chronic renal insufficiency and end stage renal disease. *Am J Kidney Dis* 1999;**33**:235–252.

11. Jungers P, Chauveau D, Choukroun G, Moynot A, Skhiri H, Houillier P, et al. Pregnancy in women with impaired renal function. *Clin Nephrol* 1997;**47**:281–288.

12. Jungers P, Houillier P, Chauveau D, Choukroun G, Moynot A, Skhiri H, et al. Pregnancy in women with reflux nephropathy. *Kidney Int* 1996;**50**:593–599.

13. Jones DC, Hayslett JP. Outcome of pregnancy in women with moderate or severe renal insufficiency. *New Engl J Med* 1996;**335**:226–232.

14. Lindheimer MD, Katz AS. Kidney function and disease in pregnancy. *Philadelphia: Lea & Febiger* 1977;146–187.

15. Holley JL, Bernardini J, Quadric KH, Greenberg A, Laifer SA. Pregnancy outcomes in a prospective matched control study of pregnancy and renal disease. *Clin Nephrol* 1996;**45**:77–82.

16. Imbasciati E, Gregorino G, Cabiddu G, Gammaro L, Ambroso G, Del Giudice A, et al. Pregnancy in CKD stages 3 to 5: Fetal and maternal outcomes. *Am J Kidney Dis* 2007;**49**:753–762.

17. Piccoli GB, Conijn A, Attini R, Biolcati M, Bossotti C, Consiglio V, Deagostini MC, Todros T. Pregnancy in chronic kidney disease: Need for a common language. *J Nephrol* 2011; **24**(03): 282–299.

18. Ramin SM, Vidaeff AC, Yeomans ER, Gilstrap LC. Chronic renal disease in pregnancy. *Obstet Gynecol* 2006;**108**:1531–1539.

19. Gallery EDM, Brown MA. Volume homeostasis in normal and hypertensive human pregnancy. *Baillieres Clin Obstet Gynaecol* 1987;**1**:835–851.

20. Chakravarty EF, Colon I, Langen ES, Nix DA, El-Sayed YY, Genovese MC, et al. Factors that predict prematurity and preeclampsia in pregnancies. *Am J Obstet Gynecol* 2005;**192**:1897–1904.

21. O'Brien E, Petrie J, Littler W, de Swiet M, Padfield PL, O'Malley K, et al. The British Hypertension Society protocol for the elevation of automated and semi-automated blood pressure measuring devices with special reference to ambulatory systems. *J Hypertens* 1990;**8**:607–619.

22. White WB, Berson AS, Robbins C, Jamieson MJ, Prisant LM, Roccella E, et al. National standard for measurement of resting and ambulatory blood pressure with automated sphygmomanometers. *Hypertension* 1993;**21**:504–509.

23. Brown MA, Buddle ML, Farrell TJ, Davis G, Jones M. Randomised trial of management of hypertensive pregnancies by Korotkoff phase IV or phase V. *Lancet* 1998;**352**:777–781.

24. Davis G, Roberts LM, Mangos G, Brown MA. Comparisons of auscultatory hybrid and automated sphygmomanometers with mercury sphygmomanometry in hypertensive and normotensive pregnant women: parallel validation studies. J Hypertension. 2014 Nov 6. [Epub ahead of print]

25. Cooper WO, Hernandez-Diaz S, Arbogast PG, Dudley JA, Dyer S, Gideon PS, et al. Major congenital malformations after first-trimester exposure to ACE inhibitors. *New Engl J Med* 2006;**354**:2443–2451.

26. Serreau R, Luton D, Macher MA, Delezoide AL, Garel C, Jacqz-Aigrain E. Developmental toxicity of the angiotensin II type 1 receptor antagonists during human pregnancy: A report of 10 cases. *BJOG* 2005;**112**:710–712.

27. Bass JK, Faix RG. Gestational therapy with an angiotensin II receptor antagonist and transient renal failure in a premature infant. *Am J Perinatol* 2006;**23**:313–317.

28. Galdo T, Gonzalez F, Espinoza M, Quintero N, Espinoza O, Herrera S, et al. Impact of pregnancy on the function of transplanted kidneys. *Transplant Proc* 2005;**37**:1577–1579.

29. Magee LA, Von Dadelszen P, Rey E, Ross S, Asztalos E, Murphy KE, et al. Less-tight versus tight control of hypertension in pregnancy. *New England Journal of Medicine*. 2015;**372**(5):407–417.

30. Davison JM, Noble MCB. Serial changes in 24 hour creatinine clearance during normal menstrual cycles and the first trimester of pregnancy. *Br J Obstet Gynaecol* 1981;**88**:10–17.

31. Akbari A, Lepage N, Keely E, Clark HD, Jaffey J, MacKinnon M, et al. Cystatin C and beta trace protein as markers of renal function in pregnancy. *BJOG* 2005;**112**:575–578.

32. Moodley J, Gangaram R, Khanyile R, Ojwang PJ. Serum cystatin C for assessment of glomerular filtration rate in hypertensive disorders of pregnancy. *Hypertens Pregnancy* 2004;**23**:309–317.

33. Ben-Haroush A, Bardin R, Erman A, Hod M, Chen R, Kaplan B, et al. Beta 2-microglobulin and hypertensive complications in pregnant women at risk. *Clin Nephrol* 2002;**58**:411–416.

34. Levey AS, Bosch JP, Lewis JB, Greene T, Rogers N, Roth D. A more accurate method to estimate glomerular filtration rate from serum creatinine: A new prediction equation. Modification of diet in renal disease study group. *Ann Intern Med* 1999;**130**:461–470.

35. Smith MC, Moran P, Ward MK, Davison JM. Assessment of glomerular filtration rate in pregnancy using the MDRD formula. *Br J Obstet Gynaecol* 2008;**115**:109–112.

36. Cockcroft DW, Gault MH. Prediction of creatinine clearance from serum creatinine. *Nephron* 1976;**16**:31–41.

37. Masuyama H, Nobumoto E, Okimoto N, Inoue S, Segawa T, Hiramatsu Y. Superimposed preeclampsia in women with chronic kidney disease. *Gynecologic and Obstetric Investigation*. 2012;**74**(4):274–281.

38. Maynard SE, Thadhani R. Pregnancy and the kidney. *Journal of the American Society of Nephrology*. 2009;**20**(1):14–22.

39. Roberts M, Lindheimer MD, Davison JM. Altered glomerular permselectivity to neutral dextrans and heteroporous membrane modelling in human pregnancy. *Am J Physiol* 1996;**270**:F338–43.

40. Milne JE, Lindheimer MD, Davison JM. Glomerular heteroporous membrane modelling in third trimester and post-partum before and during amino acid infusion. *Am J Physiol Renal Physiol* 2002:**282**:F170–5.

41. Lane C, Brown M, Dunsmuir W, Kelly J, Mangos G. Can spot urine protein/creatinine ratio replace 24 h urine protein in usual clinical nephrology? *Nephrology (Carlton)* 2006;**11**:245–249.

42. Gangaram R, Ojwang PJ, Moodley J, Maharaj D. The accuracy of urine dipsticks as a screening test for proteinuria in hypertensive disorders of pregnancy. *Hypertens Pregnancy* 2005;**24**:117–123.

43. Phelan LK, Brown MA, Davis GK, Mangos G. A prospective study of the impact of automated dipstick urinalysis on the diagnosis of pre-eclampsia. *Hypertens Pregnancy* 2004;**23**:135–132.

44. Côté A-M, Brown MA, Lam EM, Von Dalelszen P, Firoz T, Liston RM, Magee LA. Diagnostic accuracy of urinary spot protein: Creatinine ratio for proteinuria in hypertensive pregnant women: Systematic review. *BMJ*. 2008 May 3;**336**(7651):1003–1006.

45. Khandelwal M, Kumanova M, Gaughan JP, Reece EA. Role of diltiazem in pregnant women with chronic renal disease. *J Matern Fetal Neonatal Med* 2002;**12**:408–412.

46. Airoldi J, Weinstein L. Clinical significance of proteinuria in pregnancy. *Obstet Gynecol Surv* 2007;**62**:117–124.

47. Holston AM, Qian C, Yu KF, Epstein FH, Karumanchi SA, Levine RJ. Circulating angiogenic factors in gestational proteinuria without hypertension. *American Journal of Obstetrics & Gynecology* **200**(4):392.e1–.e10.

48. Morikawa M, Yamada T, Minakami H. Outcome of pregnancy in patients with isolated proteinuria. *Current Opinion in Obstetrics and Gynecology*. 2009;**21**(6):491–5 10.1097/GCO.0b013e32833040bf.

49. Osmundson SS, Lafayette RA, Bowen RA, Roque VC, Garabedian MJ, Aziz N. Maternal proteinuria in twin compared with singleton pregnancies. *Obstetrics & Gynecology*. 2014;**124**(2, PART 1):332–337.

50. Ronkainen J, Ala-Houhala M, Autio-Harmainen H, Jahnukainen T, Koskimies O, Merenmies J, et al. Long-term outcome 19 years after childhood IgA nephritis: A retrospective cohort study. *Pediatr Nephrol* 2006;**21**:1266–1273.

51. Germain S, Nelson-Piercy C. Lupus nephritis and renal disease in pregnancy. *Lupus* 2006;**15**:148–55.

52. Simmonds HA, Cameron JS, Goldsmith DJ, Fairbanks LD, Raman GV. Familial juvenile hyperuricaemic nephropathy is not a rare genetic metabolic purine disease in Britain. *Nucleosides Nucleotides Nucleic Acids* 2006;**25**:1071–1075.

53. Akbari A, Wilkes P, Lindheimer M, Lepage N, Filler G. Reference intervals for anion gap and strong ion difference in pregnancy: A pilot study. *Hypertens Pregnancy* 2007;**26**:111–119.

54. Brown MA, Wang M-X, Buddle ML, Calton MA, Cario GM, Zammit VC, et al. Albumin excretory rate in normal and hypertensive pregnancy. *Clin Sci* 1994;**86**:251–255.

55. Brown MA, Sinosich MJ, Saunders DM, Gallery EDM. Potassium regulation and progesterone aldosterone interrelationships in human pregnancy: A prospective study. *Am J Obstet Gynecol* 1986;**155**:349–353.

56. Davison JM, Sheills EA, Philips PR, Lindheimer MD. Serial evaluation of vasopressin release and thirst in human pregnancy: Role of human chorionic gonadotrophin in the osmoregulatory changes of gestation. *J Clin Invest* 1988;**81**:789–806.

57. Rowe TF, Magee K, Cunningham FG. Pregnancy and renal tubular acidosis. *Am J Perinatol* 1999;**16**:189–191.

58. Firmin CJ, Kruger TF, Davids R. Proximal renal tubular acidosis in pregnancy: A case report and literature review. *Gynecol Obstet Invest*. 2007;**63**(1):39–44. Epub 2006 Aug 10.

59. Kang DH, Finch J, Nakagawa T, Karumanchi SA, Kanellis J, Granger J, et al. Uric acid, endothelial dysfunction and pre-eclampsia: Searching for a pathogenetic link. *J Hypertension* 2004;**22**:229–235.

60. Schackis RC. Hyperuricaemia and preeclampsia: Is there a pathogenic link? *Med Hypotheses* 2004;**63**:239–244.

61. Trevisan G, Ramos JG, Martins-Costa S, Barros EJ. Pregnancy in patients with chronic renal insufficiency at Hospital de Clinicas of Porto Alegre, Brazil. *Ren Fail* 2004;**26**:29–34.

62. Schwartz MA, Wang CC, Eckert LO, Critchlow CW. Risk factors for urinary tract infection in the post-partum period. *Am J Obstet Gynecol* 1999;**181**:547–553.

63. Bukowski TP, Betrus GG, Aquilina JW, Perimutter AD. Urinary tract infections and pregnancy in women who underwent antireflux surgery in childhood. *J Urol* 1998;**159**:1286–1289.

64. Brown MA, Zammit VC, Mitar DM. Extracellular fluid volumes in pregnancy-induced hypertension. *J Hypertens* 1992;**10**:61–68.

65. Kashiwagi M, Breymann C, Huch R, Huch A. Hypertension in a pregnancy with renal anemia after recombinant human erythropoietin (rhEPO) therapy. *Arch Gynecol Obstet* 2002;**267**:54–56.

66. Askie LM, Duley L, Henderson-Smart DJ, Stewart LA, PARIS Collaborative Group. Antiplatelet agents for prevention of pre-eclampsia: A meta-analysis of individual patient data. *Lancet* 2007;**369**:1791–1798.

67. Coomarasamy A, Honest H, Papaioannou S, Gee H, Khan KS. Aspirin for prevention of pre-eclampsia in women with historical risk factors: A systematic review. *Obstet Gynecol* 2003;**101**:1319–1332.

68. Masuyama H, Nobumoto E, Okimoto N, Inoue S, Segawa T, Hiramatsu Y. Superimposed preeclampsia in women with chronic kidney disease. *Gynecologic and Obstetric Investigation* 2012;**74**(4):274–281.

69. Rolfo A, Attini R, Nuzzo A, Piazzese A, Parisi S, Ferraresi M, Todros T, Piccoli G. Chronic kidney disease may be differentially diagnosed from pre-eclampsia by serum biomarkers. *Kidney International* 2013;**83**(1):177–181.

70. Toal M, Chan C, Fallah S, Alkazaleh F, Chaddha V, Windrim RC, et al. Usefulness of a placental profile in high-risk pregnancies. *Am J Obstet Gynecol* 2007;**196**:363.e1–7.

71. Kaijomaa M, Rahkonen L, Ulander VM, Hamalainen E, Alfthan H, Markkanen H et al. Low maternal pregnancy-associated plasma protein A during the first trimester of pregnancy and pregnancy outcomes. *Int J Gynaecol Obstet* 2017;**136**(1):76–82.

72. Cararach V, Casals E, Martinez S, Carmona F, Aibar C, Quinto LI, et al. Abnormal renal function as a cause of false-positive biochemical screening for Down's syndrome. *Lancet*. 1997;**350**(9087):1295–.

73. Benachi A, Dreux S, Kaddioui-Maalej S, Czerkiewicz I, Fakhouri F, Thervet E, et al. Down syndrome maternal serum screening in patients with renal disease. *American Journal of Obstetrics and Gynecology* 2010;**203**(1).

74. Cheng PJ, Liu CM, Chang SD, Lin YT, Soong YK. Elevated second-trimester maternal serum hCG in patients undergoing haemodialysis. *Prenatal Diag* 1999;**19**(10):955–958.

75. Schulman LP, Briggs R, Phillips OP, Friedman SA, Sibai B. Renal hemodialysis and maternal serum triple analyte screening. *Fetal Diagnosis and Therapy* 1998;**13**:26–28.

76. National Institute for Health and Care Excellence. Hypertension in pregnancy: The management of hypertensive disorders in pregnancy. 2010. www.nice .org.uk/guidance/cg107

77. The Renal Association: www.renal.org/information-resources/the-uk-eckd-guide/ckd-stages#sthash .QA8XtwrS.dpbs

Chapter 6

Midwifery Issues

Floria Cheng

Introduction

Pregnancy and childbirth are viewed as rites of passage for the majority of women. Midwives enter the profession to care for women undergoing this natural process. With improved medical care and therapeutics, more women with preexisting medical conditions such as Chronic kidney disease (CKD) are now becoming pregnant. Delivering care in a very medicalized setting may pose a challenge for many midwives. The focus is on patient-centered care in the context of CKD. The woman should be the focus of her care, not her disease.

This chapter covers the theory of renal midwifery: the role of the specialist midwife, the importance of coordinated care, continuity of care and shared decision-making with a focus on "normalized" care without compromising safety of the mother and baby. There are practical tips on delivering optimal patient-focused care to meet the special needs of these women. These include: prepregnancy counseling, antenatal visits and monitoring, medication, birth planning, intrapartum care, postnatal support and breastfeeding. The midwife works in equal partnership with the multidisciplinary team to ensure the woman is the focus of her care, not her renal condition. She acts as her advocate and coordinator of care. Care is "normalized" – but without compromising the safety of the mother and her unborn child. The midwife is an integral part of the multidisciplinary team striving for a successful pregnancy outcome and a positive pregnancy and delivery experience for women with CKD.

Theory of Renal Midwifery

Role of Specialist Midwife

There are different models of midwifery care for women with medically high-risk pregnancies. Some maternity units offer joint care in the obstetric medical setting with the support of a specialist midwife. Others offer high-risk team midwifery care and the women attend separate obstetric clinics for medical care. Some receive fragmented antenatal care at antenatal clinics or community and medical care at an outpatient clinic, which may be located in a different hospital.

Ideally, women with preexisting renal disease should be cared for by a multidisciplinary team (MDT). The MDT requires, as a minimum, an obstetrician, a renal/obstetric physician and a specialist midwife, all with expertise in the management of CKD in pregnancy (see Consensus Statements).

The latest UK maternal death report from 2014 states: "Women with pre-existing medical conditions who become pregnant require a high standard of joined-up multidisciplinary care. Pregnant women who develop serious medical conditions in pregnancy will require urgent involvement of relevant specialists alongside the obstetric team. This should be at a senior level. A single identified professional should be responsible for coordinating care" [1].

It does not specify who should be the single identified professional. A specialist midwife in renal or maternal medicine with the following attributes may be the ideal person:

- Knowledgeable in CKD and pregnancy
- Flexible approach in care planning
- Easily accessible
- Proactive – attention to details
- Good communication skills with the women and MDT
- Advocate for normality and shared decision-making
- Educator to the women – pregnancy and health education
- Trainer for midwives

Women-Centered Coordinated Care

According to Maternity Services in England [2], 79 percent of women are within a 30-minute drive of both an obstetric unit and a midwifery-led unit. Women with CKD 1–2 and in general good health should be able to receive obstetric care locally. However, those with CKD 3–5 will need to travel further to a tertiary maternity unit. Antenatal care is recommended by the National Institute of Clinical Excellence (NICE) [3]: "In an uncomplicated pregnancy, there should be 10 appointments for nulliparous women and 7 appointments for parous women." It also states that women with renal disease will require additional care. For women with CKD, this may increase to 13–18 visits, and women may undergo at least five ultrasound scans. Hospitalization may be required if the renal condition deteriorates or other complications such as preeclampsia arise. This can cause huge disruption in women's daily life, including work and childcare. If possible, care should be planned around the women, and organized in a way to minimize disruption to their daily life.

The usual schedule of care for most women with CKD includes:

- Doctor appointments – obstetricians, nephrologists, obstetric physicians, etc.
- Midwives appointments
- Ultrasound scans – fetal scans and renal scan
- Glucose tolerance test – if screening criteria met
- Blood tests: routine antenatal and renal
- Antenatal classes
- Other appointment: anesthetist clinic, if required; anti-D injection if rhesus negative

Attempting to juggle patients' schedules of work, clinic/hospital visits and childcare often leads to added stress and nonattendance in clinics, potentially impacting negatively a woman's emotions and perceptions of her pregnancy. Moreover, women with CKD have increased risk of pregnancy complications such as hypertension, preeclampsia, premature birth, low birth weight and depression [4, 5]. These complications frequently result in an increased number of clinic visits or require hospital admissions.

For the women who need several different services, effective coordination and prioritization of care is needed to minimize the impact of multiple visits [6]. Whenever possible, multiple hospital appointments should be organized on the same day, e.g. ultrasound scan, glucose tolerance test, nephrologist/obstetrician and midwife appointment. Women should be empowered to arrange these appointments if possible. In turn, health professionals should try to adopt a more flexible approach and be more accommodating of their patients' schedules and other commitments. The midwife can be pivotal in organizing this schedule of care.

Some consider that midwifery care should be delivered outside the clinic or hospital setting in order to "normalize the care." This depends on the woman's preferences, but choosing to meet outside the hospital/clinic setting will create extra appointments. Moreover, the advantage of meeting on the same day is that this enables the midwife to offer timely support and further discussions that have taken place with the other health professionals and the midwife will be able to liaise with the MDT if necessary.

Continuity of Care and Trust

The number of healthcare professionals involved in antenatal care for a woman with CKD should be kept to a minimum. This helps to build a trusting relationship, and aims to reduce pain relief in labor and antenatal admission. Ideally one-to-one midwifery should be arranged. If this is not possible, a midwife should be identified as the main contact and coordinate her care.

"Individualised attention from supportive, caring and experienced midwives mattered more than anything else" [7]. Women need time and a trusting relationship to share their thoughts and concerns. They also have their own views on the safety of maternity care, which include their perception of the skills and professionalism of those providing care. Specialist midwives need to maintain the knowledge and skills for safe and effective practice as stated in the Midwives Code [8]. Those looking after women with CKD need to be knowledgeable about renal disease and comorbidities in order to assess women's health and pregnancy. Women should not feel that their midwives are unable to discuss or answer questions about their medical condition. Trust will develop when women feel safe and are reassured that their midwives understand their anxiety related to their medical concerns. This rapport is the foundation for open discussion of management and health education.

Easy accessibility via telephone or drop-ins to the midwives provides constant support and reassurance. This may impact their management as they are likely to seek help or advice sooner from their midwives when they feel unwell.

Advocate for Shared Decision-Making

Berg and Dahlberg's phenomenological study described "women's need for information was very great and was a pre-requisite for feeling participative" [9]. Women expressed a loss of control and an awareness of having an unwell, high-risk body with exaggerated responsibility, including constant worry, pressure and self-blame [10]. Even if they understand their need for specialist care, they need to be involved in the process. Shared decision-making has been hailed as the pinnacle of patient-centered care [11]. It promotes a feeling of being in control and not just being told what to do.

Miranda Dodwell thinks "this process requires a balance of power in the relationship, with the patient being empowered to contribute to the decision-making, but with no corresponding loss of professional power from the point of view of the clinician" [12].

Clinicians always think that they are sharing decision and doing the best for the patients. Patients may vary in their views about the balance of risks, benefits and side effects of treatments [6]. Every opportunity should be taken to explore women's understanding of the discussion and help them make a decision.

Those who develop renal disease during pregnancy may be resentful that their pregnancy is managed as high risk, and this has implications for their choice of birth. They need more time and support to come to terms with the change. Shared decision-making allows them to take a more active role in their care. Decision-making and partnership in care may be an unfamiliar concept for some women who take a passive role in their culture or speak little English, and they should be encouraged and assisted to take an active role in their care.

Normalized Pregnancy Care

The Maternity Service in England 2013 report states that "Pregnant women receive care from a range of health professionals. All are cared for by midwives, who act as the coordinating professional for every birth." One of its aims is for women to have a positive experience and to encourage normality in birth [13]. However, it also states, "increased complexities increase the risks of childbirth, meaning care often requires greater clinical involvement." Normalized care of a medically complicated woman does not entail the exclusion of the medical profession, but is a concerted effort to bring a semblance of normality to a woman with multiple complex comorbidities.

Some women may feel that their pregnancy care takes second place to their medical needs. Midwives can make sure that all antenatal care is delivered in a timely fashion and women have opportunities to discuss any aspects of their care. Midwives can use their medical knowledge about the effects of CKD on childbirth to emphasize normality. Care is individualized with attention to women's special needs to ensure a safe pregnancy.

Practical Issues

Although pregnancy with renal disease is labeled as "high risk," with vigilant and regular surveillance, the pregnancy outcome in most cases is good. Women should be reassured and the importance of clinic visits emphasized. The section that follows discusses practical issues in providing individualized care.

Prepregnancy Counseling

- If possible, women should meet the renal/maternal medicine specialist midwife at the prepregnancy counseling consultation.
- If no designated midwife is available, they should be given the name of the specialist midwife in the tertiary center whom they can contact once pregnancy is confirmed.
- In this meeting, the midwife can discuss further details of the following:
  - Schedule of care and hospital visits required
  - Lifestyle modification, especially if overweight
  - Medication: folic acid, aspirin and other pregnancy-compatible medication
  - Contact details for further discussion
  - Information regarding how, when and where to refer once pregnancy confirmed. Early referral to the hospital booking office is important. Self-referral is the preferred choice if available. Delay from general practitioner referrals causes undue anxiety.
  - Clarify any issues raised such as mode of delivery

First Antenatal Visit

Booking Appointment

- The booking appointment with the midwife usually takes place between 6–10 weeks' gestation in order to complete the pathway by 12+6 weeks of pregnancy for screening for sickle cell disease and thalassemia recommended by Public Health England (PHE) [14].

- Women with CKD have access to the specialist midwife, and may have attended obstetric or renal clinics before the booking appointment. If not, once CKD is identified at the booking appointment, they should be referred to the MDT. A system of clear referral pathway should be established so that pregnant women who require additional care are managed and treated by the appropriate specialist teams when problems are identified [3].
- Some women may not aware of any preexisting renal conditions. They should be referred to the obstetrician and/or nephrologist for assessment, as they may require further investigation and a different care pathway if any of the following are noted:
  - History of previous renal condition but without further renal outpatient follow-up
  - Family history of autosomal dominant polycystic kidney disease (ADPKD)
  - Recurrent urinary tract infection
  - Proteinuria at first visit and urinary tract infection excluded
  - Previous urological procedures, e.g. nephrostomies
  - Kidney donor
- Arrange genetic counseling for women with ADPKD if desired. It is an autosomal dominant disease and there is a 50 percent risk of the baby inheriting the disease if one parent is affected.

Down Syndrome Screening

- Screening for Down syndrome should be discussed at the first antenatal appointment. The Combined Screening Test which screen for Down's, Edward's and Patau's Syndrome (nuchal translucency, free β-HCG, PAPP-A) is recommended by PHE between 11+2 and 14+1 weeks. Quadruple test (alpha fetal protein, total HCG , unconjugated eostriol and inhibin A) is offered between 14+2 and 20+0 weeks of pregnancy if too late for Combined Screening Test. This test screens for Down's Syndrome only.

- For women with CKD 3–5, the nuchal translucency scan is preferable to the Combined Screening Test as there is increased risk of false positive results (see Chapter 5), and women should be counseled accordingly.
- The new noninvasive prenatal test for Down syndrome (free fetal DNA) may be the preferred choice. However, it is currently not available within the National Health Service, but this may change in the future.

Medication

Folic acid 400mcg [3] – to reduce risk of neural tube defects such as spina bifida.Those with diabetes, hypertension, previous history of preeclampsia, or family history of neural tube defect will need a higher daily dose of 5mg.

Low-dose aspirin [15] to minimize risk of preeclampsia

Vitamin D supplementation of 400 i.u (10mg) [3, 16] as recommended by the National Institute of Health and Clinical Excellence (NICE). Women with renal disease may be vitamin D deficient and require a higher dose.

Calcium supplements, e.g. Adcal D3, depend on renal condition and calcium and vitamin D levels.

Thromboprophylaxis – if they meet criteria recommended by the Royal College of Obstetricians and Gynaecologists [17] or have nephrotic syndrome. It is important that advice on injection technique and safe disposal of syringes is given.

Other considerations

Are they taking the correct dosage? Obese women weighing > 90 kg may need a higher dose of low molecular weight heparin (LMWH). For advanced CKD, reduced dose of LMWH or unfractionated heparin (UFH) may be required.

Are they agreeable to taking medication? If not, explore the underlying reason.

Do they suffer from nausea or vomiting?

Do they need to see an anesthetist prior to delivery – e.g. if on therapeutic doses of LMWH?

Women are aware of the risks posed by their pregnancies, but do not perceive risk in the same way as healthcare professionals. They will take steps to ensure the health of themselves and their infants, but these may not include following all medical recommendations [18]. Many are reluctant to take medication as they are concerned about the safety profile in pregnancy and information they obtain from the Internet. If they express doubts or admit to not taking medication, midwives should explore their concerns and refer for further counseling. They need reassurance from the specialists in the MDT about the risks and benefits of medication.

Nausea and vomiting can affect medication regimes. Psychological support and dietary advice to minimize triggers should be offered. If not resolved, anti-emetics such as cyclizine, metoclopramide, prochlorperazine and ondansetron [19] can be used. In severe cases, some women may require admission.

Chapters 5 and 7 provide further information on medication in pregnancy.

Fetal Assessment

- Fetal ultrasound scans – viability scan (if applicable), nuchal translucency scan, anomaly scan, uterine Doppler scan (if applicable) and growth scans at 28, 32 and 36 weeks. Extra scans if abnormalities detected.
- Early anomaly scan at 16 weeks' gestation for those exposed to teratogenic medication such as mycophenolate mofetil (MMF) during the first trimester.
- Fetal echocardiogram – Arrange at 16–20 weeks' gestation if anti-Ro/La antibodies positive to exclude fetal heart block with fetal heart auscultation every one to two weeks between 18–28 weeks according to local policy.

Role of Midwife in Ongoing Care in Pregnancy

- Blood pressure (BP) and urinalysis at each visit for early signs of preeclampsia
- Fetal well-being: fetal heart rate and movement, and review growth scan reports
- Review medication and monitor drug levels, e.g. tacrolimus
- Blood tests – interpret and communicate results
- Anti-D injection if rhesus negative
- Emotional and social support – discussion of any concerns during clinic visits. Additional support for women with disability, learning difficulties, mental health issues. Refer to other agencies such

as social services for child protection or for domestic violence if applicable.

- Easy accessible support via telephone contact or drop-in arrangement
- Visit women during hospital admissions to provide support

Antenatal Classes

- Encourage to attend antenatal classes especially if primigravid to build up confidence to prepare for birth and motherhood. Social support developed during antenatal classes can have a protective effect against postnatal depression.
- Not all information is applicable for woman with CKD 3–5. Delivery at an obstetric unit is recommended by NICE [20]. Home birth, delivery at a birthing center or water births are not advisable due to requirements for maternal and fetal monitoring. Women should be informed of these recommendations at an early stage of their pregnancy to avoid disappointment and give them time to plan alternative delivery.
- Encourage partner to attend classes and provide support.
- Use of good websites such as www.nhs.uk/mypregnancy for online resources.

Screening for Other Medical Complications

- Gestational diabetes – screening for gestational diabetes (GDM) as recommended by NICE [21] and for those on immunosuppressant drugs or oral steroid therapy should be arranged as per local policy. Refer to the obstetric diabetes clinic if GDM confirmed.
- Preeclampsia – blood pressure and urinalysis at each visit
- Drug toxicity – monitor drug levels, e.g. tacrolimus
- Monitor for adverse drug effects – liver function tests and white cell count
- Monitor for deterioration of renal function – urea and electrolytes, creatinine, albumin and bicarbonate and additional tests for disease activity
- Anemia– full blood count and ferritin – may need erythropoietin-stimulating agents
- Ongoing venous thromboembolism assessment – as result of deterioration of renal function and complications, including hospital admission

Communication with Healthcare Professionals and Women

- Communicate with GPs and women about abnormal results and prescription drugs.
- Attend MDT meetings.
- If fetal abnormalities or suboptimal fetal growth are detected, liaise with fetal medicine specialists for scans and coordinate these with other appointments to minimize travel to the hospital.
- If very preterm delivery is anticipated, liaise with breast milk bank coordinator for discussion of using donor milk. Arrange consultation with neonatologist and visit to neonatal unit.
- If a woman miscarries, liaise with gynecology team for medical or surgical procedure. Termination of pregnancy may be required for fetal abnormalities or severe early-onset preeclampsia.
- For women receiving dialysis, liaise with dialysis team for dialysis and clinic appointments. Ensure contact details for the obstetric team and a delivery pack are kept in the dialysis center in case of emergency.

Birth Planning

- Aim for vaginal birth. Women with CKD do not need a Caesarean section unless there are obstetric indications. Midwives can clarify any misconceptions preferably at early stage of pregnancy to allay anxiety.
- If induction of labor is required due to deterioration of renal function, preeclampsia or fetal growth restriction, continuous electronic fetal monitoring will be required. However, women can still employ natural birth techniques with support from the midwife and partner.
- Birth partner – her choice for best support during labor.
- Pain relief – All forms are available to women with CKD. If receiving thromboprophylaxis, need to discontinue 12 hours before epidural. Arrange for the woman to see an obstetric anesthetist if morbidly obese, on therapeutic LMWH or thrombocytopenic or other potential anesthetic issues.
- Support network of friends and relatives

Intrapartum Care

- Continuity of care during labor is shown to reduce use of analgesia and Caesarean section. The midwife is supportive but not intrusive.
- Telemetry monitoring is preferable if continuous fetal monitoring is required.
- With the support of the midwife, birthing environment can be modified and women encouraged to use natural birth techniques and equipment.

Postnatal Care

Immediate Care

- Continue regular observations especially BP for at least 48 hours post delivery as hypertension may reoccur or become more severe.
- Offer support in skin-to-skin contact and breastfeeding
- Fatigue can increase risk of flares/relapse of lupus and some medical conditions. Assist in care of baby and help women build up confidence in motherhood
- Monitor the baby as per local policy if born low birth weight or mother has preexisting diabetes or GDM
- Observe for signs of disease flare and postnatal depression.

Breastfeeding

- The World Health Organization (WHO) recommends exclusive breastfeeding (breast milk only, with no water, other fluids or solids) for six months, with supplemental breastfeeding continuing for two years and beyond [22].
- Encourage women to attend breastfeeding classes or workshops.
- Discussion about safety of medications in breast feeding should take place prior to delivery. Clear advice should be given based on risks and benefits of breastfeeding and the safety profile of medication. How this counseling is delivered may affect the woman's perception. Any expressed concern can undermine a woman's confidence about breastfeeding. Prednisolone, azathioprine, ciclosporin, tacrolimus and hydroxychloroquine alone or in combination are considered safe in pregnancy and breastfeeding (see Chapter 7).

- Support the woman in her chosen method of feeding. She may choose to bottle feed to avoid any uncertainty on long-term effects for the baby.
- In England from 2012 to 2013, 73.9 percent of babies were initially breastfed. By six to eight weeks of life, only 32.3 percent are totally and 14.9 percent partially breastfed [23]. All women should be offered support by professional or lay/ peer supporters, or a combination of both to breastfeed their babies to increase the duration and exclusivity of breastfeeding.
- Breast milk is especially beneficial for babies born preterm. Women should be encouraged to express breast milk and liaise with the infant nutrition specialist at the neonatal unit.
- Contact details for breastfeeding-support schemes in the community should be given prior to discharge.
- Little vitamin D is secreted into breast milk, and NICE recommends supplements for all pregnant and breastfeeding mothers [16].

Postnatal Follow-Up

- Ensure women with CKD have a follow-up appointment with the MDT or nephrologist arranged before discharge. This is important to review medication and assess renal function. Pregnancy-induced hypertension and preeclampsia usually has resolved by six weeks postpartum.
- Clear written discharge summary to all healthcare professionals with information about renal disease and specific instructions for monitoring and follow up appointment is imperative.
- Health education for those who developed CKD during pregnancy is important (see Chapter 9).

Contraception

- Contraceptive advice must be given before discharge, especially for women who have suffered complications in their pregnancy (see Chapter 3).

Conclusion

High-quality maternity care involves practices shown to be safe and effective for mothers' and babies' health and well-being and are valued by women and their families [24]. Midwives need a broad medical knowledge in order to provide comprehensive care, trusted by the woman and respected by the MDT. "The basis for genuine midwifery caring is mutual respect and confidence between different healthcare professionals, with all striving for same goal to promote mothers' well-being during pregnancy and childbirth with as little sickness, complication and intervention as possible" [25]. A positive pregnancy experience is vital to building women's confidence in motherhood and future pregnancy. Research is needed to explore the experience of pregnant women cared for in a setting where midwives and the medical team work in equal partnership.

References

1. Knight M, Kenyon S, Brocklehurst P, Neilson J, Shakespeare J, Kurinczuk JJ (eds.) on behalf of MBRRACE-UK. Saving lives, improving mothers' care – Lessons learned to inform future maternity care from the UK and Ireland Confidential Enquiries into Maternal Deaths and Morbidity 2009–12. Oxford: National Perinatal Epidemiology Unit, University of Oxford 2014.

2. Department of Health: National Audit Office. *Maternity services in England: Nov. 2013*. London: Department of Health, 2013.

3. National Institute of Clinical Excellence. NICE Guideline 62 – Antenatal care Issued: March 2008 last modified: December 2014. From: www.nice.org.uk/guidance/cg62.

4. Bar J, Ben-Rafael Z, Padoa A, Orvieto R, Boner G, Hod M. Prediction of pregnancy outcome in subgroups of women with renal disease. *Clin Nephrol.* 2000;**53**:437–444.

5. Smyth A, Radovic M, Garovic V. Women, renal disease and pregnancy. *Adv Chr Kidney Disease Dis.* 2013 Sep: **20**(5):402–410.

6. O'Flynn N, Staniszewska S. Improving the experience of care for people using NHS services: Summary of NICE guidance. *BMJ* 2012;**344**:d6422.

7. Magee H, Askham J. *Women's views about the safety in maternity care: A qualitative study*. London: King's Fund, 2007.

8. Nursing and Midwifery Council. The code: Professional standards of practice and behaviour for nurses and midwives. 2015. From: www.nmc-uk.org/Documents/NMC-Publications/revised-new-NMC-Code.pdf.

9. Berg M, Dahlberg K, A phenomenological study of women's experiences of complicated childbirth. *Midwifery* 1998; **14**:23–29.

10. Berg M. The midwife–mother relationship. In *Midwifery relationships with childbearing women at increased risk* (2nd edn.). Basingstoke: Palgrave MacMillan, 2010, chapter 10.

11. Barry MJ, Edgman-Levitan S. Shared decision making – pinnacle of patient-centred care. *New England Journal of Medicine* 2012; **366**:780–781.

12. Dodwell, M. A patient's perspective. *British Journal of Renal Medicine* 2013;**18**(1) Supplement: 6–7.

13. Department of Health. Maternity Services in England: National Audit Office 2013.

14. NHS Antenatal and Newborn Screening Programme, April 2017. Public Health England.

15. National Institute of Clinical Excellence. Hypertension in pregnancy: The management of hypertensive disorders during pregnancy. NICE guidelines [CG107] August 2010.

16. National Institute for Health and Clinical Excellence. Guidance for midwives, health visitors, pharmacists and other primary care services to improve the nutrition of pregnant and breastfeeding mothers and children in low income households. 2008.

17. Royal College of Obstetricians and Gynaecologists. Green-top Guideline No 37a: Reducing the risk of thrombosis and embolism during pregnancy and puerperium. London: Royal College of Obstetricians and Gynaecologists Press Nov 2009.

18. Lee S, Ayers S, Holden D. A metasynthesis of risk perception in women with high risk pregnancies. *Midwifery* 2014;**30**(4):403–411.

19. Jarvis S, Nelson-Piercy C. Management of nausea and vomiting in pregnancy. *BMJ* 2011;**342**:d3606.

20. National Institute for Health and Clinical Excellence (2014). "CG190: *Intrapartum care: Care of healthy women and their babies during childbirth.*" From: www.nice.org.uk/guidance/cg190.

21. National Institute for Health and Clinical Excellence. Diabetes in pregnancy: Management of diabetes and its complications from preconception to the postnatal period. London: National Institute for Health and Clinical Excellence, Feb 2015.

22. World Health Organization. *Global strategy for infant and young child feeding.* Geneva: World Health Organization, 2003.

23. NHS England. Statistical Release: Breastfeeding initiation and breastfeeding prevalence 6–8 weeks. Department of Health, Jan 2015.

24. Dodwell M, Newburn M. Normal birth as a measure of the quality of care. In *Evidence on safety, effectiveness and women's experiences.* London: National Childbirth Trust, 2010.

25. Berg, M, Dahlberg, K. Swedish midwives' care of women who are at high obstetric risk or who have obstetric complications. *Midwifery* 2001;**17**:259–266.

Drugs in Women with Renal Disease and Transplant Recipients in Pregnancy

Graham Lipkin, Asif Sarwar and Ellen Knox

Introduction

A recent study found that 80 percent of pregnant women in the United States receive prescription drugs and nearly half of these may be harmful to the fetus [1]. Almost all women known to suffer from chronic kidney disease (CKD) require antenatal drug treatment. Most of these drugs are started prepregnancy for the underlying condition or comorbidity. Medicines' optimization is therefore critical; to enhance pregnancy outcomes in women with CKD, advice should be given at the time of prepregnancy counseling. We focus on immunosuppressive agents commonly used by women in the treatment of renal disease as well as erythropoietic stimulating agents (ESAs), cinacalcet and commonly used antibiotics. Antihypertensive agents are frequently required but are covered in Chapter 8.

Prepregnancy counseling is critical to safe and effective drug use by women with known renal disease in pregnancy. Consideration of risk/benefit balance to both mother and fetus surrounding the initiation or stopping of drug treatment prepregnancy or during pregnancy is a key challenge for the multidisciplinary team caring for these women.

Search Strategy

The evidence base available to guide women in this area is limited and relies on case reports, incomplete registry data, case control series and non-controlled meta-analysis. These were identified from Entrez Pub Med search, relevant review articles, TOXbase, National Teratology Information Service (NTIS), Micromedex, the British National Formulary, reference guides [2], expert opinion and relevant pharmaceutical company pregnancy databases.

General Principles of Teratogenicity

An agent is a teratogen if its administration to the pregnant mother directly or indirectly causes structural or functional abnormalities in the fetus or in the child after birth, which may not be apparent until later life [3]. The belief that the developing fetus was protected by an effective placental barrier from adverse effects of drugs in the maternal circulation was shattered by the experience with thalidomide more than 50 years ago. Almost all drugs present in the maternal circulation reach the fetus to a greater or lesser extent.

Factors Affecting Exposure and Impact of Maternal Drugs on a Fetus

The interface comprises the uteroplacental circulation, umbilical vein and the uniquely positioned fetal liver through which all drugs must pass to reach the fetal circulation (see Figure 7.1). Fetal drug exposure and its impact are determined by a complex interplay of pharmacokinetic and pharmacodynamic factors of which many aspects are incompletely understood. These include:

i) *Timing of drug exposure in relationship to fetal development*

During the pre-embryonic stage (conception to 17 days), the "all or nothing effect" of drugs is thought to apply. Toxic damage to the dividing blastocyst will either result in its destruction, leading to miscarriage

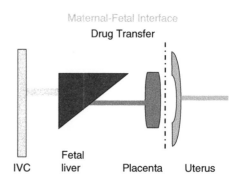

Figure 7.1 Maternal-fetal circulation and drug transfer

or, if damage is incomplete and the toxin short lived, the damaged cells may be replaced, allowing continued fetal development. Organogenesis occurs mainly during the embryonic stage, which is largely complete by the tenth week. Thus drug exposure in the first trimester is more likely to increase the rate of miscarriage or structural abnormalities (e.g. spina bifida), whereas subsequent exposure is more likely to result in growth restriction.

ii) *Factors affecting transplacental drug passage* [4]

Placental drug transfer occurs largely by diffusion across a concentration gradient. However, agents of high molecular weight such as ESAs, heparins or insulin are excluded by their size. Non-ionic and lipophilic drugs cross more easily than polar drugs. Metabolism of drugs by placental or fetal liver prior to reaching the fetal vena cava can significantly impact exposure to drugs administered to the mother. Prednisolone is extensively metabolized to inactive products by the placenta with 10 percent only reaching the fetus. Azathioprine is converted to the active metabolite 6-mercaptopurine (6-MP) by the liver. While azathioprine crosses the placenta the fetal liver has relatively low levels of the activating enzyme, inosinate pyrophosphorylase, leading to low cord levels of 6-MP, possibly protecting the fetus from toxicity [5].

iii) *Differences in susceptibility*

The background rate of congenital abnormality in the European population is 2–4 percent. It is not clear why exposure to a known teratogen at the same stage in pregnancy at the same dose will give rise to fetal malformation in some but not all pregnancies. Of note, only 20–30 percent of exposures to thalidomide during the first trimester led to fetal abnormalities [2], thus pharmacogenetic issues may be relevant.

iv) *Dose–response relationships*

Although idiosyncratic effects are described, most teratogenic effects appear dose related. Estimates of the cumulative exposure to the drug may be more important in relation to teratogenic effects than short-term transplacental transfer [4].

Guidance on Drug Use in Pregnancy

Principles of Drug Prescription in Pregnancy (BNF70)

Prepregnancy counseling: drugs can have harmful effects on a fetus at any time during pregnancy. It is important to bear this in mind when prescribing for a woman with CKD of childbearing age. Prepregnancy counseling wherever possible is of particular importance to women with renal disease who are considering pregnancy. It allows discussion of relevant risks and appropriate modification of drugs in advance of conception.

During the *first trimester*, drugs can produce congenital malformations (teratogenesis), and the period of greatest risk is from the third to the eleventh week of pregnancy.

During the *second* and *third trimesters*, drugs can affect the growth and functional development of the fetus or have toxic effects on fetal tissues. Drugs given shortly before term or during labor can have adverse effects on labor or on the neonate after delivery.

The following general principles apply to prescribing drugs in pregnancy:

- Prescribe only if expected benefit is thought to be greater than the risk to the fetus (e.g. immunosuppression in transplantation)
- Avoid all nonessential drugs in first trimester if possible
- Smallest effective dose should be used (drug level monitoring wherever possible/relevant)
- Drugs that have been extensively used in pregnancy and appear to be usually safe should be used in preference to new or untried drugs
- Contribute to the registry evidence base wherever possible

It is also worth noting that the absence of information does not imply that the drug is safe.

Alternative sources of information. Information on drugs and pregnancy is also available from the UK Teratology Information Service: www.uktis.org. The US Food and Drug Administration (FDA) had adopted a classification that codes the safety categories of drugs when used in pregnancy. These categories have limitations when applied to women with CKD in pregnancy. As from June 2015, these categories have been replaced with a narrative that provides details about the risks of the drug in:

1) pregnancy;
2) lactation;
3) females and males of reproductive potential.

Issues Specific to Patients with Renal Disease

In patients with CKD, as in normal subjects, glomerular filtration increases substantially above baseline early in pregnancy [6]. Agents excreted by the kidney may require dose increases to maintain therapeutic plasma levels. Patients with CKD may experience a marked increase in proteinuria reaching nephrotic levels, and exhibit an exaggerated fall in serum albumin during pregnancy, which impacts handling of drugs with extensive protein binding. The computation widely used to calculate eGFR outside pregnancy is not valid [7], which complicates adjustment of drug dosing in pregnancy in women with CKD.

Breastfeeding

Breastfeeding is beneficial to both mother and child; the immunological and nutritional value of breast milk to the infant is greater than that of formula feeds and breastfeeding enhances bonding.

The British National Formulary (BNF70) concludes that, although there is concern that drugs taken by the mother might affect the infant, there is very little information on this. In the absence of evidence of an effect, the potential for harm to the infant can be inferred from:

- the amount of drug or active metabolite of the drug delivered to the infant (dependent on the pharmacokinetic characteristics of the drug in the mother);
- the efficiency of absorption, distribution and elimination of the drug by the infant (infant pharmacokinetics);
- the nature of the effect of the drug on the infant (pharmacodynamic properties of the drug in the infant).

We present the view of the authoritative texts such as Briggs et al. [1] and those of the current BNF together with existing information from literature review in human studies.

Immunosuppressive Agents and Pregnancy

Continuation of immunosuppression is essential to the health of women treated by renal transplantation and in some with immunological renal disease such as lupus. These women should be advised not to stop their treatment once pregnant. The risks of stopping immunosuppressive medications in pregnancy are frequently outweighed by the benefits of continuation. The disease flare or rejection pose a greater risk to mother and fetus than most of the drugs used.

Many agents have established safety profiles in pregnancy. For those that do not, these drugs should be cautiously converted to those known to be safe in pregnancy in advance of conception. Fertility in women with advanced CKD or those treated by dialysis is reduced [8]. Renal transplantation effectively restores fertility, offering many women the chance of a successful pregnancy usually without long-term adverse impact on transplant function [9]. Nevertheless, these pregnancies are complex and preparation, including post-transplantation contraceptive advice and prepregnancy counseling, is key to reducing risk to mother and baby.

Consensus guideline statements and reviews covering the use of transplantation immunosuppression in pregnancy and those with immunological renal disease have been published, such as by the European League Against Rheumatism (EULAR) [5, 10, 11]. A meta-analysis by Deshpande et al. found that live birth and miscarriage rates in renal transplant recipients were no worse than in the American general population. However, the rates of preeclampsia, gestational diabetes, intrauterine growth restriction (IUGR) and preterm deliveries were substantially higher [9]. The increased risk of pregnancy complications is a likely consequence of the underlying disease.

• Glucocorticosteroids

The most commonly used glucocorticoids are the short-acting agents prednisolone and methylprednisolone, and the longer-acting dexamethasone and betamethasone. They easily traverse the placenta. The maternal/cord blood prednisolone ratio is 10:1, suggesting substantial protection of the fetus from maternal prednisolone exposure because of high levels of the inactivating hormone 11-beta-hydroxysteroid dehydrogenase in the placenta [5]. In comparison, dexamethasone and betamethasone reach higher concentrations in the fetus because they are less efficiently metabolized.

A meta-analysis of pregnancies with steroid exposure confirmed there was no increase in the rate of major malformations (3.6 percent versus 2.0 percent) compared with the general population and no cluster of malformations suggestive of steroid-induced teratogenicity [14]. A further study in Denmark from 2011 found no association of corticosteroids and an increased risk of cleft lip and palate malformations with exposure in pregnancy, including in the first trimester [13]. No increased teratogenic risk has been demonstrated in mothers exposed to low doses of prednisolone, though there may be an increased risk of IUGR with prolonged courses (BNF72). Cases of fetal adrenal suppression and fetal immunosuppression have been described with maternal use of higher prednisolone doses, but not where maternal prednisolone dose is kept below 15 mg/day [14].

Maternal Risks

Prolonged courses of antenatal glucocorticoids increase the risk of gestational diabetes especially when combined with other diabetogenic agents such as tacrolimus [15, 17]. They may exacerbate hypertension and fluid retention, loss of bone mineral density (also decreased by heparins) and preterm rupture of membranes [16].

Breastfeeding

Following a 10 mg oral dose, trace amounts of prednisolone are found in breast milk. Milk concentrations range from 5–25 percent of maternal blood levels [2]. A formal pharmacokinetic study on the effects of a 50 mg IV dose demonstrated only 0.025 percent recovery from breast milk, which is unlikely to be of clinical significance to the baby [18].

The consensus view is that prednisolone use in pregnancy is not associated with an increased risk of fetal malformations in usual doses. However, pregnancies in women receiving steroid therapy necessitate close maternal and fetal monitoring, including random blood glucose monitoring. Formal glucose tolerance testing at the beginning of the third trimester is recommended. It would appear that prednisolone is compatible with safe breastfeeding.

• Azathioprine

Azathioprine is used as a component of prophylaxis from rejection in solid organ transplant recipients and in patients with native renal disease, including those with systemic lupus erythromatosis (SLE) or in the maintenance stage of treatment for renal vasculitis. It is usually combined with other immunosuppressive treatment, including glucocorticoids. There is extensive experience of this drug in pregnant women.

Azathioprine freely crosses the placenta, but to be active, requires conversion to the active metabolite 6-mercaptopurine (6-MP) in the liver by the enzyme inosinate pyrophosphorylase, which is deficient in the developing fetal liver. The fetal liver metabolizes azathioprine to the inactive metabolite thiouric acid

rather than 6-mercaptopurine. A radioactive labeling study in human pregnancy reported that 64 to 93 percent of azathioprine administered to mothers appears in fetal blood as inactive metabolites [19]. It is thus possible that the fetus is to some extent protected from any teratogenic effects of azathioprine.

We rely on case series and registry data to determine adverse fetal effects in humans. No increased risk for general or specific structural defects in exposed babies has been noted in these studies, although sample size is not sufficient to rule out a small risk [20]. The reported rate of miscarriage appears similar to that of the general population. Azathioprine has been associated with dose-related myelosuppression in the fetus [21]. Maternal azathioprine dose at 32 weeks and at term correlates with cord blood leucocyte count. Fetal leucopenia is not usually a problem if maternal dose of azathioprine is less than 2 mg/kg and maternal white cell count greater than 7,500/L [14].

The National Transplant Pregnancy Registry (NTPR) in the United States evaluated 146 kidney transplant recipients who received azathioprine and prednisolone (90.4 percent), azathioprine alone (2.1 percent) or prednisolone alone (7.5 percent) [22]. Complications in the azathioprine-treated group included low birth weight and prematurity. It is likely that these adverse outcomes reflected maternal disease (renal dysfunction, hypertension, diabetes etc.) rather than the drug itself [5]. There were isolated cases of fetal abnormality that were not in excess of that expected. The UK Transplant Pregnancy Registry reported pregnancy outcomes in 209 cardiothoracic, liver and renal transplant recipients, most of whom received azathioprine. There was no increased risk of first-trimester miscarriage or fetal abnormalities [23]. Likewise no increased risk of structural abnormality is reported in babies of women treated with azathioprine during pregnancy for lupus [20].

The consensus is that azathioprine should not be suspended during pregnancy out of concern regarding teratogenicity. Women should be advised in pre-pregnancy counseling not to stop azathioprine on finding they are pregnant. Conception while taking azathioprine is not in itself grounds to recommend termination of pregnancy. There is no current evidence of teratogenicity in human pregnancy. Nevertheless women requiring azathioprine use in pregnancy for renal disease or transplantation should be considered at high risk of complications related to the underlying condition. Their care requires careful overview in a center experienced in management of these patients.

Breastfeeding

The BNF recommends women require expert neonatal review. Consensus opinion is that breastfeeding is not absolutely contraindicated [24]. A study of azathioprine-treated lactating women reported low levels of 6-mercaptopurine in only 2 of 31 breast milk samples and undetectable levels in 10 breast fed babies with no signs of immunosuppression [26]. This has been echoed in a further study that estimated an infant exposure of less than 1 percent of the maternal dose [26]. Although these studies were not in renal transplant recipients, their results are directly applicable to the transplant population.

Ciclosporine and Tacrolimus

Ciclosporine (CyA) is a novel cyclic undacapeptide with potent immunosuppressive properties. It has been widely used in the prevention of acute rejection in solid organ transplantation, as well as in the treatment of immune-mediated native renal disease. Tacrolimus has a similar mode of action and clinical toxicity profile, including nephrotoxicity and hypertension. Both drugs have a narrow therapeutic window and are associated with the development of both functional reversible and structural nephrotoxicity in humans, as well as a diabetogenic effect that is more commonly seen with tacrolimus. CyA crosses the human placenta and CyA levels in the placenta are equivalent to those in maternal blood [27]. Tacrolimus also crosses the placenta with approximately 71 percent of maternal blood levels, but low neonatal exposure is likely due to placental P-glycoprotein efflux [30].

Complex pharmacokinetic changes are seen in CyA- and tacrolimus-treated patients in pregnancy. These include increased volume of distribution due to gain in body weight, adipose tissue and raised red cell mass. Hormone-induced changes in liver metabolism and bile salt handling also have an impact. As a consequence, a mean dose increase of CyA of around 40–50 percent is frequently required to maintain therapeutic CyA levels (see Figure 7.2) [32]. Similarly, tacrolimus

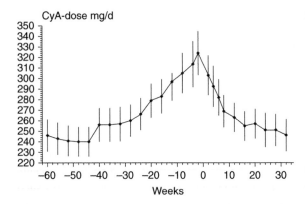

Figure 7.2 Ciclosporine dose requirements during pregnancy in CyA-treated renal transplant recipients. (Week 0 represents birth.) (from Fischer et al., *American Journal of Transplantation* 2005; **5** (11), 2732–2739) [26].

is also affected by pregnancy and the fraction of unbound tacrolimus is often increased (due to factors such as low albumin and erythrocytes). Caution should be exercised when interpreting whole blood trough levels in the setting of maternal hypoalbuminemia and anemia [30, 33]. Trough blood levels should be monitored monthly, or more frequently if drug therapy is introduced or withdrawn or if there is suspicion of toxicity or decline in renal function (the BNF should be checked or pharmacy consulted for details). Measurement of plasma or unbound tacrolimus levels have been suggested, although there is no validation of this and most units will not have access to these assays. Large inter-patient variation in tacrolimus dose changes are required to maintain stable trough whole blood concentrations in pregnancy. Many centers choose to run trough levels at the lower end of their prepregnancy target range.

Miscarriage rates in registry series for women taking calcineurin inhibitors are similar to those reported in the general population; therefore, early drug-induced fetotoxicity is unlikely (see Table 7.1).

A meta-analysis of pregnancy outcomes in solid organ transplant recipients taking CyA (n = 410) reported a nonsignificant trend to a greater malformation risk when compared to controls who received alternative immunosuppression [28]. However, the absolute rate of congenital abnormalities was 4.1 percent, which was not substantially different from the

Table 7.1 Comparison of outcome of pregnancy in ciclosporine- and prednisolone-treated renal transplant recipients

| | UK Transplant Registry [5, 20, 21] | US National Transplant Pregnancy Registry [5] | | Deshpande meta-analysis (2011) [9] | |
		Ciclosporine-treated	Steroid/ azathioprine-treated	Age <30	Age >30
Miscarriage (before 24 weeks)	11%	16%	7%	10.2%	16%

Table 7.2 Pregnancy outcomes in transplant recipients reported to the US National Transplant Pregnancy Registry [26]

	Ciclosporine (Neoral)-treated women (146 pregnancies)	Tacrolimus-treated women (70 pregnancies)
Hypertension	72%	58%
Diabetes during pregnancy	3%	10%
Miscarriage	19%	24%
Live births	79%	71%
Low birth weight	50%	50%
Newborn complications	50%	54%

general population and the finding has not been confirmed in other series. The prevalence of major structural malformations according to the NTPR was approximately 4–5 percent, similar to the incidence of 3 percent reported in pregnant women without disease [17]. Numerous single-center and registry reports have shown no evidence of an increase in structural abnormalities in babies born to transplant recipients taking ciclosporine or tacrolimus in pregnancy [5, 22, 23].

The NTPR explored the issue of whether ciclosporine treatment might be the cause of low birth weight in renal transplant recipients taking azathioprine. They ascribe the risk to known predisposing factors, including drug-treated hypertension and prematurity [23].

The maternal and fetal outcomes of tacrolimus or CyA-treated transplant recipients in pregnancy are similar [17], although gestational diabetes may be more frequently seen in those treated with tacrolimus

(Table 7.2). Babies born to women treated with tacrolimus may suffer transient renal impairment and hyperkalemia and prompt neonatal assessment may be needed [29].

An increased risk of intrahepatic cholestasis of pregnancy (ICP) has been reported in CyA-treated (but not tacrolimus-treated) renal transplant recipients, an effect possibly mediated by CyA-induced inhibition of the bile salt excretion pump[34]. Seven of 23 CyA-treated renal transplant recipients suffered this complication against a background incidence of around 1 percent.

The effects of in utero drug exposure may not be apparent at birth and subtle effects on neurocognitive or immunological function or long-term blood pressure or renal function may not be seen for more than a decade or longer. There are inconsistent reports of immunological abnormalities in babies born to transplant recipients [5]. A recent study prospectively assessed the immune profile of infants born to mothers with kidney transplants with follow-up surveillance and clinical outcomes in the first year of life [35]. Importantly, the researchers report an increased risk of severe infections requiring hospitalization among these infants compared with those born to healthy women, as well as subtle immune system perturbations. These findings emphasize the necessity of further close study of the immune system in children who might be at risk of adverse outcomes as a result of in utero exposure to immunosuppressive agents. Neurocognitive development was assessed in a follow-up study of children born to CyA-treated female transplant recipients [36]. Twenty-four percent showed some delay, but the relationship to drug treatment rather than prematurity was unclear.

Rabbits exposed to CyA in utero exhibit reduced nephron number and develop hypertension and progressive CKD in adult life [37]. Human studies in the general population show an inverse correlation between birth weight and blood pressure in later life. Preliminary data suggest renal function and blood pressure of children born to mothers treated with CyA during pregnancy appear to be normal [38]. However, long-term follow-up studies of children from these mothers are awaited.

Accumulated experience with the use of ciclosporine and tacrolimus during pregnancy supports their use where required. Currently there is no evidence of teratogenicity. European Best Practice Guidelines suggest that ciclosporine and tacrolimus may be continued during pregnancy [10]. Preterm labor and small-for-gestational-age (SGA) infants are not uncommon outcomes and pregnancy in women taking these agents should be carefully monitored. Drug dose requires review based on trough levels and gestational diabetes may occur with both drugs, although it is more common with tacrolimus treatment. Whether there will be long-term immunomodulatory or renal effects in offspring exposed to ciclosporine in utero is unknown.

Breastfeeding

The BNF comments "present in breast milk – manufacturer advises avoid." There are however, limited data on which to advise. Again several experienced units, including our own, have allowed breastfeeding in CyA-treated women and have noted no drug-related problems in their babies. Reports of breast milk CyA levels approach those in maternal blood. However, CyA was detected in only one out of six infants tested and infant development up to one year was reported as normal [39, 40]. This has been confirmed in case reports in a colitis and renal transplant patient, the latter estimating the dose that the infant is exposed to as approximately 0.33 percent of the weight-adjusted maternal dose [41, 42].

Two reports identify minimal tacrolimus transfer to the infant by breastfeeding with calculated dose exposure being between 0.02 and 0.5 percent of the mother's weight-adjusted dose [34, 36]. An observational cohort study of 14 women found that the weight-adjusted infant dose is 0.23 percent of the maternal dose. As the mothers were taking tacrolimus throughout their pregnancies, a serial reduction in infant tacrolimus levels of 15 percent per postpartum day was seen [43]. By one week postpartum no baby had detectable blood tacrolimus levels. The consensus opinion is that breastfeeding is not contraindicated. However, in this scenario the authors support breastfeeding where babies are carefully

monitored, including weekly measurement of immuno-suppressive levels in the infants [24].

• Mycophenolate Mofetil (MMF) and Enteric-Coated Mycophenolic Sodium (EC-MPS)

Mycophenolate mofetil is the ester prodrug of mycophenolic acid (MPA), a reversible inhibitor of inosine monophosphate dehydrogenase, which blocks de novo purine synthesis in T and B lymphocytes. It is licensed for the prevention of acute rejection following solid organ transplantation and has become the standard of care, usually in combination with steroids and tacrolimus, as first-line immunosuppression in renal transplantation in the United States and Europe. MMF is also indicated for treatment of severe renal manifestations of systemic lupus erthythematosis [44].

Transplacental transfer of MPA has been demonstrated in pregnant women, achieving fetal plasma levels similar to those found in the mother [45]. Mycophenolate mofetil and enteric coated-mycophenolate sodium (EC-MPS) are classified by the Medicines and Healthcare Products Regulatory Agency (MHRA) as proven teratogens in animals and in humans. They should not be initiated until a negative pregnancy test has been obtained. Effective contraception must be used before and throughout treatment.

The NTPR reported outcomes of 97 pregnancies to 68 women exposed to MMF or EC-MPS during pregnancy. A high rate of miscarriage was noted (49%), suggesting early embryo toxicity. Of the 48 live born infants, 23 percent had structural malformations, much higher than the malformation rate of 4–5 percent in non-MMF-treated patients [16]. Abnormalities reported bore similarity to those described in preclinical studies, including cleft lip and palate, microtia, diaphragmatic hernia, hypoplastic nails, shortened fingers and congenital heart defects. In a prospective study in 57 MMF-exposed pregnancies between 1998 and 2011, miscarriages occurred in 28 percent and elective abortions in 21 percent. Of the 29 live births, 62 percent were premature, 20 percent had major malformations as described earlier and 31 percent had low birth weight [46].

The management of a woman who conceives while taking MMF should be individualized and the woman counseled as to the risks of teratogenicity and the potential consequences of conversion to alternative drugs known to be safe in pregnancy, usually azathioprine. Immunosuppression drug change in pregnancy is not without some risk of toxic side effects or rejection. Each case should be assessed on its individual merits, taking into account stage of pregnancy, past history of rejection and complications. The option of termination must also be sensitively discussed. The long-term impact of exposure of the fetus to MPA at conception remains unknown.

Babies born to fathers treated with MMF or EC-MPS have not been reported as having a greater risk of adverse pregnancy outcomes. NTPR data for 152 males who fathered 208 infants showed that there was comparable rate of prematurity, low birth weight, birth defects and fetal loss rate when compared to population estimates [47], and recent post-marketing surveillance is consistent with this. However, in 2015 the UK MHRA issued the following warning for men taking MMF:

- Men (including those who have had a vasectomy) should use condoms during MMF treatment and for at least 90 days after stopping MMF treatment.
- Female partners of male patients treated with mycophenolate mofetil or mycophenolic acid should use highly effective contraception during treatment and for 90 days after the last dose [48].

A statement released by the Renal Association in 2016 recommends that potential fathers taking mycophenolate derivatives are informed of the theoretical risks of exposure to a fetus and given advice on contraception. These theoretical risks of teratogenicity should be balanced against the potential risk of exchanging this highly effective immunosuppressant for an alternative that, in the case of transplant recipients, may result in an increased risk of rejection. This can be accessed from www.renal.org/docs/default-source/default-document-library/mycophenolate-and-fathers-to-be-letter-may-2016da90a131181561659443ff000014d4d8.pdf?sfvrsn=049.

In practice, we recommend discussion of the teratogenic risk of MMF or EC-MPS and the requirement for highly effective contraception in female transplant recipients both at the time of transplant listing and before discharge post transplantation. Contraceptive advice is offered regularly post transplantation in clinic and in prepregnancy counseling. In women contemplating pregnancy, the risks of prepregnancy cessation of MMF or EC-MPS and conversion, usually to azathioprine, should be carefully discussed with a patient and her partner after first checking thiopurine S-methyltransferase (TPMT) activity to exclude abnormal metabolism of azathioprine. We advise women to defer conception for three to six months post withdrawal of MMF to ensure stable transplant function and inactive lupus.

Breastfeeding

There are no data on MPA excretion in human breast milk, although studies in rats indicate that transfer does take place (SmPC Cellcept®). There are no reports of MMF or EC-MPS use in human lactation, though theoretically the small molecular weight and moderately long half-lives of the molecules suggest that excretion in milk is likely. Therefore breastfeeding is contraindicated with MMF or EC-MPS.

• Sirolimus and Everolimus

Sirolimus (also known as rapamycin) and everolimus are potent macrocyclic immunosuppressive agents whose primary mechanism of action is inhibition of intracellular metabolic target of rapamycin (mTOR). This results in inhibition of cytokine driven T-cell proliferation. They are licensed in the United Kingdom for prevention and treatment of acute rejection following solid organ transplantation (SmPC Rapamune®). The safety of these agents in pregnancy has not been determined.

Studies in animals indicate transplacental drug transfer and fetotoxicity, reduced fetal weight and delayed ossification in rats. Embryo toxicity was increased when sirolimus was coadministered with ciclosporine, consistent with the well-recognized increased nephrotoxicity in this setting [1].

It appears that sirolimus is associated with gonadal toxicity in both sexes, reducing fertility. Sirolimus significantly reduces sperm counts and motility in males aged 20–40 years post renal transplant, and this translated to a lower actual pregnancy rate in sirolimus-treated males (5.9/1,000 patient years versus 92.9/1,000 patient years). Women treated with sirolimus have a much higher risk of oligomenorrhea and possibly ovarian cysts [50, 51].

The NTPR reported the outcomes of 18 transplant (12 kidney, 1 kidney/pancreas, 2 cardiac and 3 liver) recipients exposed to sirolimus during pregnancy with 19 pregnancies. There were 13 live births and 6 miscarriages. There were 3 live births with defects, but 2 of these also had MMF exposure [52]. A report of 7 women taking sirolimus, which was discontinued on diagnosis of pregnancy (within the first 6 weeks), resulted in 3 miscarriages and 4 live births. One possibly unrelated structural abnormality was reported in a patient switched to sirolimus at 24 weeks [53]. Everolimus has been reported to cause toxicities in animals at doses lower than those used in humans (SmPC for Rapamune®). There have been few case reports of pregnancies with everolimus throughout pregnancy.

Sirolimus and everolimus are powerful inhibitors of growth, associated with impaired wound healing post transplant or subsequent surgery [54]. The placental mTOR-signaling pathway regulates the trafficking of the amino acid leucine in human pregnancies complicated by intrauterine growth restriction [55]. Whether further observational data suggest a role of sirolimus in SGA babies remains to be determined. Another potential risk of mTOR inhibition is poor healing of caesarean section scars. Impaired healing of surgical wounds is well described in other surgical situations.

Breastfeeding

In animals, sirolimus and everolimus are excreted in breast milk. There are currently no data on breast milk transfer in lactating women treated with sirolimus or everolimus. We advise against breastfeeding.

• Therapeutic Antibodies

Therapeutic antibodies are increasingly used in the management of renal transplant recipients and in those with other causes of CKD.

Rituximab is a monoclonal antibody that binds specifically to transmembrane CD20 on B-lymphocytes. As rituximab is an IgG1 k construct, it is likely to cross the placenta, especially in the last four weeks of gestation. The half-life of rituximab is approximately 22 days and maternal B-cell depletion may occur for up to six months post treatment. Experience outside transplantation indicates B-cell lymphopenia in newborns exposed to rituximab in utero [56, 57]. Of the 90 live births exposed to rituximab, 76 percent were born at term and the incidence of congenital malformations was not increased (2.2 percent). Twelve percent of babies had hematological abnormalities (B-cell depletion, neutropenia, lymphopenia, thrombocytopenia or anemia). Eleven pregnancies had enough data for paternal exposure evaluation. There were two miscarriages, seven live births and two still ongoing at the time of publishing [58]. The significance of in utero and postnatal B cell depletion remains to be determined. The risk–benefit balance of use of rituximab in pregnancy must be individualized. Ideally pregnancy should be avoided for 12 months after rituximab, but may be needed to manage aggressive or refractory disease.

Belatacept is licensed for the prevention of rejection in renal transplant recipients. Belatacept is a fusion protein of human IgG1 that blocks T-cell co-stimulation. There are no data on the use of belatacept in human pregnancy. However, in rats, fetal mortality was increased although pups did not display malformations (SmPC for belatacept). The manufacturer advises avoidance of pregnancy for at least eight weeks after the last injection.

Eculizumab is a monoclonal antibody that inhibits C5 in the complement cascade and is used in the long-term treatment of patients with paroxysmal nocturnal hemoglobinuria (PNH) and treatment of atypical hemolytic uremia syndrome. Some data exist in pregnant women receiving eculizumab for prophylaxis of atypical hemolytic uremic syndrome (aHUS), There are two case reports using eculizumab in pregnancies at 26 weeks' gestation with no adverse outcomes to the infants [59, 60]. A recent retrospective study of 75 pregnancies receiving long-term treatment with eculizumab for PNH found a 29 percent rate of premature births with no apparent increase in adverse outcomes to mothers or infants [61]. Eculizumab dosing or frequency had to be increased in half of the patients.

Breastfeeding Human IgG is excreted into breast milk, but does not appear in the infant circulation [1]. This was confirmed by Kelly et al. in 10 breastfed infants [61]. Therefore biologic therapies are not contraindicated in breastfeeding mothers. It is likely that the antibodies are destroyed by acid and enzymes in the infant's gastrointestinal tract, preventing systemic absorption.

Leflunomide

Leflunomide is an immunosuppressant that has been used off-label in renal transplant recipients as an adjunctive treatment for BK virus nephropathy. It has a long half-life of two weeks and complete elimination may take up to two years. A report described 16 women exposed during the first trimester and 29 women prior to conception where all women underwent a "rapid elimination procedure" involving cholestyramine on discovery of pregnancy or before conception. First-trimester exposure was associated with preterm births [62]. A continuation to this study in 2010 examined 250 pregnancy outcomes. Ninety-five percent of patients underwent the rapid elimination procedure. There was no difference in major malformations or miscarriages, but minor malformations were more common, though no pattern was seen [63].

Erythropoietic-Stimulating Agents (ESAs) and Intravenous Iron in Pregnancy

• Erythropoietic-Stimulating Agents

A greater increase in intravascular volume compared to red cell mass in normal pregnancy results in physiologic anemia (hemoglobin<105 g/L) (see Figure 7.3), the nadir being 30 to 34 weeks of gestation. Increased plasma erythropoietin (EPO) produced by the healthy kidney induces the rise in red cell mass [64]. There is a high risk of anemia in pregnant patients with CKD where EPO production is limited [65]. Exogenous erythropoietic-stimulating agents (ESA), which do not cross the placenta or increase fetal hemoglobin, have been widely used in pregnancy complicated by the anemia of CKD. They effectively increase hemoglobin levels and reduce transfusion requirement [14, 66, 67, 68, 69].

The most frequent and serious side effect of ESAs outside pregnancy is new onset or worsening of

existing hypertension. As pregnancy itself is frequently associated with worsening blood pressure control, any additional impact of EPO is difficult to assess. A significant dose increase in the order of at least 50 percent compared to prepregnancy dosing is required to maintain hematocrit [72]. Reports of hypertension clearly related to EPO in pregnancy are sparse [72]. Hou reported no difference in pregnancy outcome from 19 dialysis patients treated with EPO as compared with 11 contemporary patients who were not [14], though it has been reported that 25 percent to 50 percent of women with CKD develop some form of preeclampsia. Anemia frequently complicates renal transplant pregnancies in which serum endogenous EPO is inappropriately low and the rate of erythropoiesis is blunted [65]. Treatment with ESA is effective in renal transplant recipients. The role, if any, of erythropoietin in the development or worsening of hypertension in pregnancy remains unclear [72, 73].

Target hemoglobin of 100-110 g/L is recommended and ESA doses should be adjusted to approach Hb target slowly as in the nonpregnant population. Close antenatal blood pressure monitoring is mandatory in these patients.

Breastfeeding

Erythropoietin is a normal constituent of human breast milk and appears to play an important role in the development of infants' gastrointestinal system, central nervous system and immunity [72]. There are no data on the newer longer-acting ESAs (methoxy polyethylene glycol-epoetin beta) in human breastfeeding. The authors cautiously allow breastfeeding in ESA-treated women.

• Intravenous Iron

Intravenous iron may better overcome functional iron deficiency and lead to a greater erythopoietic response with ESA treatment in CKD outside pregnancy. A systematic review of IV iron for treatment of anemia in normal pregnancy notes a limited evidence base [74]. Antenatal IV iron (mainly iron sucrose [Venofer®]) and iron carboxymaltose (Ferinject®) reduce the need for postpartum blood transfusions when compared to oral iron [75, 76]. Their use is contraindicated if there is a history of anaphylaxis to parenteral iron, during the first trimester, during infection and in chronic liver disease. This advice is based largely around the risk to the pregnancy of anaphylaxis (EMEA and MHRA recommendation)

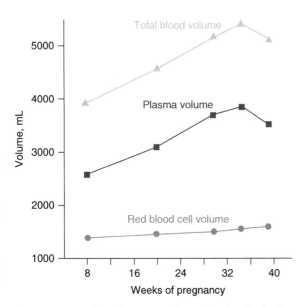

Figure 7.3 Physiological changes in plasma, blood and red cell volume in normal pregnancy (taken from UpToDate www.uptodate.com/contents/image?imageKey=OBGYN%2F61948&topicKey=OBGYN%2F443&search=physiological%20changes%20in%20pregnancy&source=outline_link&selectedTitle=1~150).

when using iron dextran, Cosmofer®, although it can occur with any preparation and should only be administered in an environment with full resuscitation facilities [77]. The authors use iron sucrose or iron carboxymaltose, which are associated with a lower risk of allergic reactions outside pregnancy.

Cinacalcet

Cinacalcet is used for the management of tertiary hyperparathyroidism in women with CKD. Nadarasa et al. reported a patient with parathyroid carcinoma, treated prepregnancy and antenatally in two pregnancies with the delivery of two healthy infants [78]. Further case reports describe the successful use of cinacalcet in the third trimester [79, 80]. Although these are encouraging reports, the role of the calcium-sensing receptor in pregnancy is not yet fully understood and thus cinacalcet should be withdrawn if possible prepregnancy.

Antibiotics in Pregnancy (see Table 7.3)

• Penicillins and Cephalosporin antibiotics

The UK teratology information service (UKTIS) advises that penicillins and cephalosporins are not teratogenic and should be considered as first-line agents for suitable bacterial infections in pregnancy. They are preferred agents in non-allergic individuals for first-line therapy while awaiting microbiological sensitivity. Some antibiotics have limited evidence of safety in pregnancy and the risk-to-benefit ratio can be difficult to ascertain. Nevertheless, it should be borne in mind that inadequately treated infection in pregnancy constitutes a significant risk to mother and baby.

• Co-amoxiclav

There is no evidence of teratogenicity of this agent in pregnancy. Concerns were raised late in pregnancy by the ORACLE study [81] and confirmed in a Cochrane review in 2013, where 22 random controlled trials of different antibiotics involving 6,872 infants were analyzed [82]. Co-amoxiclav was associated with an increased risk of neonatal necrotizing enterocolitis (risk ratio 4.72). However, the increased risk was not seen with intact membranes and was associated with co-amoxiclav administered at the time of delivery [83]. Co-amoxiclav should be avoided near term if an alternative antibiotic is considered suitable.

Table 7.3 Summary of antibiotic use in pregnancy where required

Antibiotic	First trimester	Second trimester	Third trimester	Comments
Cephalosporins	Safe	Safe	Safe	
Penicillins	Safe	Safe	Safe	
Macrolides	Probably safe	Probably safe	Probably safe	
Co-amoxiclav	Probably safe	Probably safe	Avoid after 36 weeks	Increased risk of necrotizing enterocolitis if membranes ruptured
Nitrofurantoin	Can use	Can use	Do not use beyond week 36 or at term	Increase risk of neonatal hemolysis after 36 weeks
Trimethoprim	Avoid	Use with caution	Use with caution	Risk of neural tube defects with first-trimester use (give high-dose folic acid)
Ciprofloxacin	Not recommended	Use with caution (see comments)	Use with caution (see comments)	
Meropenem and ertapenem	Use with caution	Use with caution	Use with caution	Limited experience

Breastfeeding

Co-amoxiclav is considered compatible with breastfeeding, though the infant should be monitored for any signs of gastrointestinal adverse events. Prospective data from 67 women exposed to co-amoxiclav during lactation found that 22 percent of infants had adverse events, as reported by mothers, which increased with dosage [84]. No pattern was seen and adverse effects were considered minor and self-limiting.

• Macrolide antibiotics

The macrolide antibiotics include azithromycin, clarithromycin, erythromycin, spiramycin and telithromycin. Limited data are available on the use of macrolides in human pregnancy, but those which have been published do not suggest a clear increased risk of adverse pregnancy outcome. An increased incidence of cardiovascular defects and pyloric stenosis have been suggested for macrolides as a class, although causality has not been established. Erythromycin is considered safe and is used in the prophylaxis of infection following preterm labor [81].

• Nitrofurantoin

A meta-analysis of nitrofurantoin exposures indicated it was a safe option in the first two trimesters of pregnancy [85]. In the later stages of pregnancy nitrofurantoin has been associated with a risk of hemolytic anemia in newborns, including those who are glucose-6-phosphate-dehydrogenase (G6PD) deficient, if nitrofurantoin is administered close to delivery [1]. Therefore, as a precaution, nitrofurantoin should not be used beyond week 38 or if labor is imminent [86]. A large case-controlled study in 22,000 patients found that although clinical doses (<400 mg per day) were not teratogenic, neural tube defects and clubfoot occurred at a higher rate in mothers exposed to nitrofurantoin [87]. The MHRA advises nitrofurantoin may be considered with caution in patients with impaired renal function for no more than three to seven days if there are multi-drug-resistant organisms that require treatment.

Breastfeeding

Studies have found that nitrofurantoin is excreted in breast milk, and although the amounts are considered low, adverse events may be experienced by infants younger than one year or in those with G6PD deficiency [1].

• Trimethoprim

Trimethoprim is a selective inhibitor of dihydrofolate reductase that prevents folic acid synthesis in bacteria, thereby preventing bacterial DNA replication. There has been concern that trimethoprim might increase the risk of neural tube defects if administered in the first trimester. Trimethoprim crosses the placenta and Scottish Intercollegiate Guideline Network (SIGN) guidance on treatment of urinary tract infections in pregnancy (SIGN 88) advises that it should not be used for pregnant women with established folate deficiency, with low dietary folate intake, or taking other folate antagonists, such as antiepileptics [88]. The authors avoid the use of trimethoprim in the first trimester of pregnancy. A recent study has reported an increased overall risk of congenital malformations, and specifically of cardiac and limb defects, among offspring of women who were dispensed trimethoprim in the 12 weeks prior to pregnancy. Studies of use in the first trimester have reported an increased risk of neural tube defects, cleft lip/palate and cardiac defects. As such it is recommended that any mother who has had exposure to trimethoprim in the first trimester should also receive folate supplementation (see www.uktis.org).

Breastfeeding

There have been reports of milk concentrations of 1.2 to 5.5mcg/mL in mothers taking up to 640 mg trimethoprim daily, with an average milk-to-plasma ratio of 1.26 [89, 90, 91]. These studies were conducted with trimethoprim-sulfamethoxazole, with no adverse effects noted in the nursing infants.

Fluoroquinolones

Fluoroquinolone antibiotics are broad-spectrum anti-infective agents, which act by inhibiting bacterial DNA gyrase. They are known to cross the placenta, but experience of their use in pregnancy is limited. They are not known to be fetotoxic in animals. A small number of reports of ciprofloxacin use in human pregnancy do not demonstrate an increased rate of congenital abnormalities or a common pattern of malformations, though it may be prudent to avoid use in the first trimester. Inadvertent use would not be considered grounds for termination (UKTIS, 2012). A multicenter study looking at fluoroquinolones in pregnancy reported on data from 105 pregnancies exposed to ciprofloxacin found no differences in prematurity, spontaneous abortion or major malformations when compared to controls [92]. Data from 666 cases with a known outcome showed a 4.8 percent malformation rate with ciprofloxacin, which was considered equivalent to the background rate with no patterns noted [93].

Experience of the use of fluoroquinolones is less than with other more commonly used antibiotics and as such these agents should normally be avoided in pregnancy unless the benefits of treating susceptible infection outweigh potential risks.

Breastfeeding

Ciprofloxacin is excreted in breast milk, with the milk-to-serum ratio varying from 0.85–2.14 following an oral dose of 750 mg [1]. There have been a number of reports of ciprofloxacin being used safely in breastfeeding, though one report described pseudomembranous colitis in a two-month-old nursing infant whose mother self-administered ciprofloxacin (doses not specified) [94]. The infant was being treated for necrotizing enterocolitis one month prior to the event, and therefore the isolated findings should be interpreted with caution.

• Meropenem and ertapenem

There is a lack of data on the use of carbapenems in pregnancy. A report from 2013 on a Japanese lady with a brain abscess describes the use of 3 g meropenem daily with no adverse effects to the infant when delivered [95]. Extrapolating data from other drugs with beta-lactam structures reassuringly suggests that these antibiotics may be safe, though the lack of specific outcomes means they should be used with a degree of caution [1].

Breastfeeding

There are very few data, though extrapolating from other beta-lactams, no adverse events other than oral thrush or self-limiting gastrointestinal disturbances are expected.

References

1. McCarthy M. Use of prescription drugs is common during pregnancy, US study finds. *BMJ* 2015; **351**: h4421.

2. Briggs GG, Freeman RK, Yaffe SJ. *Drugs in pregnancy and lactation: A reference guide to fetal and neonatal risk.* 7th edn. Philadelphia, PA; London: Lippincott Williams & Wilkins, 2005.

3. Koren G, Pastuszak A, Ito S. Drugs in pregnancy. *N Engl J Med* 1998; **338**(16): 1128–1137.

4. Garbis H, Elefant E, Diav-Citrin O, Mastroiacovo P, Schaefer C, Vial T, et al. Pregnancy outcome after exposure to ranitidine and other H2-blockers: A collaborative study of the European Network of Teratology Information Services. *Reprod Toxicol* 2005; **19**(4): 453–458.

5. McKay DB, Josephson MA. Pregnancy in recipients of solid organs – effects on mother and child. *N Engl J Med* 2006; **354**(12): 1281–1293.

6. Fischer MJ. Chronic kidney disease and pregnancy: Maternal and fetal outcomes. *Adv Chronic Kidney Dis* 2007; **14**(2): 132–145.

7. Levey AS, Bosch JP, Lewis JB, Greene T, Rogers N, Roth D. A more accurate method to estimate glomerular filtration rate from serum creatinine: A new prediction equation. Modification of Diet in Renal Disease Study Group. *Ann Intern Med* 1999; **130**(6): 461–470.

8. Watnick S, Rueda J. Reproduction and contraception after kidney transplantation. *Current Opinion in Obstetrics and Gynaecology* 2008; **19**(3): 308–318.

9. Deshpande, NA et al. Pregnancy outcomes in kidney transplant recipients: A systematic review and meta-analysis. *American Journal of Transplantation* 2011; **11**(11): 2388–2404.

10. European Best Practice Guidelines for Renal Transplantation. Section IV: Long-Term Management of the Transplant Recipient. IV.10. Pregnancy in renal transplant recipients. *Nephrol Dial Transplant* 2002; **17** Suppl. 4: 50–55.

11. Götestam Skorpen C, et al. The EULAR points to consider for use of antirheumatic drugs before pregnancy, and during pregnancy and lactation. *Annals of the Rheumatic Diseases* 2016; **75**: 795–810.

12. Park-Wyllie L, et al. Birth defects after maternal exposure to corticosteroids: Prospective cohort study and meta-analysis of epidemiological studies. *Teratology* 2000; **62**(6): 385–392.

13. Hviid A, Molgaard-Nielsen D. Corticosteroid use during pregnancy and risk of orofacial clefts. *Canadian Medical Association Journal* 2011; **183**(7): 796–804.

14. Hou S. Pregnancy in chronic renal insufficiency and end-stage renal disease. *Am J Kidney Dis* 1999; **33**(2): 235–252.

15. Empson M, Lassere M, Craig J, Scott J. Prevention of recurrent miscarriage for women with antiphospholipid antibody or lupus anticoagulant. *Cochrane Database Syst Rev* 2005; (**2**): CD002859.

16. Ostensen M, Khamashta M, Lockshin M, Parke A, Brucato A, Carp H, et al. Anti-inflammatory and immunosuppressive drugs and reproduction. *Arthritis Res Ther* 2006; **8**(3): 209.

17. Armenti VT, Radomski JS, Moritz MJ, Philips LZ, McGrory CH, Coscia LA. Report from the National Transplantation Pregnancy Registry (NTPR): Outcomes of pregnancy after transplantation. *Clin Transpl* 2000; 123–134.

18. Greenberger PA, Odeh YK, Frederiksen MC, Atkinson AJ, Jr. Pharmacokinetics of prednisolone transfer to breast milk. *Clin Pharmacol Ther* 1993; **53** (3): 324–328.

19. Saarikoski S, Seppala M. Immunosuppression during pregnancy: Transmission of azathioprine and its metabolites from the mother to the fetus. *Am J Obstet Gynecol* 1973; **115**(8): 1100–1106.

20. Chambers CD, Tutuncu ZN, Johnson D, Jones KL. Human pregnancy safety for agents used to treat rheumatoid arthritis: Adequacy of available information and strategies for developing post-marketing data. *Arthritis Res Ther* 2006; **8**(4): 215.

21. Davison JM, Dellagrammatikas H, Parkin JM. Maternal azathioprine therapy and depressed haemopoiesis in the babies of renal allograft patients. *Br J Obstet Gynaecol* 1985; **92**(3): 233–239.

22. Armenti VT, Ahlswede KM, Ahlswede BA, Jarrell BE, Moritz MJ, Burke JF. National Transplantation Pregnancy Registry – outcomes of 154 pregnancies in ciclosporine-treated female kidney transplant recipients. *Transplantation* 1994; **57**(4): 502–506.

23. Sibanda N, Briggs JD, Davison JM, Johnson RJ, Rudge CJ. Pregnancy after organ transplantation: A report from the UK Transplant Pregnancy Registry. *Transplantation* 2007; **83**(10): 1301–1307.

24. McKay DB, Josephson MA, Armenti VT, August P, Coscia LA, Davis CL, et al. Reproduction and transplantation: Report on the AST Consensus Conference on Reproductive Issues and Transplantation. *Am J Transplant* 2005; **5**(7): 1592–1529.

25. Sau A, Clarke S, Bass J, Kaiser A, Marinaki A, Nelson-Piercy C. Azathioprine and breastfeeding: Is it safe? *Bjog* 2007; **114**(4): 498–501.

26. Christensen LA, Dahlerup JF, Nielsen M, Fallingborg, J, Schmiegelow K. Azathioprine treatment during lactation. *Ailment Pharmacol Ther* 2008; **28**: 1209–1213.

27. Venkataramanan R, Koneru B, Wang CC, Burckart GJ, Caritis SN, Starzl TE. Ciclosporine and its metabolites in mother and baby. *Transplantation* 1988; **46**(3): 468–469.

28. Bar Oz B, Hackman R, Einarson T, Koren G. Pregnancy outcome after ciclosporine therapy during pregnancy: A meta-analysis. *Transplantation* 2001; **71** (8): 1051–1055.

29. Satchell S, Moppett, J, Quinn, M, Nicholls, A. Pregnancy, tacrolimus, and renal transplantation: Survival of a 358-g baby (letter). *Nephrol Dial Transplant* 2000; **15**(12): 2065–2066.

30. Hebert M, Zheng S, Hays K, Shen D, Davis C, Umans J, Miodovnik M, Thummel K, Easterling T. Interpreting tacrolimus concentrations during pregnancy and postpartum. *Transplantation* 2013; **95** (7): 908–915.

31. Armenti VT, Radomski JS, Moritz MJ, Gaughan WJ, Hecker WP, Lavelanet A, et al. Report from the National Transplantation Pregnancy Registry (NTPR): Outcomes of pregnancy after transplantation. *Clin Transpl* 2004: 103–114.

32. Fischer T, Neumayer HH, Fischer R, Barenbrock M, Schobel HP, Lattrell BC, et al. Effect of pregnancy on long-term kidney function in renal transplant recipients treated with ciclosporine and with azathioprine. *Am J Transplant* 2005; **5**(11): 2732–2739.

33. Zheng S, Easterling T, Umans J, Miodovnik M, Calamia J, Thummel K, Shen D, Davis C, Herbert M. Pharmacokinetics of tacrolimus during pregnancy. *Ther Drug Monit* 2012; **34**(6): 660–670.

34. Day C, Hewins P, Sheikh L, Kilby M, McPake D, Lipkin G. Cholestasis in pregnancy associated with ciclosporin therapy in renal transplant recipients. *Transpl Int* 2006; **19**(12): 1026–1029.

35. Ono E, et al. Immunophenotypic profile and increased risk of hospital admission for infection in infants born to female kidney transplant recipients. *American Journal of Transplantation*; **15**(6): 1654–1665.

36. Stanley CW, Gottlieb R, Zager R, Eisenberg J, Richmond R, Moritz MJ, et al. Developmental well-being in offspring of women receiving ciclosporine post-renal transplant. *Transplant Proc* 1999; **31**(1–2): 241–242.

37. Tendron-Franzin A, Gouyon JB, Guignard JP, Decramer S, Justrabo E, Gilbert T, et al. Long-term effects of in utero exposure to cyclosporin A on renal function in the rabbit. *J Am Soc Nephrol* 2004; **15**(10): 2687–2693.

38. Giudice PL, Dubourg L, Hadj-Aissa A, Said MH, Claris O, Audra P, et al. Renal function of children exposed to cyclosporin in utero. *Nephrol Dial Transplant* 2000; **15**(10): 1575–1579.

39. Munoz-Flores-Thiagarajan KD, Easterling T, Davis C, Bond EF. Breast-feeding by a ciclosporine-treated mother. *Obstet Gynecol* 2001; **97**(5 Pt 2): 816–818.

40. Moretti ME, Sgro M, Johnson DW, Sauve RS, Woolgar MJ, Taddio A, et al. Ciclosporine excretion into breast milk. *Transplantation* 2003; **75**(12): 2144–2146.

41. Lahiff C, Moss A. Ciclosporine in the management of severe ulcerative colitis while breast-feeding. *Inflamm Bowel Dis* 2011; **17**(7): E78.

42. Osadchy A, Koren G. Ciclosporine and lactation: When the mother is willing to breastfeed. *Ther Drug Monit* 2011; **33**(2): 147–148.

43. Bramham K, Chusney, G, Lee J, Lightstone L, Nelson-Piercy C. Breastfeeding and tacrolimus: Serial monitoring in breast-fed and bottle-fed infants. *Clin J Am Soc Nephrol* 2013; **8**(4): 563–567.

44. D'Cruz DP, Khamashta MA, Hughes GR. Systemic lupus erythematosus. *Lancet* 2007; **369**(9561): 587–596.

45. Tjeertes IF, Bastiaans DE, van Ganzewinkel CJ, Zegers SH. Neonatal anemia and hydrops fetalis after maternal mycophenolate mofetil use. *J Perinatol* 2007; **27**(1): 62–64.

46. Hoeltzenbein M, Elefant E, Vial T, Finkel-Pekarsky V, Stephens S, Clementi M, Allignol A, Weber-Schoendorfer C, Schaefer C. Teratogenicity of mycophenolate confirmed in a prospective study of the European Network of Teratology Information Services. *Am J Med Genet* 2012; Part A; **158**(3): 588–596.

47. Jones A, Clary M, McDermott E, Coscia L, Constantinescu S, Moritz M, Armenti V. Outcomes of pregnancies fathered by solid-organ transplant recipients exposed to mycophenolic acid products. *Prog Transplant* 2013; **23**(2): 153–157.

48. Medicines and Healthcare Products Regulatory Agency. Drug Safety Update: Mycophenolate mofetil, mycophenolic acid new pregnancy-prevention advice for women and men. Published December 14, 2015. www.gov.uk/drug-safety-update/mycophenolate-mofetil-mycophenolic-acid-new-pregnancy-prevention-advice-for-women-and-men.

49. Hall M, et al. Recommendations for men taking mycophenolate derivatives and pregnancy following MHRA recommendations. Published November 5, 2016. www.renal.org/docs/default-source/default-document-library/mycophenolate-and-fathers-to-be-letter-may-2016da90a131181561659443ff000014d4d8.pdf?sfvrsn=0.

50. Zuber J, Anglicheau D, Elie C, Bererhi L, Timsit M, Mamzer-Bruneei L, Ciroldi M, Martinez F, Snanoudj R, Hiesse C, Kreis, Eustach F, Laborde K, Thervet E, Legendre C. Sirolimus may reduce fertility in male renal transplant recipients. *Am J Transplant* 2008; **8**(7): 1471–1479.

51. Braun M. et al. Ovarian toxicity from sirolimus. *N Engl J Med* 2012; **366**: 1062–1064.

52. Coscia L, Constantinescu S, Moritz M, Frank A, Ramirez C, Maley W, Doria C, McGrory C, Armenti V.

Report from the National Transplantation Pregnancy Registry (NTPR): Outcomes of pregnancy after transplantation. Los Angeles. *Clinical Transplants*, 2010; 65–85.

53. Sifontis NM, Coscia LA, Constantinescu S, Lavelanet AF, Moritz MJ, Armenti VT. Pregnancy outcomes in solid organ transplant recipients with exposure to mycophenolate mofetil or sirolimus. *Transplantation* 2006; **82**(12): 1698–1702.

54. Valente JF, Hricik D, Weigel K, Seaman D, Knauss T, Siegel CT, et al. Comparison of sirolimus vs. mycophenolate mofetil on surgical complications and wound healing in adult kidney transplantation. *Am J Transplant* 2003; **3**(9): 1128–1134.

55. Roos S, Jansson N, Palmberg I, Saljo K, Powell TL, Jansson T. Mammalian target of rapamycin in the human placenta regulates leucine transport and is down-regulated in restricted fetal growth. *J Physiol* 2007; **582**(Pt 1): 449–459.

56. Ton E, Tekstra J, Hellmann P, Nuver-Zwart I, Bijlsma J. Safety of rituximab therapy during twins' pregnancy. *Rheumatology* 2011; **50**(4): 806–808.

57. Brian L, Jentoft M, Porrata L, Boyce T, Witzig T. Single-agent rituximab for primary CNS lymphoma during pregnancy as a bridge to definitive management. *Journal of Clin Oncol* 2014; **32**(7): e14–e17.

58. Chakraverty E, Murray E, Kelman A, Farmer P. Pregnancy outcomes after maternal exposure to rituximab. *Blood* 2011; **117**(5): 1499–1506.

59. Ardissino G, Ossola M, Baffero G, Rigotti A, Cugno M. Eculizumab for atypical hemolytic uremic syndrome in pregnancy. *Obstet Gynaecol* 2013; **122**(2): 487–489.

60. Mussoni M, Veneziano A, Boetti L, Tassi C, Calisesi C, Nucci S, Rigotto A, Panzini I, Ardissino G. Innovative therapeutic approach: Sequential treatment with plasma exchange and eculizumab in a pregnant woman affected by atypical hemolytic-uremic syndrome. *Transfus Apher Sci* 2014; **51**(2): 134–136.

61. Kelly R et al. Eculizumab in pregnant patients with paroxysmal nocturnal haemoglobulinuria. *New England Journal of Medicine* 2015; **373**: 1032–1039.

62. Cassina M, Johnson D, Robinson L, Braddock S, Xu R, Jiminez J, Mirrasoul N, Salas E, Luo Y, Jones K, Chambers C. Pregnancy outcome in women exposed to leflunomide before or during pregnancy. *Arthritis Rheum* 2012; **64**(7): 2085–2094.

63. Chambers C, Johnson D, Robinson L, Braddock S, Xu R, Lopez-Jimenez J, Mirrasoul N, Salas E, Luo Y, Jin S, Jones K. Organisations of Teratology Information Specialists Collaborative Research Group: Birth outcomes in women who have taken leflunomide

during pregnancy. *Arthritis Rheum* 2010; **62**: 1494–1503.

64. Milman N, Graudal N, Nielsen OJ, Agger AO. Serum erythropoietin during normal pregnancy: Relationship to hemoglobin and iron status markers and impact of iron supplementation in a longitudinal, placebo-controlled study on 118 women. *Int J Hematol* 1997; **66**(2): 159–168.

65. Magee L, Von Dadelszen P, Darley J, Beguin Y. Erythropoiesis and renal transplant pregnancy. *Clin Transplant* 2000; **14**(2): 127–135.

66. Schneider H, Malek A. Lack of permeability of the human placenta for erythropoietin. *J Perinat Med* 1995; **23**(1–2): 71–76.

67. Hou SH. Frequency and outcome of pregnancy in women on dialysis. *Am J Kidney Dis* 1994; **23**(1): 60–63.

68. Szurkowski M, Wiecek A, Kokot F, Daniel K. Safety and efficiency of recombinant human erythropoietin treatment in anemic pregnant women with a kidney transplant. *Nephron* 1994; **67**(2): 242–243.

69. Okundaye I, Abrinko P, Hou S. Registry of pregnancy in dialysis patients. *Am J Kidney Dis* 1998; **31**(5): 766–764.

70. Chao AS, Huang JY, Lien R, Kung FT, Chen PJ, Hsieh PC. Pregnancy in women who undergo long-term hemodialysis. *Am J Obstet Gynecol* 2002; **187**(1): 152–156.

71. Toma H, Tanabe K, Tokumoto T, Kobayashi C, Yagisawa T. Pregnancy in women receiving renal dialysis or transplantation in Japan: a nationwide survey. *Nephrol Dial Transplant* 1999; **14**(6): 1511–1516.

72. Sienas L, Wong T, Collins R, Smith J. Contemporary uses of erythropoietin in pregnancy: A literature review. *Obs and Gyn Survey* 2013; **68**(8): 594–602.

73. Kashiwagi M, Breymann C, Huch R, Huch A. Hypertension in a pregnancy with renal anemia after recombinant human erythropoietin (rhEPO) therapy. *Arch Gynecol Obstet* 2002; **267**(1): 54–56.

74. Thorp M, Pulliam J. Use of recombinant erythropoietin in a pregnant renal transplant recipient. *Am J Nephrol* 1998; **18**(5): 448–451.

75. Reveiz L, Gyte GM, Cuervo LG. Treatments for iron-deficiency anaemia in pregnancy. *Cochrane Database Syst Rev* 2007; **2**: CD003094.

76. Al R, Unlubilgin E, Kandemir O, Yalvac S, Cakir L, Haberal, A. Intravenous versus oral iron for treatment of anemia in pregnancy: A randomized trial. *Obstetrics and Gynecology* 2005; **106**(6): 1335–1340.

77. Bhandal N, Russell R. Intravenous versus oral therapy for postpartum. *BJOG*. 2006; **113**: 1248–1252.

78. European Medicines Agency (EMEA). Assessment report for: Iron containing intravenous (IV) medicinal products. [Online] *EMEA* 2013. www.ema.europa.eu/d ocs/en_GB/document_library/Referrals_document/ IV_iron_31/WC500150771.pdf.

79. Nadarasa K, Bailey M, Chahal H, Raja O, Bhat R, Gayle C, Grossman A, Druce M. The use of cinacalcet in pregnancy to treat a complex case of parathyroid carcinoma. *Endocrinol Diabetes Metab Case Rep.* 2014; **2014**: 140056.

80. Edling K, Korenman S, Janzen C, Sohsman M, Apple S, Bhuta S, Yeh M. A pregnant dilemma: Primary hyperparathyroidism due to parathyromatosis in pregnancy. *Endocr Pract.* 2014; **20**(2): e14–7.

81. Horjus C, Groot I, Telting D, Van Setten P, Van Sorge A, Kovacs C, Hermus A, de Boer H. Cinacalcet for hyperparathyroidism in pregnancy and puerperium. *J Pediatr Endocrinol Metab.* 2009; **22**(8): 741–749.

82. Kenyon S, Taylor DJ, Tarnow-Mordi WO, ORACLE Collaborative Group. ORACLE–antibiotics for preterm prelabour rupture of the membranes: Short-term and long-term outcomes. *Acta Paediatr Suppl.* 2002; **91**(437): 12–15.

83. Kenyon S, Boulvain M, Neilson JP. Antibiotics for preterm rupture of membranes. *Cochrane Database Syst Rev.* 2013; **12**: CD001058.

84. Williams M, Spencer R. Caesarean section: Summary of updated NICE guidance. *BMJ* 2011; **343**: d7108.

85. Benyamini L, Merlob P, Stahl B, et al. The safety of amoxicillin/clavulanic acid and cefuroxime during lactation. *Ther Drug Monit.* 2005; **27**: 499–502.

86. Ben David S, Einarson T, Ben David Y, et al. The safety of nitrofurantoin during the first trimester of pregnancy: Meta-analysis. *Fundam Clin Pharmacol* 1995; **9**: 503–507.

87. Apgar V: Drugs in pregnancy. *JAMA* 1964; **190**: 840.

88. Czeizel AE, Rockenbauer M, Sorensen HT, et al. Nitrofurantoin and congenital abnormalities. *Eur J Obstet Gynecol Reprod Biol* 2001; **95**: 119–126.

89. Scottish Intercollegiate Guidelines Network (SIGN): *Management of suspected bacterial urinary tract infections in adults.* Edinburgh: SIGN, 2012 (SIGN guidance No. 88) [Online]. www.sign.ac.uk.

90. Pagliaro LA, Levin RH: *Problems in pediatric drug therapy.* Hamilton, IL: Drug Intell Publications, 1979.

91. Miller RD, Salter AJ. The passage of trimethoprim/ sulphamethoxazole into breast milk and its significance. *Progress in chemotherapy: Proceedings of the Eighth International Congress of Chemotherapy,* Athens, 1973, 687–691.

92. Anon. Committee on Drugs & American Academy of Pediatrics: The transfer of drugs and other chemicals into human milk. *Pediatrics* 1994; **93**, 137–150.

93. Loebstein R, Addis A, Ho E, et al. Pregnancy outcome following gestational exposure to fluoroquinolones: A multicenter prospective controlled study. *Antimicrob Agents Chemother* 1998; **42**(6): 1336–1339.

94. Schaefer C, et al. Pregnancy outcome after prenatal quinolone exposure: evaluation of a case registry of the European Network of Teratology Information Services (ENTIS). *European Journal of Obstetrics & Gynecology and Reproductive Biology* 1996; **69**(2): 83–89.

95. Harmon T, Burkhart G. Perforated pseudomembranous colitis in the breast-fed infant. *J Ped Surg* 1992; **27**(6): 744–746.

96. Yoshida M, Matsuda H, Furuya K. Successful prognosis of brain abscess during pregnancy. *J Reprod Infertil.* 2013; **14**(3): 152–155.

8

Management of Hypertension in Renal Disease in Pregnancy

Jenny Myers and Graham Lipkin

Introduction

Chronic kidney disease (CKD) is a common cause of secondary hypertension in women of reproductive age. In the nonpregnant state, CKD is defined either as kidney damage (which is confirmed by renal biopsy or secondary markers of damage) or as the presence of glomerular filtration rate (GFR) of less than 60 ml/minute/1.73 m² for a period of greater than three months [1]. CKD is strongly associated with hypertension and the greater the severity of renal impairment, the higher the risk. In end-stage renal disease, 80 percent of patients have associated hypertension.

The prevalence of hypertension varies somewhat with the etiology of the underlying renal disease, with approximately 40 percent prevalence in chronic interstitial nephritis, IgA nephropathy and in the nonpregnant population, whereas rates of above 60 percent are associated with diabetic nephropathy, autosomal dominant polycystic kidney disease and focal segmental glomerulosclerosis [2].

In general, in the nonpregnant, and probably the pre-pregnant, population control of hypertension is relatively poor. Studies have suggested that around 40 percent of patients with recognized hypertension fail to achieve a target blood pressure of <140/90mmHg. Studies investigating this phenomenon within cohorts of patients with CKD indicate that control rates are lower still [3, 4]. Up to 40 percent of newly diagnosed hypertensive patients will discontinue their medication within the first year, with only 40 percent of patients continuing their therapy over the next decade [5].

Large epidemiological studies of nonpregnant subjects with CKD have demonstrated increased cardiovascular mortality even in moderate renal failure [6]. A meta-analysis of 85 publications demonstrated that the threshold for an increase in cardiovascular risk occurs when the GFR falls below 75 ml/minute, with the risk increasing steeply with a further

reduction in GFR [7]. When subjects with CKD start dialysis, the cardiovascular mortality rate increases 5- to 10-fold and those with established end-stage renal disease have an increased risk of 100-fold [8].

However, hypertension is just one risk factor in subjects with CKD. Dyslipidemia, insulin resistance, anemia, hyperhomocysteinemia, reduced nitric oxide availability and chronic inflammation also add to the cardiovascular risk in these individuals.

In the Multiple Risk Factor Intervention Trial (MRFIT), blood pressure was noted to be a strong predictor of worsening renal disease with primary hypertensive nephrosclerosis (with associated hyalinization and sclerosis of afferent renal arterioles) being a significant cause of chronic renal impairment [9]. Many factors may exist in an individual (of reproductive age or not) that may be responsible for blood pressure elevation (Table 8.1). The added mortality and cardiovascular risk induced by hypertension are significant and the effects of blood pressure control

Table 8.1 Possible mechanisms for hypertension in subjects with chronic kidney disease

- Preexisting essential hypertension
- Extracellular fluid volume expansion
- Renin-angiotensin-aldosterone system stimulation
- Increased activity of the sympathetic nervous system
- Increased BMI
- Erythropoietin administration
- PTH secretion and increased intracellular calcium concentrations
- Calcification of the arterial tree
- Renal artery disease
- Alterations in endothelial derived factors (i.e. nitric oxide, endothelin, prostaglandins)
- Chronic allograft dysfunction
- Cadaveric allografts (especially if donor has family history of hypertension)
- Immunosuppressive pharmacotherapy (i.e. ciclosporine, tacrolimus and corticosteroids)

through dialysis and antihypertensive medication are very important.

Hypertension in Pregnancy

Hypertension is the commonest medical disorder of pregnancy, affecting 10 percent of all pregnancies, of which 10–20 percent of cases will comprise women with chronic hypertension [10]. In 2008, population data from the United States reported a prevalence of primary and secondary hypertension of 1.52 percent and 0.24 percent, respectively [11]. Hypertension is a significant cause of maternal morbidity and mortality both worldwide and within the United Kingdom [12]. Severe hypertension is a common indication for level 2 high-dependency care during pregnancy and in the immediate postnatal period. Hypertensive disease in pregnancy contributes to around 12 percent of maternal deaths worldwide. In general, hypertension in pregnancy is associated with significantly increased perinatal mortality and morbidity with an increased risk of preterm delivery, intrauterine growth restriction and placental abruption [13].

Preexisting or chronic hypertension, defined as hypertension identified prior to pregnancy or before 20 weeks' gestation [14], is one of the most rapidly growing causes of hypertension in pregnancy. A combination of factors appears important in this rise in prevalence, including the postponement of childbearing to a more advanced age, often coupled with obesity and insulin resistance. Although less common than essential hypertension in women of reproductive age, three forms of secondary hypertension require exclusion. These include endocrine causes, such as phaechromocytoma and primary hyperaldosteronism, cardiac causes such as aortic coarctation and renal causes, including CKD and renovascular hypertension. It is estimated that 10 percent of women presenting with hypertension in pregnancy will have secondary hypertension [11] with renal disease accounting for 8 percent of these cases.

Many apparently healthy young women may not have had any blood pressure assessment prior to pregnancy. The physiological mechanisms of gestational blood pressure alteration and increased vasodilatation in the second trimester may mask chronic hypertension. This will then only be revealed in the second half of pregnancy and may be difficult to differentiate from gestational hypertension or preeclampsia. Indeed, a recent review of renal biopsy data in women close to pregnancy reiterated

the fact that a small but significant number of women with preeclampsia have underlying preexisting renal disease with hypertension mistaken as severe preeclampsia [15].

Pregnancy Complications Associated with Chronic Hypertension and Kidney Disease

Chronic hypertension and underlying kidney disease are important risk factors for a number of pregnancy complications including preeclampsia, fetal growth restriction (FGR), placental abruption, stillbirth, premature delivery and caesarean section. A recent meta-analysis that included 55 studies from 25 countries (795,221 pregnancies complicated by chronic hypertension) reported an incidence of perinatal mortality of 4 percent and preeclampsia, preterm delivery and neonatal unit admission of 26 percent, 28 percent and 21 percent, respectively [13]. In comparison to US population data, there was an 8-fold increased risk of developing preeclampsia, a 2.7-fold increased risk of a low birth weight infant (< 2,500g) and a 4-fold increased risk of perinatal death amongst women with chronic hypertension in comparison to the background population. Approximately half of the studies excluded women with secondary hypertension and/or renal disease and a subgroup analysis for women with underlying kidney disease was not possible in this meta-analysis.

There is a paucity of data detailing pregnancy complication risks in women with hypertension secondary to kidney disease, but evidence would suggest that the coexistence of hypertension and impaired renal function significantly increases the risk of pregnancy complications. A large US population database study (1995–2008) reported outcomes for 81,795 pregnancies complicated by secondary hypertension (including all causes), of which 6,614 had chronic hypertension and renal disease [11]. Compared to hospital deliveries without chronic hypertension, the odds ratios (ORs) for preeclampsia, stillbirth and abnormal fetal growth were 27.87 (24.85–31.25), 7.29 (5.59–9.52) and 7.94 (6.67–9.44). Interestingly, these were dramatically higher than the risks associated with chronic kidney disease without associated hypertension (preeclampsia 3.28 [3.10–3.47], stillbirth 1.74 [1.51–2.02] and abnormal fetal growth 2.29 [2.12–2.49]). In addition, in comparison to the

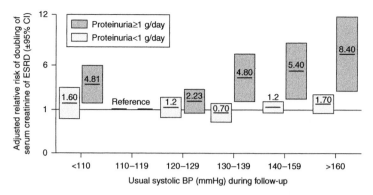

Figure 8.1 (a) Duration of pregnancy in those women without hypertension (untreated diastolic BP < 90mmHg) according to maternal serum creatinine (mg/dL); (b) Duration of pregnancy in those women with hypertension (treated, or diastolic BP > 90mmHg), according to maternal serum creatinine (mg/dL); after Ferraro et al. [16]

other reported categories of secondary hypertension (preexisting diabetes, collagen vascular disease and thyroid disorders), the risks for pregnancy complications were highest in the renal hypertension group.

A UK retrospective study of 270 women (301 pregnancies) from the maternity hospitals in Birmingham, Leicester and Hammersmith in London compared pregnancy outcomes in women with chronic kidney disease to a control cohort of 113,782 women without renal disease (CORD Study; published as abstract at BMFMS 2005) [16]. Chronic hypertension (with diastolic blood pressures of 90 mmHg or higher [in those treated or untreated]) was independently associated with perinatal death, and both chronic hypertension (OR 3.6 [1.8–7.5]) and renal impairment (5.7 [1.8–18]) with preterm delivery in multivariate analysis. Kaplan Meier curves indicate that hypertension is associated with poorer outcomes in terms of gestation of delivery, whatever the severity of chronic renal impairment (i.e. serum creatinine) (Figure 8.1). This perinatal risk increased in parallel with greater degrees of baseline maternal renal dysfunction.

One of the challenges facing obstetricians and renal physicians caring for women with chronic hypertension and/or kidney disease in pregnancy is the ability to make an accurate diagnosis of preeclampsia, often termed "superimposed preeclampsia."

Superimposed preeclampsia frequently occurs preterm in women with underlying medical disease [17], and there is a strong association with placental dysfunction often manifest as FGR [18]. There is an increased risk of development of the severe features of preeclampsia, often because pregnancies are managed expectantly to gain gestational benefit for the fetus and to reduce the consequences of a very premature delivery. The severe consequences of preeclampsia

(pulmonary edema, acute renal failure, ventilation) and severe hypertension (cerebrovascular complications) are therefore more common in women with underlying hypertension and kidney disease [11].

More recently, the measurement of serum or plasma angiogenic markers is emerging as a tool with the potential to aid the diagnosis of preeclampsia [19]. Abnormal placental development and function is central to the pathophysiology of preeclampsia, particularly disease that develops before 34 weeks. Over the past decade, compelling in vitro and in vivo evidence has provided support for the hypothesis that dysregulation of several angiogenic factors is characteristic of preeclampsia. There are now several tests that measure a number of these markers, soluble fms-like tyrosine kinase-1 (sflt) and placental growth factor (PlGF). Several studies have reported the potential benefit of these tests as diagnostic and prognostic markers for the condition and these may be particularly helpful in differentiating between worsening hypertension and/or proteinuria associated with placental disease [20–22]. In one such study, a low PlGF was able to identify women who required delivery for preeclampsia within 14 days of testing with a high degree of accuracy [23].

Several prospective studies are under way that will assess the clinical utility of these tests [24, 25], and it is anticipated that these tests will aid the diagnosis of preterm preeclampsia and placental disease in women with chronic hypertension and kidney disease in the future [26].

Other potential risks associated with hypertension in pregnancy stem from the known risks of hypertensive disease (i.e. cerebral hemorrhage, heart failure, hypertensive encephalopathy, retinopathy, acute renal failure). Despite these risks, treatment targets for women with chronic hypertension during pregnancy remain controversial [27]. Beneficial effects of treatment appear to be limited to prevention of maternal morbidity and depend upon the severity of the disease.

Measurement of Blood Pressure during Pregnancy

Accurate measurement of blood pressure in pregnancy is key to the management of hypertensive disorders. Despite clear recommendations by the National Institute for Health and Care Excellence (NICE), blood pressure measurement in clinical practice is often not performed accurately using the auscultatory technique. Several factors contribute to the acquisition of inaccurate measurements, including the use of faulty equipment, inadequate training and time constraints. Observational studies that have assessed the calibration of blood pressure devices have demonstrated that 20–25 percent of devices used in hospital and clinic settings had unacceptable calibration errors [28]. In addition, it has been estimated that only 10 percent of midwives and obstetricians routinely record blood pressure to the nearest 2 mmHg [29], and that 78 percent of readings obtained by clinicians in the antenatal clinic setting ended in a zero [30]. This concept also extends to threshold avoidance, where the observer adjusts the BP reading to avoid thresholds that entail making a diagnosis or requiring intervention.

In recent years, there has been a shift toward the use of automated BP devices, which rely on detecting changes in the amplitude of the intra-arterial oscillometric waveforms produced during cuff deflation to determine BP. An enormous number of devices are available on the market, but very few have been validated for use in pregnancy. A list of currently validated devices is available at www.dableducational.org/sphyg momanometers/devices_1_clinical.html#ClinTable.

This is particularly relevant as there has been concern that automated devices may underestimate blood pressure in women with preeclampsia [31]. For those devices that have been validated for use in pregnancy, the obvious advantage is a reduction in observer error and threshold avoidance.

Automated, ambulatory BP devices have been recommended outside of pregnancy to confirm a diagnosis of hypertension prior to instigation of treatment [32], and it is likely that this mode of monitoring could be used with great advantage to women with chronic hypertension and kidney disease in pregnancy. In the home setting, ambulatory readings enable differentiation between true white-coat hypertension and sustained hypertension and allow assessment of patterns of BP variation throughout the day. Ambulatory blood pressure monitoring is well tolerated with high rates of compliance [33], and the use of ambulatory monitoring could be expanded in the obstetric population. Self-monitoring using validated automated devices would also provide a simpler, cheaper and potentially more acceptable tool for women with chronic hypertension. Self-monitoring can deliver many of the advantages of ambulatory monitoring, while also improving surveillance and potentially reducing scheduled visits [34].

Treatment of Hypertension

Goals of Antihypertensive Treatment in Kidney Disease: Nonpregnant Patients

In nonpregnant individuals with CKD and hypertension, treatment objectives are prevention of cardiovascular events (the most frequent complication of CKD) and prevention or amelioration of further renal deterioration. Guidelines produced by the Joint National Committee in the United States (JNC8) [35], the European Society of Hypertension and the European Society of Cardiology [36] relaxed blood pressure targets for nonpregnant patients with CKD and hypertension to less than 140/90 mmHg. This differs from previous guidelines, which had stipulated that patients with CKD and hypertension should aim for a blood pressure <130/80mm Hg. Previous recommendations were based on analyses of long-term clinical trials in patients with diabetic and non-diabetic kidney disease that demonstrated that lowering blood pressure was associated with greater preservation of kidney function. This evidence has been reexamined and added to in the updated guidelines. The guideline groups have concluded that there is insufficient evidence to support lower blood pressure targets in these patients and that the specific effects of renin-angiotensin system blockers cannot be determined. Three trials conducted in CKD patients did not demonstrate any significant differences in end-stage renal disease or death from patients randomized to a higher target (140 mmHg) [37–39]. Recent meta-analyses have also not demonstrated that different BP targets in patients with CKD translate to

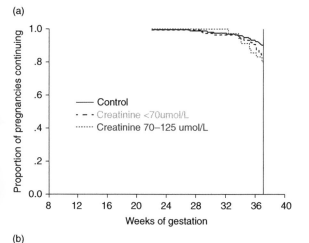

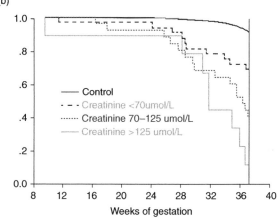

Figure 8.2 Relative risk of kidney disease progression based upon current level of systolic blood pressure and urine protein excretion. Based upon a meta-analysis of 11 RCTs (reference group for each is a systolic blood pressure of 110–119mmHg); reproduced with permission from Sarafidis and Bakris (Sarafidis PA and Bakris GL. Kidney disease and hypertension. Chapter 49: 607–619 in *Comprehensive hypertension* (ed. Yip GY and Hall JE), Mosby Elsevier, 2007 original figure in [47].

definitive benefits from achieving lower BP goals in terms of cardiovascular or renal events [40, 41]. However, in long-term observational follow-up studies following two of these trials, there was a trend toward reduced risk of renal progression, which was more evident in patients with proteinuria [42, 43]. The KDIGO CKD Guideline Development Work Group recommend that adults with urine albumin excretion of ≥30 mg/24 hours (or equivalent) should be treated with BP-lowering drugs to maintain a BP that is consistently ≤130/80 mmHg [44].

It has been proposed that there is a J-shaped relationship between over-treatment of blood pressure and cardiovascular and renal risk. This is plausible, as physiology has shown that there is a low, as well as high, blood pressure threshold for organ blood flow autoregulation [45]. This concept is potentially important in pregnancy because of the potential effect of blood pressure lowering on placental perfusion and fetal growth [46].

In adults with CKD it is important to manage both components of hypertension – hypervolemia and vasoconstriction. In patients with CKD who are not on dialysis, it is commonplace to initiate antihypertensive therapy with a renin-angiotensin-aldosterone blocker to minimize vasoconstriction (except some structural vascular changes) and some of the sympathetic hyperactivity [36]. Residual hypertension often indicates the hypervolemic component and this can be treated using diuretics. Figure 8.2 summarizes the long-term outcome studies that demonstrate long-term attenuation of renal impairment with treatment of hypertension in CKD [47].

The management of hypertension outside of pregnancy is highly relevant for obstetricians and renal physicians providing care for women before, during and after pregnancy as women of reproductive age will frequently be prescribed antihypertensive regimens, some of which are not suitable during pregnancy. Ideally women of reproductive age who are taking antihypertensive medication should be aware of the implications of these treatments in preparation for pregnancy and appropriate advice about changing to alternative medications, where necessary, in early pregnancy should be provided [48]. While there is only limited evidence to support the hypothesis that treatment of severe hypertension (diastolic > 110mmHg) in early pregnancy influences pregnancy outcome [49], it is likely that avoidance of severe hypertension in the periconceptual period and in early pregnancy when the placenta is developing has a positive impact on pregnancy outcomes.

Treatment of Uncomplicated Hypertension in Pregnancy

Blood pressure targets for women with uncomplicated chronic hypertension in pregnancy have long been debated, and until recently the quality of evidence to guide management has been of poor quality [50]. The use of antihypertensive treatments to normalize blood pressure has been associated with a reduction in maternal morbidity, particularly a reduction in severe hypertension, but there have long been concerns that "over-treatment" of blood pressure may be associated with worse perinatal outcomes, particularly related to fetal growth [46, 51]. A meta-regression of available data concluded that fetal growth was significantly impaired by the reduction in mean arterial pressure induced by antihypertensive therapy: a 10 mmHg fall in maternal mean arterial pressure was associated with a 145 g decrease in birth weight. However, this study is potentially affected by the biases of observational studies. In contrast, the Cochrane review did not find an increased risk of having a small-for-gestational-age (SGA) baby (RR 0.97; 95 percent CI 0.80–1.17) in those receiving antihypertensive treatment compared with placebo [52].

The CHIPS trial aimed to determine whether "tight" control (target diastolic 85mmHg) versus "less-tight" control (target diastolic 100mmHg) was associated with worse perinatal outcomes [27]. The study included women with uncomplicated chronic hypertension and non-proteinuric gestational hypertension, but not those with CKD. The target blood pressure difference between the two groups set at the start of the trial was 5mmHg; the achieved differences were 5.8 mmHg in systolic and 4.6 mmHg in diastolic blood pressure. The primary outcome of the study was a composite of pregnancy loss or high-level neonatal intensive care for more than 48 hours; this outcome was not different between the groups (31.4 versus 30.7 percent). In addition, gestation at delivery (36.8 versus 37.2 weeks) and the number of SGA infants (16.1 versus 19.7 percent [<10th centile] 4.7 versus 5.3 percent [<3rd centile]) was not different between the less tight and tight control groups. Serious maternal complications, placental abruption and the development of preeclampsia were also not different between the groups; however, the risk of developing severe hypertension was significantly higher in the less tight control group (40.6 versus 27.5 percent) in agreement with the meta-analysis of previous trials.

The conclusion of the CHIPS trial therefore is that there is no increased risk of adverse perinatal outcome associated with a target blood pressure of 85mmHg. In the CHIPS trial the women randomized to the "tight" and "less-tight" control groups actually achieved mean systolic and diastolic blood pressures (between randomization and delivery) of 138.8±0.5 versus 133.1±0.5 mm Hg and 89.9±0.3 versus

85.3±0.3 mm Hg, respectively. The evidence would therefore support a slightly lower blood pressure target from women with uncomplicated hypertension than has previously been recommended (<150/80-100mmHg) [14] on the basis that there is a significant reduction in the risk of severe maternal hypertension, which in turn is associated with an increased frequency of hospital admission, high-dependency care and most importantly cerebrovascular hemorrhage [53]. Antihypertensive therapy should therefore be considered in women with blood pressure measurements persistently above 140mmHg and/or 90mmHg. The potential risk of over-treatment persists; however, treating diastolic blood pressure to below 80 mmHg should be avoided. Severe hypertension (blood pressure ≥ 160/110 mmHg) should be treated urgently to protect the mother from serious complications, such as stroke, heart failure or renal failure.

Treatment of Secondary Hypertension in Pregnancy

Women with secondary hypertension, particularly those with CKD and collagen vascular disease, are at increased risk of developing pregnancy complications associated with superimposed preeclampsia and adverse perinatal outcomes [11, 54]. To date there have been no randomized controlled trials of antihypertensive treatments that have focused on this group specifically. Management of hypertension in this group is particularly problematic given the conflict between maternal and fetal well-being. While there is no evidence to guide absolute blood pressure targets in these women, given that the risk of placental dysfunction and preeclampsia is highest in this group, it is possible that the potential risk of FGR associated with "over-treatment" is also highest in this group. There has been a tendency in recent years, given the motivation to reduce the risk of long-term renal decline and preserve cardiovascular health, to treat hypertension more aggressively in women with CKD, particularly those with significant proteinuria. While there is good evidence to support maintaining blood pressure below 140/90mmHg, there is not sufficient evidence to provide guidance for a lower blood pressure target during pregnancy. Common sense would dictate, however, that artificial lowering of blood pressure below 75mmHg is unlikely to be of any benefit to the mother or fetus.

Antihypertensive Agents

All antihypertensive drugs cross the placenta. There are no data from large, well-designed randomized trials on which to base a recommendation for use of one drug over another. Data regarding both comparative efficacy in improving pregnancy outcome and fetal safety are inadequate for almost all antihypertensive drugs. Commonly used oral antihypertensive drugs prescribed in pregnancy are summarized in Table 8.2 and discussed further in Chapter 7.

Labetalol

Labetalol, the most widely used beta-adrenergic blocker in pregnancy, is not selective, having some alpha-blockade effects. Labetalol has a good safety profile in pregnancy and is considered safe for use throughout pregnancy. Although there is limited published evidence describing first trimester use there has been no association with congenital anomalies [14]. One small RCT did not demonstrate a significantly increased risk of SGA infants or other pregnancy

Table 8.2 Oral antihypertensive medications commonly used to treat chronic hypertension in pregnancy

Drug	Dose	Fetal concerns	Comments
First line			
Labetalol (α- and β-blocker)	200mg–2.4g/d in two to four divided doses	Limited information regarding first-trimester use; no reports of increased congenital anomalies Rare mild neonatal hypotension in first 24 hours of life Very rare hypoglycemia	Recommended by NICE as first line
Nifedipine	10–120 mg/d of a modified-release preparation	Human data suggests low risk	Less experience with other calcium entry blockers
Methyldopa	0.5–3.0 g/d in two to three divided doses	No documented association with congenital anomalies	Maternal side effects often limit use
2nd line			
Hydralazine	50–100 mg/d in two divided doses	No reports linking hydralazine with congenital defects	Neonatal thrombocytopenia and bleeding secondary to hydralazine ingestion throughout the third trimester have been reported in three infants. This, however, may have been due to maternal hypertension.
Other agents			
Doxazosin (α blocker)	2–8mg/day	No information available	
Loop diuretics		Furosemide has been used in the second and third trimesters without fetal or newborn adverse effects	Limited information first trimester
Thiazide diuretics	Depends on specific agent	Limited information Possible association with congenital abnormalities (chlorothiazide)	Concerns regarding neonatal hypoglycemia, neonatal hypovolemia and maternal/fetal serum electrolyte imbalances

Table 8.2 (cont.)

Drug	Dose	Fetal concerns	Comments
Atenolol (β-blocker)	25–50mg/day	No obvious association with congenital abnormalities Low birth weight/placental weight Decreased fetal heart rate described	Not usually recommended for use in pregnancy, but may be useful post delivery
Contraindicated			
ACE inhibitors and AT1 receptor antagonists			Use after first trimester can lead to fetopathy, oligohydramnios, growth retardation, and neonatal anuric renal failure, which may be fatal

complications compared to women treated with methyldopa or placebo [55]. However, concern remains that treatment with beta-blockers compared to no treatment is associated with an increased risk of SGA infants as demonstrated by the recent Cochrane review [50]. This analysis does not differentiate between different beta-blockers, however, and the strongest association with FGR appears to be with atenolol [56–58]. One of the disadvantages of labetalol is that it requires multiple dosing regimes due to its short half-life of six to eight hours.

Calcium Channel Blockers

Experience with calcium channel blockers has been accumulating over the past decade, and these agents appear safe for use in pregnancy [14]. Nifedipine is available in various modified-release/long-acting preparations suitable for once or twice daily dosing (20mg–120mg/day). The recent Cochrane review did not demonstrate any increased risk of SGA with calcium channel blockers versus no treatment [50]. Although more contemporary calcium antagonists such as amlodipine are widely used in nonpregnant individuals with hypertension, there is no published data to guide their use in pregnancy. Non-dihydropyridine calcium antagonists such as verapamil and diltiazem have also been used, although most reports in the literature are of small numbers of women.

Methyldopa

Methyldopa, historically one of the most widely used drugs in pregnant women, is a centrally acting compound with a very good safety record for use in pregnancy [14]. At low doses it is well tolerated and has the longest follow-up of childhood development following in utero exposure [59]. The disadvantage of methyldopa is that it is a mild antihypertensive drug with a short half-life requiring multiple daily doses. In comparison to other agents it is less effective in terms of the prevention of severe hypertension and has a worse side effect profile at higher doses [50], particularly related to depression and sedation.

ACE-Inhibitors and Angiotensin Receptor Blockers

In nonpregnant adults there is good evidence that for individuals with hypertension and CKD, ACE-inhibitors and angiotensin II antagonists are beneficial in achieving good blood pressure control but also ameliorating renal damage [47]. Unfortunately, these drugs have been associated with a significant risk of fetotoxic effects [60, 61] and should therefore be discontinued once a pregnancy is confirmed [14]. For women planning a pregnancy who are currently taking ACE-inhibitors, a risk–benefit assessment should be undertaken and appropriate prepregnancy information provided [48]. In women where there is clear benefit, in terms of renal preservation, associated with continuing the ACE-inhibitor, women can be advised that this can be safely continued until a pregnancy is confirmed with a view to switching to an alternative antihypertensive (where necessary) as early as possible in the first trimester [62].

Diuretics

The NICE guidelines [14] recommend that women taking chlorothiazide diuretics should be informed that there may be an increased risk of congenital abnormality and neonatal complications if these drugs are taken during pregnancy. It would be usual, therefore, to discontinue these drugs unless the benefits were considered to outweigh risk. Loop diuretics may be used to treat fluid overload in women where severe edema is particularly problematic but would not usually be used first line for hypertension alone.

Other Management Issues Related to the Management of Hypertension in Pregnancy

Maternal Evaluation

Baseline tests for women with hypertension in pregnancy should include urinalysis, urine culture, serum creatinine, glucose and electrolytes [54]. A renal ultrasound scan should also be considered. These tests will effectively exclude many causes of previously unrecognized secondary hypertension, such as renal disease, and will also identify important comorbidities, such as diabetes mellitus. If qualitative testing for urine protein is negative, quantitative testing is not necessary. Women who develop evidence of proteinuria on a urine dipstick should have a quantitative test for urine protein, usually a protein-to-creatinine ratio. An electrocardiogram and echocardiogram should be considered in women with long-standing hypertension.

Prevention of Pregnancy Complications

Antihypertensive therapy and lowering blood pressure alone per se do not prevent preeclampsia [14]. It is thus important to consider the evidence for preventative strategies that may be adjuvant to antihypertensive treatment in pregnant women with preexisting hypertension and renal disease in the prevention of subsequent pregnancy complications related to placental disease.

Aspirin

Many studies have investigated the benefit of low-dose aspirin for the prevention of preeclampsia. The Cochrane review included 18 studies of high-risk women (n = 4,121) and reported a relative risk of 0.75 (95 percent CI 0.66 to 0.85) [63]. An individual patient data meta-analysis also demonstrated a significant benefit of aspirin for the prevention of preeclampsia (RR 0.90; 95 percent CI 0.84 to 0.97), but did not find that the benefit was greater in women with underlying medical conditions [64]. The 2010 NICE guidelines therefore recommend that women with CKD and/or hypertension should be advised to take 75mg aspirin from 12 weeks' gestation until birth of the baby [14].

Since publication of the NICE guidelines a meta-analyses has also been published that concluded that there is a larger benefit from aspirin if commenced prior to 16 weeks' gestation [65], particularly in women with risk factors for developing the condition, including chronic kidney disease and hypertension.

Calcium

A systematic review of 12 trials concluded that calcium supplementation is associated with a reduced risk of preeclampsia; this effect was greatest for women at high risk and for those with low baseline calcium intake [66]. However, where calcium intake is known to be adequate, there is no statistically significant reduction in risk and therefore a recommendation for the routine use of additional calcium in women at risk of preeclampsia cannot be justified in a UK setting at present [14].

Antioxidants

Overwhelming data supports a contribution of oxidative stress to the pathophysiology of preeclampsia, but several trials have now demonstrated that treatment with prophylactic vitamin C and E does not reduce the risk of preeclampsia in high- or low-risk women [67–71]. These should therefore not be recommended.

Identification of Pregnancy Complications

Antepartum assessment is directed toward monitoring and optimizing blood pressure control and identifying super-imposed preeclampsia and/or FGR. This is best accomplished by frequent (two to four times weekly) antenatal visits for monitoring maternal blood pressure, proteinuria and assessments of fetal growth and well-being [14]. Additional assessments, such as uterine artery Doppler [72–74], may also identify those pregnancies most likely to be complicated by superimposed placental disease, but these have not been recommended as part of routine care as they do not necessarily change clinical care pathways.

Conclusion

Women with CKD and hypertension are at significant risk of increased maternal morbidity and mortality from the sequelae of severe hypertension and pre-clampsia, and at high risk of perinatal morbidity and mortality attributable in the main to placental dysfunction. In this high-risk group, avoidance of severe hypertension is important and there is good rationale to maintain blood pressure between 120–139/70-85mmHg; however, no evidence remains to guide the optimal lower treatment targets in women with hypertension and chronic kidney disease. The diagnosis of superimposed preeclampsia is particularly challenging in this group and emerging diagnostic tests are likely to aid the diagnosis of pre-term placental disease in this group in the future.

References

1. K/DOQI clinical practice guidelines on hypertension and antihypertensive agents in chronic kidney disease. *American journal of kidney diseases: The official journal of the National Kidney Foundation.* 2004; **43**: S1–290.

2. Mailloux LU, Haley WE. Hypertension in the ESRD patient: Pathophysiology, therapy, outcomes, and future directions. *American journal of kidney diseases: The official journal of the National Kidney Foundation.* 1998; **32**: 705–719.

3. Ong KL, Cheung BM, Man YB, Lau CP, Lam KS. Prevalence, awareness, treatment, and control of hypertension among United States adults 1999–2004. *Hypertension.* 2007; **49**: 69–75.

4. Sarafidis PA, Li S, Chen SC, Collins AJ, Brown WW, Klag MJ, Bakris GL. Hypertension awareness, treatment, and control in chronic kidney disease. *The American journal of medicine.* 2008; **121**: 332–340.

5. Van Wijk BL, Klungel OH, Heerdink ER, de Boer A. Rate and determinants of 10-year persistence with antihypertensive drugs. *Journal of hypertension.* 2005; **23**: 2101–2107.

6. Sarnak MJ, Levey AS, Schoolwerth AC, Coresh J, Culleton B, Hamm LL, McCullough PA, Kasiske BL, Kelepouris E, Klag MJ, Parfrey P, Pfeffer M, Raij L, Spinosa DJ, Wilson PW. Kidney disease as a risk factor for development of cardiovascular disease: A statement from the American Heart Association Councils on Kidney in Cardiovascular Disease, High Blood Pressure Research, Clinical Cardiology, and Epidemiology and Prevention. *Circulation.* 2003; **108**: 2154–2169.

7. Vanholder R, Massy Z, Argiles A, Spasovski G, Verbeke F, Lameire N. Chronic kidney disease as cause of cardiovascular morbidity and mortality. *Nephrology, dialysis, transplantation: Official publication of the European Dialysis and Transplant Association – European Renal Association.* 2005; **20**: 1048–1056.

8. Baigent C, Burbury K, Wheeler D. Premature cardiovascular disease in chronic renal failure. *Lancet.* 2000; **356**: 147–152.

9. Klag MJ, Whelton PK, Randall BL, Neaton JD, Brancati FL, Ford CE, Shulman NB, Stamler J. Blood pressure and end-stage renal disease in men. *The New England journal of medicine.* 1996; **334**: 13–18.

10. Saftlas AF, Olson DR, Franks AL, Atrash HK, Pokras R. Epidemiology of preeclampsia and eclampsia in the United States, 1979–1986. *Am J Obstet Gynecol.* 1990; **163**: 460–465.

11. Bateman BT, Bansil P, Hernandez-Diaz S, Mhyre JM, Callaghan WM, Kuklina EV. Prevalence, trends, and outcomes of chronic hypertension: A nationwide sample of delivery admissions. *American journal of obstetrics and gynecology.* 2012; **206**: 134 e1–8.

12. Knight MKS, Brocklehurst P, Neilson J, Shakespeare J, Kurinczuk JJ (eds.) on behalf of MBRRACEUK. 2014. *Saving lives, improving mothers' care – Lessons learned to inform future maternity care from the UK and Ireland Confidential Enquiries into Maternal Deaths and Morbidity 2009–12*; 2014.

13. Bramham K, Parnell B, Nelson-Piercy C, Seed PT, Poston L, Chappell LC. Chronic hypertension and pregnancy outcomes: Systematic review and meta-analysis. *Bmj.* 2014; **348**: g2301.

14. NICE. Hypertension in pregnancy. http://guidanceniceorguk/CG107. 2010.

15. Day C, Hewins P, Hildebrand S, Sheikh L, Taylor G, Kilby M, Lipkin G. The role of renal biopsy in women with kidney disease identified in pregnancy. *Nephrology, dialysis, transplantation: Official publication of the European Dialysis and Transplant Association – European Renal Association.* 2008; **23**: 201–206.

16. Ferraro A, Somerset DA, Lipkin G, Al-Jayyousi R, Carr S, Brunskill N, Kilby MD. Pregnancy in women with pre-existing renal disease: Maternal and fetal outcome. *Journal of Obstetrics and Gynaecology.* 2005; **25**: S13.

17. Tuuli MG, Rampersad R, Stamilio D, Macones G, Odibo AO. Perinatal outcomes in women with preeclampsia and superimposed preeclampsia: Do they differ? *American journal of obstetrics and gynecology.* 2011; **204**: 508 e1–7.

18. Chappell LC, Enye S, Seed P, Briley AL, Poston L, Shennan AH. Adverse perinatal outcomes and risk

factors for preeclampsia in women with chronic hypertension: A prospective study. *Hypertension*. 2008; **51**: 1002–1009.

19. Staff AC, Benton SJ, von Dadelszen P, Roberts JM, Taylor RN, Powers RW, Charnock-Jones DS, Redman CW. Redefining preeclampsia using placenta-derived biomarkers. *Hypertension*. 2013/03/06 ed; 2013.

20. Verlohren S, Galindo A, Schlembach D, Zeisler H, Herraiz I, Moertl MG, Pape J, Dudenhausen JW, Denk B, Stepan H. An automated method for the determination of the sFlt-1/PlGF ratio in the assessment of preeclampsia. *Am J Obstet Gynecol*. 2010; **202**: 161 e1–e11.

21. Verlohren S, Herraiz I, Lapaire O, Schlembach D, Moertl M, Zeisler H, Calda P, Holzgreve W, Galindo A, Engels T, Denk B, Stepan H. The sFlt-1/PlGF ratio in different types of hypertensive pregnancy disorders and its prognostic potential in preeclamptic patients. *American journal of obstetrics and gynecology*. 2012; **206**: 58 e1–8.

22. Benton SJ, Hu Y, Xie F, Kupfer K, Lee SW, Magee LA, von Dadelszen P. Angiogenic factors as diagnostic tests for preeclampsia: A performance comparison between two commercial immunoassays. *Am J Obstet Gynecol*. 2011.

23. Chappell LC, Duckworth S, Seed PT, Griffin M, Myers J, Mackillop L, Simpson N, Waugh J, Anumba D, Kenny LC, Redman CW, Shennan AH. Diagnostic accuracy of placental growth factor in women with suspected preeclampsia: A prospective multicenter study. *Circulation*. 2013; **128**: 2121–2131.

24. Hund M, Verhagen-Kamerbeek W, Reim M, Messinger D, van der Does R, Stepan H. Influence of the sFlt-1/PlGF ratio on clinical decision-making in women with suspected preeclampsia – the PreOS study protocol. *Hypertension in Pregnancy*. 2015; **34**: 102–115.

25. Hund M, Allegranza D, Schoedl M, Dilba P, Verhagen-Kamerbeek W, Stepan H. Multicenter prospective clinical study to evaluate the prediction of short-term outcome in pregnant women with suspected preeclampsia (PROGNOSIS): Study protocol. *BMC pregnancy and childbirth*. 2014; **14**: 324.

26. Bramham K, Seed PT, Lightstone L, Nelson-Piercy C, Gill C, Webster P, Poston L, Chappell LC. Diagnostic and predictive biomarkers for pre-eclampsia in patients with established hypertension and chronic kidney disease. *Kidney international*. 2016; **89**: 874–885.

27. Magee LA, von Dadelszen P, Rey E, Ross S, Asztalos E, Murphy KE, Menzies J, Sanchez J, Singer J, Gafni A, Gruslin A, Helewa M, Hutton E, Lee SK, Lee T, Logan AG, Ganzevoort W, Welch R, Thornton JG,

Moutquin JM. Less-tight versus tight control of hypertension in pregnancy. *The New England journal of medicine*. 2015; **372**: 407–417.

28. de Greeff A, Lorde I, Wilton A, Seed P, Coleman AJ, Shennan AH. Calibration accuracy of hospital-based non-invasive blood pressure measuring devices. *Journal of human hypertension*. 2010; **24**: 58–63.

29. Perry IJ, Wilkinson LS, Shinton RA, Beevers DG. Conflicting views on the measurement of blood pressure in pregnancy. *British journal of obstetrics and gynaecology*. 1991; **98**: 241–243.

30. Wen SW, Kramer MS, Hoey J, Hanley JA, Usher RH. Terminal digit preference, random error, and bias in routine clinical measurement of blood pressure. *Journal of clinical epidemiology*. 1993; **46**: 1187–1193.

31. Natarajan P, Shennan AH, Penny J, Halligan AW, de Swiet M, Anthony J. Comparison of auscultatory and oscillometric automated blood pressure monitors in the setting of preeclampsia. *Am J Obstet Gynecol*. 1999; **181**: 1203–1210.

32. NICE. Hypertension. http://guidanceniceorguk/ CG127. 2011.

33. Hermida RC, Ayala DE, Iglesias M. Circadian rhythm of blood pressure challenges office values as the "gold standard" in the diagnosis of gestational hypertension. *Chronobiology international*. 2003; **20**: 135–156.

34. Ross-McGill H, Hewison J, Hirst J, Dowswell T, Holt A, Brunskill P, Thornton JG. Antenatal home blood pressure monitoring: A pilot randomised controlled trial. *BJOG: An international journal of obstetrics and gynaecology*. 2000; **107**: 217–221.

35. James PA, Oparil S, Carter BL, Cushman WC, Dennison-Himmelfarb C, Handler J, Lackland DT, LeFevre ML, MacKenzie TD, Ogedegbe O, Smith SC, Jr., Svetkey LP, Taler SJ, Townsend RR, Wright JT, Jr., Narva AS, Ortiz E. 2014 evidence-based guideline for the management of high blood pressure in adults: Report from the panel members appointed to the Eighth Joint National Committee (JNC 8). *Jama*. 2014; **311**: 507–520.

36. Mancia G, Fagard R, Narkiewicz K, Redon J, Zanchetti A, Bohm M, Christiaens T, Cifkova R, De Backer G, Dominiczak A, Galderisi M, Grobbee DE, Jaarsma T, Kirchhof P, Kjeldsen SE, Laurent S, Manolis AJ, Nilsson PM, Ruilope LM, Schmieder RE, Sirnes PA, Sleight P, Viigimaa M, Waeber B, Zannad F, Burnier M, Ambrosioni E, Caufield M, Coca A, Olsen MH, Tsioufis C, van de Borne P, Zamorano JL, Achenbach S, Baumgartner H, Bax JJ, Bueno H, Dean V, Deaton C, Erol C, Ferrari R, Hasdai D, Hoes AW, Knuuti J, Kolh P, Lancellotti P, Linhart A, Nihoyannopoulos P, Piepoli MF, Ponikowski P, Tamargo JL, Tendera M, Torbicki A, Wijns W, Windecker S, Clement DL, Gillebert TC, Rosei EA,

Anker SD, Bauersachs J, Hitij JB, Caulfield M, De Buyzere M, De Geest S, Derumeaux GA, Erdine S, Farsang C, Funck-Brentano C, Gerc V, Germano G, Gielen S, Haller H, Jordan J, Kahan T, Komajda M, Lovic D, Mahrholdt H, Ostergren J, Parati G, Perk J, Polonia J, Popescu BA, Reiner Z, Ryden L, Sirenko Y, Stanton A, Struijker-Boudier H, Vlachopoulos C, Volpe M, Wood DA. 2013 ESH/ESC guidelines for the management of arterial hypertension: The Task Force for the Management of Arterial Hypertension of the European Society of Hypertension (ESH) and of the European Society of Cardiology (ESC). *European heart journal*. 2013; **34**: 2159–2219.

37. Klahr S, Levey AS, Beck GJ, Caggiula AW, Hunsicker L, Kusek JW, Striker G. The effects of dietary protein restriction and blood-pressure control on the progression of chronic renal disease: Modification of Diet in Renal Disease Study Group. *The New England journal of medicine*. 1994; **330**: 877–884.

38. Wright JT, Jr., Bakris G, Greene T, Agodoa LY, Appel LJ, Charleston J, Cheek D, Douglas-Baltimore JG, Gassman J, Glassock R, Hebert L, Jamerson K, Lewis J, Phillips RA, Toto RD, Middleton JP, Rostand SG. Effect of blood pressure lowering and antihypertensive drug class on progression of hypertensive kidney disease: Results from the AASK trial. *Jama*. 2002; **288**: 2421–2431.

39. Ruggenenti P, Perna A, Loriga G, Ganeva M, Ene-Iordache B, Turturro M, Lesti M, Perticucci E, Chakarski IN, Leonardis D, Garini G, Sessa A, Basile C, Alpa M, Scanziani R, Sorba G, Zoccali C, Remuzzi G. Blood-pressure control for renoprotection in patients with non-diabetic chronic renal disease (REIN-2): Multicentre, randomised controlled trial. *Lancet*. 2005; **365**: 939–946.

40. Arguedas JA, Perez MI, Wright JM. Treatment blood pressure targets for hypertension. *The Cochrane database of systematic reviews*. 2009; CD004349.

41. Upadhyay A, Earley A, Haynes SM, Uhlig K. Systematic review: Blood pressure target in chronic kidney disease and proteinuria as an effect modifier. *Annals of internal medicine*. 2011; **154**: 541–548.

42. Sarnak MJ, Greene T, Wang X, Beck G, Kusek JW, Collins AJ, Levey AS. The effect of a lower target blood pressure on the progression of kidney disease: Long-term follow-up of the modification of diet in renal disease study. *Annals of internal medicine*. 2005; **142**: 342–351.

43. Appel LJ, Wright JT, Jr., Greene T, Agodoa LY, Astor BC, Bakris GL, Cleveland WH, Charleston J, Contreras G, Faulkner ML, Gabbai FB, Gassman JJ, Hebert LA, Jamerson KA, Kopple JD, Kusek JW, Lash JP, Lea JP, Lewis JB, Lipkowitz MS, Massry SG, Miller ER, Norris K, Phillips RA, Pogue VA, Randall OS, Rostand SG, Smogorzewski MJ, Toto RD, Wang X. Intensive blood-pressure control in hypertensive chronic kidney disease. *The New England journal of medicine*. 2010; **363**: 918–929.

44. Stevens PE, Levin A. Evaluation and management of chronic kidney disease: Synopsis of the kidney disease: Improving global outcomes 2012 clinical practice guideline. *Annals of internal medicine*. 2013; **158**: 825–830.

45. Zanchetti A. Blood pressure targets of antihypertensive treatment: Up and down the J-shaped curve. *European heart journal*. 2010; **31**: 2837–2840.

46. von Dadelszen P, Ornstein MP, Bull SB, Logan AG, Koren G, Magee LA. Fall in mean arterial pressure and fetal growth restriction in pregnancy hypertension: A meta-analysis. *Lancet*. 2000; **355**: 87–92.

47. Jafar TH, Stark PC, Schmid CH, Landa M, Maschio G, de Jong PE, de Zeeuw D, Shahinfar S, Toto R, Levey AS. Progression of chronic kidney disease: The role of blood pressure control, proteinuria, and angiotensin-converting enzyme inhibition: A patient-level meta-analysis. *Annals of internal medicine*. 2003; **139**: 244–252.

48. NICE. Hypertension in pregnancy. NICE quality standard 35. www.niceorguk/guidance/qs35/resour ces/guidance-hypertension-in-pregnancy-pdf. 2013.

49. Landesman R, Holze E, Scherr L. Fetal mortality in essential hypertension. *Obstetrics and gynecology*. 1955; **6**: 354–365.

50. Abalos E, Duley L, Steyn DW. Antihypertensive drug therapy for mild to moderate hypertension during pregnancy. *The Cochrane database of systematic reviews*. 2014; **2**: CD002252.

51. Magee LA, von Dadelszen P, Chan S, Gafni A, Gruslin A, Helewa M, Hewson S, Kavuma E, Lee SK, Logan AG, McKay D, Moutquin JM, Ohlsson A, Rey E, Ross S, Singer J, Willan AR, Hannah ME. The Control of Hypertension in Pregnancy Study pilot trial. *BJOG: An international journal of obstetrics and gynaecology*. 2007; **114**: 770, e13–20.

52. von Dadelszen P, Magee LA. Fall in mean arterial pressure and fetal growth restriction in pregnancy hypertension: An updated metaregression analysis. *Journal of obstetrics and gynaecology Canada : JOGC = Journal d'obstetrique et gynecologie du Canada : JOGC*. 2002; **24**: 941–945.

53. Martin JN, Jr., Thigpen BD, Moore RC, Rose CH, Cushman J, May W. Stroke and severe preeclampsia and eclampsia: A paradigm shift focusing on systolic blood pressure. *Obstet Gynecol*. 2005; **105**: 246–254.

54. Sibai BM, Lindheimer M, Hauth J, Caritis S, VanDorsten P, Klebanoff M, MacPherson C, Landon M, Miodovnik M, Paul R, Meis P, Dombrowski M. Risk factors for preeclampsia,

abruptio placentae, and adverse neonatal outcomes among women with chronic hypertension. National Institute of Child Health and Human Development Network of Maternal-Fetal Medicine Units. *N Engl J Med*. 1998; **339**: 667–671.

55. Sibai BM, Mabie WC, Shamsa F, Villar MA, Anderson GD. A comparison of no medication versus methyldopa or labetalol in chronic hypertension during pregnancy. *American journal of obstetrics and gynecology*. 1990; **162**: 960–966; discussion 6–7.

56. Montan S, Ingemarsson I, Marsal K, Sjoberg NO. Randomised controlled trial of atenolol and pindolol in human pregnancy: Effects on fetal haemodynamics. *Bmj*. 1992; **304**: 946–949.

57. Butters L, Kennedy S, Rubin PC. Atenolol in essential hypertension during pregnancy. *Bmj*. 1990; **301**: 587–589.

58. Lydakis C, Lip GY, Beevers M, Beevers DG. Atenolol and fetal growth in pregnancies complicated by hypertension. *American journal of hypertension*. 1999; **12**: 541–547.

59. Redman CW. Controlled trials of antihypertensive drugs in pregnancy. *American journal of kidney diseases: The official journal of the National Kidney Foundation*. 1991; **17**: 149–153.

60. Piper JM, Ray WA, Rosa FW. Pregnancy outcome following exposure to angiotensin-converting enzyme inhibitors. *Obstetrics and gynecology*. 1992; **80**: 429–432.

61. Velazquez-Armenta EY, Han JY, Choi JS, Yang KM, Nava-Ocampo AA. Angiotensin II receptor blockers in pregnancy: A case report and systematic review of the literature. *Hypertension in Pregnancy*. 2007; **26**: 51–66.

62. Li DK, Yang C, Andrade S, Tavares V, Ferber JR. Maternal exposure to angiotensin converting enzyme inhibitors in the first trimester and risk of malformations in offspring: A retrospective cohort study. *Bmj*. 2011; **343**: d5931.

63. Duley L, Henderson-Smart DJ, Meher S, King JF. Antiplatelet agents for preventing pre-eclampsia and its complications. *Cochrane Database Syst Rev*. 2007; CD004659.

64. Askie LM, Duley L, Henderson-Smart DJ, Stewart LA. Antiplatelet agents for prevention of pre-eclampsia: A meta-analysis of individual patient data. *Lancet*. 2007; **369**: 1791–1798.

65. Bujold E, Roberge S, Lacasse Y, Bureau M, Audibert F, Marcoux S, Forest JC, Giguere Y. Prevention of preeclampsia and intrauterine growth restriction with aspirin started in early pregnancy: A meta-analysis. *Obstet Gynecol*. 2010; **116**: 402–414.

66. Hofmeyr GJ, Duley L, Atallah A. Dietary calcium supplementation for prevention of pre-eclampsia and related problems: A systematic review and commentary. *BJOG: An international journal of obstetrics and gynaecology*. 2007; **114**: 933–943.

67. McCance DR, Holmes VA, Maresh MJ, Patterson CC, Walker JD, Pearson DW, Young IS. Vitamins C and E for prevention of pre-eclampsia in women with type 1 diabetes (DAPIT): A randomised placebo-controlled trial. *Lancet*. 2010; **376**: 259–266.

68. Poston L, Briley AL, Seed PT, Kelly FJ, Shennan AH. Vitamin C and vitamin E in pregnant women at risk for pre-eclampsia (VIP trial): Randomised placebo-controlled trial. *Lancet*. 2006; **367**: 1145–1154.

69. Rumbold AR, Crowther CA, Haslam RR, Dekker GA, Robinson JS. Vitamins C and E and the risks of preeclampsia and perinatal complications. *N Engl J Med*. 2006; **354**: 1796–1806.

70. Spinnato JA, 2nd, Freire S, Pinto ESJL, Cunha Rudge MV, Martins-Costa S, Koch MA, Goco N, Santos Cde B, Cecatti JG, Costa R, Ramos JG, Moss N, Sibai BM. Antioxidant therapy to prevent preeclampsia: A randomized controlled trial. *Obstet Gynecol*. 2007; **110**: 1311–1318.

71. Villar J, Purwar M, Merialdi M, Zavaleta N, Thi Nhu Ngoc N, Anthony J, De Greeff A, Poston L, Shennan A. World Health Organisation multicentre randomised trial of supplementation with vitamins C and E among pregnant women at high risk for pre-eclampsia in populations of low nutritional status from developing countries. *BJOG: An international journal of obstetrics and gynaecology*. 2009; **116**: 780–788.

72. Cnossen JS, Morris RK, ter Riet G, Mol BW, van der Post JA, Coomarasamy A, Zwinderman AH, Robson SC, Bindels PJ, Kleijnen J, Khan KS. Use of uterine artery Doppler ultrasonography to predict pre-eclampsia and intrauterine growth restriction: A systematic review and bivariable meta-analysis. *Cmaj*. 2008; **178**: 701–711.

73. Roncaglia N, Crippa I, Locatelli A, Cameroni I, Orsenigo F, Vergani P, Ghidini A. Prediction of superimposed preeclampsia using uterine artery Doppler velocimetry in women with chronic hypertension. *Prenatal diagnosis*. 2008; **28**: 710–714.

74. Shaker OG, Shehata H. Early prediction of preeclampsia in high-risk women. *J Womens Health (Larchmt)*. 2011; **20**: 539–544.

Chapter

9

Postpartum Follow-Up of Antenatally Identified Renal Problems

Al Ferraro and Liz Lightstone

Introduction

The estimated prevalence of chronic kidney disease (CKD) is 6–10 percent in women aged 20 to 49 years [1]. Many are asymptomatic and many are undiagnosed. For many women, it is pregnancy-related screening tests, in particular blood pressure checks and urinalysis for protein, that reveal the first evidence of an underlying renal condition. Such antenatal screening has long been nearly universally applied, though the National Institute for Health and Care Excellence (NICE) now recommends it is done at every antenatal appointment [2]. While a renal biochemical profile is not a part of routine antenatal screening, it is usually undertaken in women who are found to have urine abnormalities, those with hypertension, preeclampsia, recurrent urine infections or unexplained severe anemia – all of which are more common in individuals with underlying CKD. A renal biochemical profile is also frequently undertaken in pregnant women presenting with other significant intercurrent illness (whether or not a pregnancy-restricted illness) – and a proportion of these people will have acute kidney injury (AKI).

Interpretation of renal-related results in pregnancy is often confounded by the normal physiological and anatomical changes of pregnancy, which render many of the "standard" normal ranges irrelevant or unreliable (see Chapter 1). Examples include kidney size and morphology, systemic blood pressure, serum creatinine, eGFR [3] and the threshold for "normal" levels of proteinuria. Pregnancy-specific normal ranges have been published for some parameters [4, 5], but, in practice, there is often considerable uncertainty about the severity, or even the existence, of any true underlying renal condition if it is first suspected due to antenatal tests. Nonetheless, it is important to note that acute and substantial changes in serum creatinine still reflect a reciprocal change in underlying maternal renal function.

When pregnancy-related screening tests are undertaken only later in pregnancy, additional ambiguity and concerns can arise. It can be impossible to tell whether hypertension or newly identified biochemical abnormalities are due to emerging complications of pregnancy (e.g. preeclampsia), underlying CKD or a combination of both. Furthermore, there is significant variability in the rate at which pregnancy-related changes resolve postpartum. After preeclampsia, 54 percent and 39 percent have persisting hypertension at six weeks and three months postpartum, respectively [6]. In the same cohort, the prevalence of persistent proteinuria (greater than 0.3 g/day) was 21 percent and 14 percent at the corresponding time points, even though it resolved by two years postpartum in all but 2 percent. In those with some degree of underlying renal disease, it is even less clear how quickly superimposed pregnancy-related changes will resolve, if at all.

Thus, for women recently delivered from pregnancies marred by the identification of possible underlying CKD, it is often unclear a) whether there is significant underlying disease; b) by whom they should be followed up postpartum; and c) how much "watchful waiting" can be afforded. Such clinical judgments are often best undertaken by nephrologists and experienced obstetricians, in the context of an established multidisciplinary team, where decisions are based on the antenatal presentation and the evolution and severity of the identified abnormalities.

Women found to have a renal problem should have a renal diagnosis made. Ideally this occurs during pregnancy, but where not practical, certainly postpartum. During pregnancy this may be a simple matter of the patient having a renal ultrasound that demonstrates scarred kidneys in a woman with recurrent urinary tract infections (UTIs) and hypertension – supporting a diagnosis of reflux nephropathy. In other instances, diagnosis may not be confirmed during pregnancy because of the requirement for tests (e.g. certain forms of imaging) that pose an unacceptable risk to the mother or the baby. A woman who presents with modest proteinuria in early pregnancy with no hypertension, normal function and no markers of systemic disease would not warrant a renal biopsy during pregnancy as diagnosis will not alter management. However, if the proteinuria persists postpartum, then she may well merit biopsy to determine diagnosis and prognosis, not least for future pregnancies (see later in this chapter).

In summary, all women found to have a kidney problem during pregnancy should be informed of it, and of the need for postpartum diagnostic tests and follow-up. They need to be advised of its significance, which depends on the diagnosis, the stage of kidney disease and the level of associated hypertension and/or proteinuria.

Follow-Up Plans

All women with newly identified or suspected CKD should be followed up at least once postpartum to: a) evaluate proteinuria and renal function when not pregnant; b) to ensure appropriate diagnostic tests are requested; and, most important, c) to ensure a proper care pathway is identified that is clear to both the patient and her primary care physician. This first follow-up appointment would normally be with a nephrologist, perhaps acting as part of a multidisciplinary renal/obstetric outpatient clinic. Important medications can be reviewed and optimized with respect to renoprotection, especially instituting therapy with ACE inhibitors or angiotensin 2 receptor blockers.

The scenario to avoid is that of a woman who presents with end-stage renal failure later in life and volunteers that she was noted to have hypertension and proteinuria in each of her pregnancies previously but was never seen postpartum, nor advised that she had significant kidney disease or that she needed any follow-up. It is always tragic to consider that she may have had preventable renal failure or, at the very least, missed opportunities for risk factor management and preemptive transplantation.

Who Should Follow Up the Patient?

NICE recommends that those with a urine albumin-creatinine ratio (ACR) > 70 mg/mmol (not attributable to diabetes), or those with an ACR > 30 mg/mmol

and with hematuria should be referred to a nephrologist [7]. For reasons discussed earlier, these thresholds are not directly applicable within pregnancy, but it seems reasonable to apply them to women presenting with renal abnormalities before 20 weeks' gestation.

Women who are found to have abnormal renal function in pregnancy (bearing in mind the significant rise in GFR and fall in serum creatinine seen during pregnancy in women with normal kidney function) should have their renal function, and associated urinary indices, checked soon after delivery and again at six weeks. NICE does not recommend referral to nephrology for all those with low-level proteinuria, and not all those with CKD. However, we would advocate that referral to a nephrologist should at least be considered in women with antenatally defined renal problems that persist postpartum given that a) evidence of CKD is unusual in women of childbearing age, and b) confirmed CKD is of potential significance for any subsequent pregnancy (as a risk factor for preeclampsia, it should trigger consideration of aspirin from 12 weeks' gestation in future pregnancies) [8].

NICE recommends monitoring anyone who has suffered AKI for at least two to three years for the emergence of CKD [7], but does not specify this follow-up should be with a nephrologist. In most cases, primary care monitoring is sufficient. This can reasonably be applied to women who suffered a significant antenatal (or puerperal) AKI, but nephrology input may be warranted in some cases (see later in this chapter).

NICE recommends that women who develop gestational hypertension or preeclampsia should be offered a medical review at six to eight weeks postpartum [8]. Where such women have an ongoing need for antihypertensive treatment at six to eight weeks postpartum, a referral for specialist assessment of their hypertension is recommended. It follows that if there is evidence or suspicion of a preexisting renal condition, then a nephrology referral also seems appropriate at that stage. Underlying CKD may be particularly likely in the context of early-onset preeclampsia (i.e. that which required delivery before 34 weeks).

Consistent with this, NICE also recommends that, after preeclampsia, women should have dipstick urinalysis at the postnatal review [8]. Where persistent proteinuria (+1 or more) is found, a further check of proteinuria should be undertaken at three months postpartum. Based on this, and renal function testing, nephrology referral should be considered. In practice, a proportion of such patients may have already come to the attention of renal services during pregnancy and thus may have be seen by nephrologists (or obstetrician experienced in renal medicine) for their six-week postpartum review. Some patients with previous preeclampsia and with non-resolving proteinuria eventually warrant a renal biopsy to exclude other causes of proteinuria. Nonetheless, if the renal function is acceptable and stable and there are no other concerning features during follow-up in a nephrology clinic, it is our practice to defer renal biopsy until six months postpartum. A recent publication, using cases identified from UK biopsy registries, describes the range of diagnoses made in such women [9]. Of note, the same paper reports that the prognosis may be poorer for women obtaining a diagnosis in a postpartum situation; their rate of GFR decline appeared to be faster than in women with otherwise comparable levels of creatinine and proteinuria. While the mechanisms behind this observation are yet to be fully unpacked, it serves to emphasize the importance of appropriate postpartum review and investigations and follow-up.

If an episode of AKI was clearly associated with severe preeclampsia and resolves rapidly postpartum, then it may well not be necessary to refer to nephrology. Conversely, if renal function has been unstable toward the end of pregnancy, e.g. with a rapid rise in creatinine or proteinuria, then women should be seen and assessed very soon postpartum and again within a couple of weeks, preferably following discussion with a nephrologist during the perinatal period. Women can lose all their renal function in a matter of weeks after delivery in certain conditions, particularly where serum creatinine was already significantly raised. A blanket policy of not seeing women until six weeks postpartum will miss such patients [10]. Similarly, delivery may have been expedited to allow safe renal biopsy and diagnosis in a woman suspected of having active nephritis, e.g. associated with SLE. These women need to be aware before delivery that the nephrologists wish to make a diagnosis as soon as is practical and safe postpartum. The key is not letting the patient disappear back into the community before follow-up plans have been established, documented and communicated to the patient, her family and all relevant medical and nursing personnel. It is often

difficult to persuade a mother who perhaps has a vulnerable preterm baby that she also needs to be looked after and investigated; however, it is important to do so.

In some other chronic and stable settings, it may be reasonable to refer women directly back to their GPs for continuing care but with advice about monitoring and referring to clinical practice guidelines (RCGP, Renal Association and NICE or local guidance). These patients would include those found to have preserved renal function with minimal proteinuria or isolated microscopic hematuria or mild hypertension. These women will likely still warrant a renal ultrasound scan to exclude structural abnormalities (if not already done in pregnancy) and future regular assessments of proteinuria, hematuria and renal function. Women found to have anatomical evidence of reflux nephropathy (scarred/dysplastic kidneys) and recurrent UTIs, but with normal or mildly impaired function can be monitored by their GPs in the longer term, through the practice CKD register.

These women do need to be advised they have kidney abnormalities that put them at higher risk of developing high blood pressure or preeclampsia in a future pregnancy, and possibly a higher risk of cardiovascular disease. They should be advised to stop smoking, as it is an independent risk factor for progression of kidney disease regardless of contributing to cardiovascular risk. As the two most important determinants of progression to kidney failure are blood pressure control and degree of proteinuria, women need to be advised of the importance of monitoring and treating proteinuria and hypertension – aiming for a systolic blood pressure between 120–139 mmHg and a diastolic BP less than 90 mmHg, as per NICE [7].

If both proteinuria and hypertension are present, the ideal first-line agent would be an ACE inhibitor or an angiotensin 2 receptor blocker [7]. Enalapril, captopril and fosinopril are compatible with breastfeeding (except with preterm babies) (see Chapter 7), and suitable contraception should be advised, if appropriate (see Chapter 3).

Even in a patient group that is at lower risk of future complications (by renal standards), such general advice may be best delivered through a postpartum appointment at a multidisciplinary renal-obstetric clinic, or in a one-off nephrology clinic appointment, rather than in primary care. This will depend on local arrangements and the patient's personal circumstances.

Clearly all of this also needs to be explained to GPs at the time of discharge from renal/obstetric follow-up. Important, it is also worth giving some guidance as to when referral back to a nephrologist would be warranted – namely, if proteinuria rises significantly, renal function deteriorates or hypertension becomes difficult to manage, as per NICE [7].

Some women who are found to have kidney disease in pregnancy might also be under the care of other hospital physicians for long-term conditions. The most notable of these is diabetes. Diabetic nephropathy is now the commonest cause of renal failure in the UK and is rising rapidly due to the epidemic of type 2 diabetes. Some women will present with their type 2 diabetes for the first time in pregnancy, and they may already have complications such as retinopathy and nephropathy. It is imperative that such patients are firmly embedded in a good diabetic care pathway postpartum to slow their progression to end stage [11]. Furthermore, physicians looking after their diabetes need to be aware of changes in their renal state during pregnancy as risk factor management will need optimizing postpartum. Women with type 1 diabetes are likely to be embedded in a diabetic service already, but may have fallen out of the system during adolescence, thus postpartum reassessment allows the opportunity to reestablish specialist care.

Women with a connective tissue disease may have had a renal flare for the first time in pregnancy and will need long-term renal follow-up. Though a preemptive increase in medication at the time of delivery is not normally warranted, women with autoimmune disease also need to be kept under close watch as their disease can flare and progress rapidly postpartum. They are often reluctant to start immunosuppression during pregnancy or when breastfeeding (even though hydroxychloroquine, prednisolone, azathioprine, ciclosporin and tacrolimus are all considered safe in both situations, albeit with doses that may need to be reviewed and adjusted). Irrespective of breastfeeding, postpartum medication adjustments may be needed, requiring close communication with their rheumatologist and/or GP. Where appropriate, it is important that a) the diagnosis is secured with a renal biopsy, if not already obtained during pregnancy; and b) clear discussions are had at an early stage postpartum about the risks of under-treating active disease [12].

Newly Diagnosed Kidney Disease with a Heritable Component

Women need to be informed not only about how their kidney disease might impact future pregnancies, but also how it might affect their new baby. Many renal diseases have a heritable component. This may be difficult to face for the first time during pregnancy and requires review postpartum to allow a full discussion of the implications for her and her child. For instance, a woman in her mid-20s may well be unaware she has autosomal dominant polycystic kidney disease (ADPKD) – she is likely to have normal function, may have 1+ blood only on urine dipstick and may have no family history. However, she is very likely to develop significant hypertension early on in pregnancy, is at higher risk of preeclampsia, and because of minor urine abnormalities may have a renal ultrasound that confirms the diagnosis. It can be distressing to discover one has a heritable renal disease at any time, but more so when pregnant. These women need to understand what the disease means for them, the risk it poses to their offspring (a one in two chance of inheriting ADPKD) and when it is likely to manifest in them (young adulthood at the earliest). Sometimes the discussions are harder – a woman may present with microscopic hematuria but with a history of kidney disease among the men in her family; it is likely she is a carrier for x-linked Alport syndrome in which affected males often require dialysis/transplantation by their late teens. Such women may well want genetic counseling as well as consideration of screening of their male offspring.

Vesicoureteric reflux (VUR) is commonly diagnosed in pregnancy. Individuals who may have been entirely asymptomatic before conception may develop pregnancy-related recurrent UTIs, modest proteinuria and hypertension. VUR has a strong heritable component and is probably autosomal dominant in a large number of cases (see Chapter 12). Hence, women found to have reflux nephropathy should be advised that their children (newborn or older children) are at risk of developing the same condition, and furthermore, that if diagnosed early, then some complications may be prevented. Clinical pathways for referral and assessment vary – not least because there is no consensus on optimal strategies for the diagnosis and management of VUR [13]. Nonetheless, it is the responsibility of the obstetricians and physicians who make the diagnosis in the mother to ensure that she is signposted to the appropriate services [14].

Conclusion

Pregnancy provides an opportunity to identify women with undiagnosed renal disease, but the opportunity is wasted if they are not appropriately followed up postpartum [15]. The key to safe long-term care is to empower the women. They should be offered information explaining the basics of kidney disease, the importance of making a diagnosis and future monitoring of renal function, blood pressure and urine abnormalities. Above all, they need to be told that they require continued follow-up. In the first instance, virtually all need a postpartum review in hospital to establish stability of renal function and levels of ongoing proteinuria (or not), to ensure appropriate diagnostic tests have been done or are planned and to give some advice about future pregnancy. At the postpartum appointment it is crucial to define who will follow up the patient thereafter. Where disease is mild and stable, this follow-up can be in primary care, but where there are diagnostic dilemmas, significant disease or inherited conditions this should be with a nephrologist.

References

1. Mills KT, Xu Y, Zhang W, Bundy JD, Chen C-S, Kelly TN, Chen J, He, J (2015). A systematic analysis of world-wide population-based data on the global burden of chronic kidney disease in 2010. *Kidney Int.* **88**(5): 950–957.

2. NICE Clinical Guideline 62. Antenatal care. Accessed at www.nice.org.uk/guidance/cg62 on October 8, 2014.

3. Smith MC, Moran P, Ward MK, Davison JM (2008). Assessment of glomerular filtration rate during pregnancy using the MDRD formula. *BJOG* **115**(1): 109–112.

4. Larsson A, Palm M, Hansson L, Axelsson O (2008). Reference values for clinical chemistry tests during normal pregnancy. *BJOG* **115**; 874–881.

5. Klajnbard A, Szecsi PB, Colov NP, Andersen MR, Jørgensen M, Bjørngaard B, Barfoed A, Haahr K, Stender S. (2010). Laboratory reference intervals during pregnancy, delivery and the early postpartum period. *Clin Chem Lab Med* **48**(2): 237–248.

6. Berks D, Steegers EAP, Molas M, Visser W (2009). Resolution of hypertension and proteinuria after preeclampsia. *Obstet Gynecol.* **114**, 1307–1314.

7. NICE Clinical Guideline 182. Chronic kidney disease: Early identification and management of chronic kidney disease in adults in primary and secondary care. Accessed at www.nice.org.uk/guidance/cg182 on October 8, 2014.

8. NICE CG 107. Hypertension in pregnancy: The management of hypertensive disorders during pregnancy. Accessed at www.nice.org.uk/guidance/cg107 on October 8, 2014.

9. Webster P, Webster, LM, Cook T, Horsfield C, Seed, PT, Vaz R, Santos C, Lydon, I, Homsy M, Lightstone L, Bramham K (2016). A multicenter cohort study of histologic findings and long-term outcomes of kidney disease in women who have been pregnant. *CJASN* **12**(3): 408–416.

10. Jones DC, Hayslett JP (1996). Outcome of pregnancy in women with moderate or severe renal insufficiency. *N Engl J Med* **335**(4): 226–232.

11. Landon MB (2007). Diabetic nephropathy and pregnancy.*Clin Obstet Gynaecol.* **50**: 998–1006.

12. Molad Y, Borkowski T, Monselise A, Ben-Haroush A, Sulkes J, Hod M, Feldberg D, Bar J (2005). Maternal and fetal outcome of lupus pregnancy: A prospective study of 29 pregnancies. *Lupus* **14**(2): 145–151.

13. Tekgul S, Riedmiller H, Hoebeke P, Kocvar R, Nijman RJ, Radmayr C, Stein R, Dogan HS (2012). European Association of Urology guidelines on vesicoureteral reflux in children. *Eur Urol.* **62**(3): 534–542.

14. Gargollo PC, Diamond DA (2007). Therapy insight: What nephrologists need to know about primary vesicoureteral reflux. *Nat Clin Pract Nephrol.* **3**(10): 551–563.

15. Thomas MC (2007). Early detection of patients with kidney disease. *Nephrology,* **12**: S37–S40.

Pregnancy and Dialysis

Kainat Shahid, Liam Plant and Michele Hladunewich

Introduction

For women with end-stage renal disease (ESRD) on dialysis, pregnancy remains an uncommon event. Although pregnancy outcomes have improved since the first reported case in 1971 [1], miscarriage, stillbirth, premature delivery and neonatal death remain substantial risks. Strategies such as "enhanced" dialysis regimens to improve fetal outcomes are themselves not without the potential to cause harm. Furthermore, experience in managing these patients is sporadic. Pregnancy in such women, therefore, poses a formidable challenge to renal physicians, obstetricians, neonatologists and the renal multidisciplinary staff. Given the more favorable experience of pregnancy in renal transplant patients, transplantation may be considered as the ideal means to facilitate conception and delivery in patients with ESRD. Unfortunately, a lack of potential living donors, anti-human leukocyte antigen (HLA) sensitization and waiting times for cadaveric donation potentially extending beyond the reproductive window may limit transplantation as a viable reproductive option for many young women. As such, knowledge about the many issues surrounding pregnancy on dialysis is necessary for the practicing nephrologist as well as for the obstetric community.

Incidence of Pregnancy in ESRD

The earliest registry data come from the European Dialysis and Transplant Association published in the 1970s, which comprised data from 67 centers in 19 countries [2]. There were only 16 pregnancies reported among approximately 8,500 women on dialysis aged 15 to 44 years, a pregnancy rate of < 0.002 per woman on dialysis. In 1996, a comprehensive national survey in Belgium from all of its 32 dialysis centers included 1,472 women of childbearing age and reported an incidence of pregnancy beyond the first trimester of 0.3 per 100 patient-years [3].

Similarly low rates were reported in a nationwide Japanese survey, again from 1996, which revealed a conception rate of only 0.44 percent among 38,889 women [4]. Further observational data collated from dialysis centers in the United States from 1992 to 1995 reported a higher pregnancy rate (2.2 percent) among 6,230 women of childbearing age on dialysis [5]. Within the same survey, 1,699 women were on peritoneal dialysis, of which only 1.1 percent conceived.

More recent data suggest conception rates may be improving over time. Higher pregnancy rates of 7.9 percent (9 pregnant patients among 113 dialysis patients of childbearing age) were reported from a survey of dialysis units in Saudi Arabia in 2003 [6]. All women who conceived were on conventional hemodialysis, with no pregnancies reported among women on peritoneal dialysis. A more contemporary survey of nocturnal dialysis patients from Canada, conducted from 2001 to 2006, revealed a higher conception rate of 15.9 percent, with seven pregnancies among 45 women of childbearing age [7]. The trend toward improving conception rates by era is also reflected in the Australia and New Zealand Dialysis and Transplant (ANZDATA) registry [8]. The registry reported a notably progressive increase in pregnancy rates from 0.03 percent (1976–1985) to 0.05 percent (1986–1995) and then 0.6 percent (1996–2008). Again, patients on peritoneal dialysis were found to have a lower rate of conception (0.1 percent). Similarly, a recently published systematic review and meta-regression analysis noted a sizable increase in the number of reported cases of pregnancy in women on hemodialysis (n = 616 between 2000 and 2014) [9] compared with a similar systematic review completed less than a decade earlier (n = 90 between 2000 and 2008) [10].

Overall, published data still indicate low rates of conception in women on dialysis. The etiology of diminished fertility can be multifactorial. Menstrual irregularities are common, with more than half of women on dialysis experiencing amenorrhea. Of those who continue to menstruate, cycles tend to be anovulatory due to lack of a luteal surge in luteinizing hormone [11]. Hyperprolactinemia and a higher incidence of subclinical hypothyroidism may further compound reproductive dysfunction [12]. Estradiol and progesterone levels tend to be low, impeding proliferation of the endometrial bed for implantation [13]. In addition to hormonal dysregulation, sexual dysfunction frequently affects pre-menopausal women with ESRD, with a reported prevalence as high as 84 percent [14]. Medications, nutritional status, anemia, fatigue, altered body image and depression may all contribute to sexual dysfunction in this group.

Recent work has focused on potential methods of improving conception rates in dialysis patients. Increasing erythropoietin use, the use of high-flux dialyzers and, particularly, more intensive hemodialysis may all potentially ameliorate reproductive dysfunction [7]. Recognition of sexual dysfunction and subsequent counseling of patients may further improve pregnancy rates. Published data on the use of assisted reproduction in dialysis patients are sparse and further study is warranted. The cause for lower rates of conception in women on peritoneal dialysis remains unclear. Possibilities include damage to the ovum from hypertonic dextrose solutions, along with mechanical interference of ovum transit due to a fluid-filled peritoneal space [15]. It is contentious whether women on peritoneal dialysis should switch modality when wishing to conceive.

Outcomes of Pregnancy in ESRD

Pregnancy outcomes over time are summarized in Table 10.1. The first reported successful pregnancy in a hemodialysis patient resulted in a relatively uncomplicated pregnancy with delivery at term of a healthy infant weighing 1,950 grams [1]. However, poor fetal outcomes with low live birth rates and high premature delivery rates were consistently noted in subsequent series from the early 1980s to the 1990s. In 1980, the European Dialysis and Transplant Association reported that only 23 percent of 115 pregnancies in dialysis patients ended with live births [2]. During the 1990s, the authors of the Registry of Pregnancy in Dialysis Patients reported an infant survival rate of 42 percent [5]. The Belgian national survey from 1998 indicated that approximately 50 percent of pregnancies in dialyzed patients were

successful [3]. Since 1995, a trend toward increased numbers of successful deliveries has been reported with live birth rates of 80 percent or greater [8, 16–21]. Despite the improved live birth rates, premature deliveries remain common with reported mean gestational ages at delivery of approximately 32 weeks' gestation with birth weights tending to be below 2,200 grams [8, 16–21]. Maternal mortality is fortunately not noted to be higher than in the general population [5].

Recently, the ANZDATA registry has provided valuable insights into pregnancy outcomes in a sizable cohort of young women, as well as the effects of residual renal function on pregnancy outcomes in women on dialysis. In an observational outcomes study of 49 pregnancies derived from 23,700 person-years of follow-up, 79 percent of women who conceived achieved a live birth, although 53.4 percent were premature and 65 percent of a low birth weight [8]. While conception was more likely in younger women and in those on hemodialysis, live birth rates were not related to age or dialysis modality. Another analysis compared pregnancy outcomes based on the use of dialysis prior to or after conception in 73 women between 2001 and 2011 [22]. Women who had conceived before dialysis initiation had significantly higher live birth rates than women already established on dialysis (91 percent versus 63 percent), but ultimately delivered infants with a similar gestational age and birth weight. This difference in live birth rates reflected a higher incidence of early pregnancy loss in women already established on dialysis at the time of conception, with similar outcomes observed once beyond 20 weeks of gestation. The ANZDATA registry reflects other large studies that also demonstrate higher live birth rates in women conceiving prior to initiation of dialysis, most likely due to the presence of higher residual renal function [3, 5, 20].

Retrospective data have also suggested that maintenance of lower pre-dialysis urea levels promotes longer gestation and increases likelihood of successful pregnancy [23]. Nocturnal hemodialysis, providing intensive renal replacement therapy for eight hours during sleep for three to six nights per week augments clearance of "uremic toxins" with improved control of phosphorus, extracellular volume status and blood pressure. A prescription of nocturnal hemodialysis has been demonstrated in the setting of a descriptive cohort study to improve fertility and pregnancy outcomes, delivering neonates with a mean gestational

Table 10.1 Outcomes of Pregnancy in End Stage Renal Disease

Period	Country of Origin	N	Spontaneous Abortion*	Stillbirth*	Neonatal Death*	Live Birth	Weight (g)†**	Gestational Age (wk)†
1980	Europe [2]	16	38%	NR	NR	23%	1900 (800–2500)	32
1992–1995	United States [5]	244 HD, 59 PD	32%	6%	8%	42%	84% < 1500g	33.8
1988–1998	Italy [56]	5	NR	20%	0	80%	1431 ± 738	28.6 ± 4
1986–2007	Japan [23]	28	12%	4%	18%	64%	1414 ± 759	28.3 ± 9
1992–2003	Saudi Arabia [6]	12	25%	0	17%	58%	1700 (1115–2300)	31.5 [27–36]
1995–2001	France [16]	7	NR	0	17%	83%	1495 (660–1920)	31 [24–34]
1995–2004	Singapore [17]	10 HD, 1 PD	18%	0	0	82%	1390 ± 705	31 [26–36]
2000–2002	Turkey [18]	7	14%	0	14%	86%	1400 (420–2640)	32 [26–36]
2000–2004	Germany [19]	5	NR	0	0	100%	1765 ± 554	32.8 ± 3.3
1988–2008	Brazil (20)	52	NR	8%	6%	87%	1554 ± 663	32.7 ± 3.1
1966–2008	Australia/NZ [8]	49	6%	10%	5%	79%	2131 (800–4200)	33.5 [26–41]
2000–2013	Canada [21]	22	5%	5%	5%	86%	2118 ± 857	36 [32–37]

Where NZ is New Zealand, NR is not reported, * percentage when excluding elective abortions, ** reported mean weights of live births only, † Data are presented as mean ± SD (or range), depending on available data in the original report age of 36.2 weeks and birth weight of 2,418 grams [7]. Extending these findings, a recent comparison of Canadian and US cohorts has indicated a dose response between dialysis intensity and pregnancy outcomes, reporting live birth rates of 48 percent in women dialyzed ≤ 20 hours per week compared with 85 percent in women dialyzed ≥ 36 hours per week, with an associated increased gestational age and greater infant birth weight seen in those more intensely dialyzed women [21].

With respect to dialysis modality, historical literature suggests that infant survival rates are similar in women treated with hemodialysis or peritoneal dialysis [5, 24]. Several reports, spanning from the early 1980s to this decade, indicate successful pregnancy while receiving chronic ambulatory peritoneal dialysis [25–30]. However, many of these patients conceived prior to dialysis initiation and tended to have higher residual renal function with creatinine clearances between 5–15 ml/min, which was likely a significant contributing factor toward successful outcomes. Additionally, the comparisons were between peritoneal dialysis and *standard*-intensity hemodialysis. Registry data from the United States have failed to support an advantage with peritoneal dialysis [5, 31], and a later single-center case series actually noted worse outcomes [24]. Further, the aforementioned systematic review and meta-regression analysis noted a significantly higher rate of small-for-gestational-age (SGA) babies among peritoneal versus hemodialysis patients at 67 percent compared to 31 percent, respectively (p = 0.015) [9]. Unique challenges with peritoneal dialysis during pregnancy include the potential difficulties with catheter drainage and migration [30], limitations in fill volumes [26, 29, 32] and risk of catheter-induced traumatic injury in the face of an expanding uterus [33, 34]. Preterm delivery and stillbirth have also been documented secondary to acute peritonitis [27, 35]. Presently, it is reasonable to conclude that there is no evidence to support the use of peritoneal dialysis in pregnancy in preference to hemodialysis, and in our practice we would consider switching a woman who conceived on peritoneal dialysis to an intensive regimen of hemodialysis where possible.

Overall, more recent studies indicating improved outcomes for women who commence dialysis in pregnancy, along with growing evidence to support an intensive dialysis approach, prompt a shift toward a more positive attitude in counseling women

considering motherhood [10]. A coordinated approach combining the efforts of nephrologists, obstetricians, neonatologists, nurse specialists and nutritionists remains central to achieving this previously inaccessible goal.

Potential Pregnancy Complications in Women with ESRD

Women on dialysis are prone to the complications of both pregnancy and ESRD alike with the additional risks of an intensified hemodialysis regimen that is intended to improve pregnancy outcomes, but that may introduce new complications. Reported complications are summarized in Table 10.2.

The major maternal complications are hypertension and preeclampsia. Increased blood pressure has been reported in 30–80 percent of cases [7, 16, 36]. ESRD is associated with increased endothelial dysfunction and preeclampsia has been reported in approximately 20 percent of cases [8, 17, 20], to much higher rates in several other series [6, 18]. However, these may be over- or underestimations as the diagnosis of preeclampsia is challenging in these patients, most of whom are already hypertensive, have proteinuria or are anuric. These complications have been noted to be less frequent in series utilizing intensified dialysis regimens [7, 19, 21].

Anemia with increased erythropoietin and iron requirements is reported almost universally [3, 7, 19, 21]. In addition to the demands of placental and fetal growth, requirements in dialysis patients may be higher due to blood loss in hemodialysis circuits and potential erythropoietin resistance due to inflammatory cytokines. The need for supplementary blood transfusions is frequently reported [19, 20]. Anti-HLA sensitization from transfusions and as result of pregnancy may become a significant issue in dialysis patients who may be awaiting transplantation in the future.

Arguably the most detrimental impact on fetal outcomes remains the increased risk of preterm birth and low birth weight (LBW). Although fetal growth restriction is reported, the principal reason for LBW has been premature birth with a weight appropriate for the duration of gestation. Along with preeclampsia necessitating urgent delivery, polyhydramnios, acute shifts in maternal volume status and shortened cervix can all lead to increased risk of preterm labor.

Table 10.2 Potential Pregnancy Complications in Women with End-Stage Renal Disease

Period	Country of Origin	N	Hypertension	Preeclampsia/ HELLP	Poly-hydramnios	Fetal Growth Restriction	Preterm Delivery*	Conception prior to Dialysis	Dialysis Time (weekly)	Pre-dialysis Urea (mmol/L)
1992–1995	United States [5]	244 HD 59 PD	81%	NR	NR	28%	84%	22%	NR	NR
1988–1998	Italy [56]	5	20%	NR	100%	NR	100%	0	14–27 h	18–36
1986–2007	Japan [23]	28	39%	NR	39%	NR	92%	15%	18.2 ± 3.9 h	18 ± 4.9
1992–2003	Saudi Arabia [6]	12	NR	67%	42%	70%	100%	42%	4–6 times	Target < 18
1995–2001	France [16]	7	50%	NR	83%	33%	100%	0	15–24 h	21
1995–2004	Singapore [17]	10 HD 1 PD	64%	18%	18%	27%	100%	0	3h, 6 times	Target < 20
2000–2002	Turkey [18]	7	NR	43%	28%	14%	100%	43%	20 (16–24) h	Target< 21.5
2000–2004	Germany [19]	5	40%	0	40%	80%	80%	0	28.6 ± 6.3 h	13 ± 5
1988–2008	Brazil [20]	52	70%	19%	40%	NR	85%	54%	18.4 (12–24) h	31 ± 9.8
1966–2008	Australia/NZ [8]	49	NR	19%	5%	NR	53%	51%	NR	NR
2000–2013	Canada [7, 21]	22	18%	5%	5%	14%	53%	18%	43 ± 6 h	9.9

HD: hemodialysis; PD: peritoneal dialysis; HELLP: hemolysis, elevated liver enzymes, low platelets syndrome; NZ: New Zealand; NR: not reported. *Preterm defined by < 37 weeks of gestation

Increased frequency of polyhydramnios has been reported in almost all series, ranging from 18 percent to 60 percent of pregnancies [6, 17, 19, 20, 23, 36]. It is possibly a sequela to the raised maternal urea concentration that drives fetal solute diuresis with a subsequent expansion of the amniotic fluid volume. Additionally, amniotic volume closely reflects maternal volume status in women treated by hemodialysis. While reduced ultrafiltration can lead to polyhydramnios, maternal intravascular depletion may precipitate oligohydramnios. Acute shifts in maternal volume status during dialysis can also result in compromised uteroplacental and fetal perfusion, provoking fetal growth restriction or fetal distress, necessitating an early delivery. The umbilical artery pulsatility index and fetal heart rate both exhibit substantial variation after dialysis treatment [37]. However, when strategies to minimize fluid shifts are deliberately applied, these adverse effects are not observed [38, 39].

Dialysis-induced reductions in serum progesterone may increase the risk of preterm labor, as low progesterone activity is associated with increased uterine contractility and cervical ripening [40]. However, the degree to which progesterone is lowered is subject to patient-specific variability. Furthermore, for pregnant women on hemodialysis, there seems to be little demonstrable association between progesterone levels and uterine contractions [41]. There is an increased rate of cervical shortening reported in women on intensified dialysis, with 3 out of 5

pregnant women in a German cohort [19] and 4 out of 21 pregnancies in a Canadian cohort [21] suffering from cervical insufficiency. The precise contribution to cervical shortening by progesterone lowering from intensive dialysis remains unclear.

Preterm labor can reflect any combination of these factors and seeking to minimize their impact has underscored contemporary strategies developed to support pregnancies in women on dialysis.

Management of the Pregnant Hemodialysis Patient

The ultimate goal of a successful pregnancy is the well-being of both mother and infant. Fetal outcomes are influenced by several aspects of care from preconception to the neonatal period (Figure 10.1). As such, management of the pregnant patient necessitates a comprehensive multidisciplinary approach to optimize all dialysis and obstetric considerations (Table 10.3).

Information Sharing and Counseling

Recognition of the impact of ESRD on reproductive health is an essential prerequisite to providing supportive care to young women with ESRD. All young women on dialysis should be offered systematic information on reproductive health issues supplemented as needed with further counseling. Sharing accurate information with women about

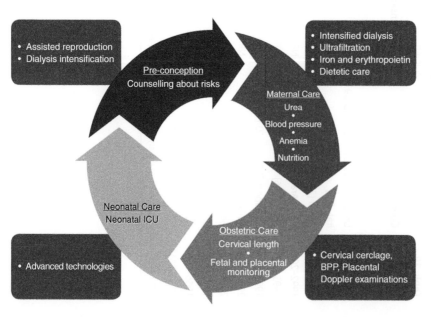

Figure 10.1 Factors influencing fetal outcomes and strategies for their optimization. Reprinted with permission from *Seminars in Nephrology*.

Table 10.3 Recommendations for a Systematic Protocol for the Management of Pregnant Women on Hemodialysis

Activation of multidisciplinary team including nephrologists, dialysis nurses, high-risk obstetricians, neonatologists, pharmacists, social workers and dieticians	
Medication Review	• Stop angiotensin-converting enzyme inhibitors, angiotensin receptor blockers, statins
Intensification of Dialysis Treatment	• > 36 hours/week or as necessary to target near normal physiology in a adequately nourished patient
Hypertension	• Target blood pressure < 140/90 mmHg post dialysis
Volume Status	• Monthly, then weekly volume assessments using blood pressure, edema and fetal ultrasound as a guide
Electrolytes	• Dialysate potassium concentration: 3–3.5 mmol/l
	• Dialysate bicarbonate concentration: 25 mmol/l
	• Dialysate calcium concentration: 1.5–1.75 mmol/l
	• Sodium phosphate (fleet enema) to dialysate as needed
Vitamins, Minerals and Diet	• Double dose of multivitamin
	• Folic acid 5 mg daily
	• Unrestricted diet
	• Daily protein intake 1.5–1.8 g/kg/day
Anemia	• Intravenous and/or oral iron to maintain normal stores
	• Erythropoietin-stimulating agent to target a hemoglobin of 110 g/l
Fetal assessment and follow-up	• Cautious interpretation of all screening tests
	• Ultrasound to measure cervical length and assess for anomalies at 18–20 weeks
	• Placental ultrasound with Doppler assessment at 22 weeks
	• Weekly ultrasound and biophysical profile from 26 weeks until delivery
	• Consultation with neonatologist
Emotional support	• Regular mental health assessments to diagnose difficulty coping during pregnancy or postpartum depression

Adapted from the Toronto Pregnancy and Kidney Disease (PreKid) Clinic Protocol [46]

outcomes should empower informed choices with regards to both contraception and pregnancy. Given the more favorable experience of pregnancy outcomes in the transplant population [42], all suitable patients should be encouraged to explore living donor options and be activated on the waiting list for cadaveric transplantation at the earliest opportunity. Switching to a more intensified hemodialysis regimen to improve chances of conception may also be considered. At the same time, the potential for anti-HLA sensitization if conception occurs while on dialysis also needs to be discussed. Data with respect to the utilization of assisted reproduction services are sparse and require further study.

Early Diagnosis and Rapid Activation of a Multidisciplinary Care Plan

Pregnancy in patients with ESRD is often diagnosed late due to the amenorrhea and anovulatory cycles that are characteristic in this patient population. Furthermore, hormonal diagnosis is also more complex, as reduced renal clearance of human chorionic gonadotropin (hCG) can lead to false-positive serum pregnancy tests in women with ESRD [43]. High iron and erythropoietin requirements may be initial clues to pregnancy. Early diagnosis is essential to expedite review and adjustment of medications (e.g. discontinuation of angiotensin-converting enzyme inhibitors [ACEi], angiotensin receptor blockers [ARBs] and statins), implementation of a systematic intensified dialysis protocol and formulation of a multidisciplinary care plan involving health care providers with expertise in high-risk pregnancy.

Changes in the Dialysis Regimen

Observational studies from the past decade of pregnant women on dialysis have shown improved outcomes with more intensive hemodialysis [7, 19, 21]. This may be mediated by increased urea clearance, improved blood pressure control, decreased fluctuations in volume status, decreased endothelial dysfunction, improved phosphate control and the alleviation of dietary restrictions, resulting in better nutrition.

The most noteworthy benefit of intensive dialysis may be related to improved urea clearance. Increased maternal urea results in fetal solute diuresis, and subsequent polyhydramnios. Historically, a pre-dialysis urea below 17.9 mmol/L (50 mg/dl) was recommended as the target [44]. In support of this was a series from 2009 of 28 pregnant women receiving hemodialysis with 18 surviving infants, in which urea levels were found to be negatively correlated with gestational age [23]. A pre-dialysis urea level of 17.1 mmol/L (48 mg/dl) corresponded to a gestational age of 32 weeks and fetal birth weight of 1,500 grams. In a series of seven pregnant women on nocturnal hemodialysis, dialysis time was increased to 48±5 hours per week with much lower pre-dialysis urea concentrations (mean 9.9 mmol/L) maintained throughout the pregnancy [7]. The mean gestational age was 36.2±3.0 weeks, suggesting that targeting lower pre-dialysis urea levels may improve pregnancy outcomes. A dose-related response between dialysis intensity and pregnancy outcomes has been described [21], with live birth rates of 85 percent achieved in women dialyzed ≥ 36 hours per week, with an associated older gestational age (36 weeks) and birth weight (2,118 grams). Current best evidence supports delivering a greater amount of hemodialysis than the standard accepted with traditional regimens, with a focus on restoring the commonly measured laboratory values closer to normal maternal physiology. At least 36 hours of hemodialysis weekly appears necessary for women with ESRD without residual kidney function, whereas women with residual renal function may not require as many hours of hemodialysis. Potential barriers such as distance from the dialysis center, problems with vascular access, personal tolerance and availability of local resources may limit the delivery of highly intensified dialysis. Still, the escalation of dialysis regimen

intensity should be implemented as soon as conception is confirmed whenever possible.

Intensifying peritoneal dialysis is typically achieved through an increase in dialysate volume and number of exchanges, though there are fewer reports to guide this modality in general [45]. It seems likely that a higher peritoneal dialysis dose is beneficial, with increased frequency of exchanges, but a growing gravid uterus may progressively limit exchange volumes as the pregnancy advances.

Changes in Fluid Balance Management

Attentive management of fluid balance is of particular importance in anuric patients and is intimately integrated within the dialysis regimen. More frequent hemodialysis can improve control of salt and water balance, and thus, blood pressure, protecting both mother and fetus from the dangers of uncontrolled hypertension and potentially obviating the need for medication. A target blood pressure of <140/90 mmHg following dialysis has been recommended [46]. Preventing large shifts in maternal fluid volume is paramount to preventing the attendant hazards of polyhydramnios, oligohydramnios and diminished fetal perfusion. Daily treatment with more limited ultrafiltration volumes offers optimal control in this regard. Appropriate monitoring of amniotic fluid volume and uteroplacental circulation via ultrasound can help inform the optimal dialysis fluid management [38]. Weight gain is an integral component of pregnancy, and thus, target post-dialysis dry weight needs to be adjusted on a continuing basis. An adequately nourished woman can be expected to gain approximately 1–1.5 kg in the first trimester with a subsequent weight gain of about 0.5 kg per week until delivery. Astute ongoing clinical examination, balancing nutritional status, blood pressure and amniotic fluid volume to customize target weight, is essential.

Electrolyte Management

Intensification of dialysis can lead to reductions in phosphate, calcium and potassium levels [7]. Prolonged dialysis often leads to hypophosphatemia and total body phosphate depletion. Cessation of phosphate binders, a phosphate-rich diet and even addition of phosphate to the dialysate bath is often required to maintain normal serum phosphate levels [46]. The potassium bath often requires an increase to 3 mmol/L to avoid hypokalemia [46].

Pregnancy is associated with an increase in intestinal calcium absorption, parathyroid hormone-related protein (PTHrp), and placental conversion of 25-OH vitamin D to 1,25-OH vitamin D, all of which can lead to hypercalcemia. However, with frequent prolonged dialysis, patients are commonly in negative calcium balance. As a result, the dialysate calcium bath often needs to be increased up to 1.75mmol/L so that adequate calcium exists for fetal skeletal development during the third trimester [46].

Serum magnesium concentrations are typically normal or high in dialysis patients, but this may not be the case in intensively dialyzed patients. In the absence of urinary excretion, there is also an inherent danger of iatrogenic hypermagnesemia with standard-dose magnesium infusions used for the prevention and management of eclampsia. Dose reductions in magnesium infusions and close monitoring with serial levels are essential.

Progesterone-induced hyperventilation in pregnancy leads to respiratory alkalosis. A lack of renal compensation in ESRD patients, compounded by emesis during pregnancy, may lead to persistent alkalemia. This may require a reduction in the dialysate bicarbonate bath to 25 mmol/L [46] to maintain a physiological serum bicarbonate during pregnancy (18–21mmol/L).

Frequent assessment of all electrolyte levels is required for close monitoring and adjustments.

Ensuring Good Maternal Nutrition

More frequent dialysis permits alleviation of dietary and fluid restrictions that are otherwise standard with less intense regimens. A trained dietician should provide nutritional supervision. The recommended protein intake of pregnant women in the general population is 1.1g/kg/day. However, ESRD patients already require a higher protein intake of about 1.4g/kg/day to account for protein losses during dialysis. Therefore, an increase in dietary protein intake up to 1.8g/kg/day has been suggested for pregnant dialysis patients [46]. As water-soluble vitamins and minerals can be removed with the more intensive regimens, generous folate supplementation of up to 5mg/day is suggested along with doubling of daily multivitamin supplementation [46].

Intensified Anemia Management

Anemia management also demands escalation in order to maintain a target hemoglobin of 110 g/L.

Requirements for exogenous erythropoietin increase by 50–100 percent due to erythropoietin resistance possibly mediated by cytokine production during pregnancy. Given its large molecular size and lack of erythropoietin receptors on the human placenta [47], it is unlikely to cross the placenta.

The estimated iron requirement in pregnancy is approximately 0.8 mg/day in the first trimester, 4 to 5 mg/day in the second trimester, and >6 mg/day in the third trimester [48]. In addition, there is an estimated 1–3 g yearly loss of iron on hemodialysis. As a result, maintaining adequate iron stores to support optimal erythropoiesis commonly requires parenteral supplementation, usually necessitating a greater than 30–50 percent increase in intravenous iron dosing [46].

Anticoagulation

As frequent circuit clotting and loss of blood can worsen anemia, it is important to maintain good extracorporeal-circuit anticoagulation during dialysis. Pregnancy is a hypercoagulable state and there may be requirements for increased doses of heparin. Heparin is non-teratogenic and does not cross the placenta [49]. However, a recent study demonstrated that heparin can increase serum sFlt-1 levels up to 25-fold during dialysis [50]. What effect this may have with respect to the risk of preeclampsia is unknown.

Fetal and Maternal Obstetric Monitoring

Fetal monitoring comprises careful screening for congenital anomalies and follow-up of fetal growth. The first-trimester screens for Down syndrome and trisomy 18 involve measurement of maternal serum beta human chorionic gonadotropin (β-hCG), maternal serum pregnancy-associated plasma protein-A (PAPP-A) and an ultrasound measurement of nuchal translucency (NT) between 9 and 13 weeks of gestation. Both serum markers can be elevated in dialysis patients; β-hCG is inversely correlated with creatinine clearance [51] and PAPP-A levels can be augmented by the intravenous administration of heparin [52]. As a result, a positive screen becomes difficult to interpret. The maternal serum screen or the quadruple test, performed during 15 to 18 weeks of gestation, consists of total hCG, α-fetoprotein, inhibin A and unconjugated estriol (uE3). Unconjugated estriol levels are low in dialysis patients, thereby also decreasing the reliability of the test [53]. Definitive fetal chromosomal analysis (karyotyping) by chorionic villus sampling (CVS) or amniocentesis, or maternal cell free DNA sequencing may be required to aid the diagnostic process. As α-fetoprotein is not dependent on renal clearance [54], it can still be used to assess the risk for neural tube defects. Most centers perform a second ultrasound at 18–20 weeks to further screen for anomalies.

Monitoring of fetal growth with weekly ultrasounds after 26 weeks of gestation has been recommended to follow biophysical profile (BPP) scores, the amniotic fluid index and biometry (estimated fetal weight) [46]. Decreased amniotic fluid volume and index may indicate over aggressive ultrafiltration, allowing for readjustment of the target weight to higher levels. Conversely, increased amniotic fluid index or polyhydramnios may prompt increased ultrafiltration, or assessment of dialysis efficiency to target lower pre-dialysis urea levels. Assessment of uterine–umbilical artery blood flow and continuous fetal heart rate tracings may be performed before, during and after dialysis sessions, to further guide ultrafiltration [38]. Some authors suggest that such fetal heart rate monitoring should be performed during each dialysis after 25 weeks of gestation [19], but this is not routine or practical in many centers.

A placental ultrasound to assess placental length, thickness and placental cord insertion along with uterine and umbilical artery Doppler studies to quantify pulsatility indices are performed in some centers at approximately 22 weeks of gestation. Abnormal pulsatility indices along with fetal growth restriction, in addition to high blood pressure and hematological alterations that may be suggestive of hemolytic anemia with elevated liver enzymes and low platelets (HELLP) syndrome can point toward the development of preeclampsia [46].

Increased rates of cervical insufficiency have been incidentally noted during ultrasound surveillance in patients on intensified hemodialysis [7, 19, 21]. Shortened cervical length is deemed an important predictor of preterm delivery, and affected women may benefit from cervical cerclage. Vaginal progesterone has been shown to decrease spontaneous preterm birth in women with asymptomatic second-trimester cervical shortening [55]. Whether this benefit may be extrapolated to the pregnant dialysis population is unknown. The joint involvement of expert nephrologists and obstetricians is essential in the interpretation and management of the aforementioned measures of surveillance.

Conclusion

Pregnancy outcomes have improved over the past 30 years, at least in those pregnancies continuing beyond the first trimester, with a shift toward more hope and enthusiasm. However, many unresolved issues persist. Even with fastidious implementation of strategies such as those detailed in this chapter, the risk of preterm birth and morbidity remains significant.

With low conception rates, pregnancy in a hemodialysis patient is a rare challenge for individual renal units. The experiences reported earlier can and should help formulate a local "pregnancy in dialysis protocol" constructed by renal and obstetric units in partnership. It would seem reasonable to base this upon the strategies reported from case series published in the new millennium modified as necessary to match local resources and expertise (Table 10.3).

Undoubtedly, the most important aspect of management is meticulous attention to detail by a skilled multidisciplinary team. Those focusing on the renal replacement therapy need to achieve excellence in the many elements detailed earlier. Obstetricians and midwives will need to perform far more frequent assessments of maternal and fetal well-being, as they will face many challenges. Finally, neonatologists will need to be prepared for the birth of preterm low birth weight infants and ensure provision of neonatal intensive care facilities at the delivery center.

References

1. Confortini P, Galanti G, Ancona G, Giongo A, Bruschi E, Orenzini E. Full term pregnancy and successful delivery in a patient on chronic hemodialysis. *Proc Eur Dial Transplant Assoc.* 1971(8):74–80.

2. Successful pregnancies in women treated by dialysis and kidney transplantation: Report from the Registration Committee of the European Dialysis and Transplant Association. *British journal of obstetrics and gynaecology.* 1980;**87**(10):839–845.

3. Bagon JA, Vernaeve H, De Muylder X, Lafontaine JJ, Martens J, Van Roost G. Pregnancy and dialysis. *American journal of kidney diseases: The official journal of the National Kidney Foundation.* 1998;**31**(5):756–765.

4. Toma H, Tanabe K, Tokumoto T, Kobayashi C, Yagisawa T. Pregnancy in women receiving renal dialysis or transplantation in Japan: A nationwide survey. *Nephrology, dialysis, transplantation: Official publication of the European Dialysis and Transplant Association – European Renal Association.* 1999;**14**(6):1511–1516.

5. Okundaye I, Abrinko P, Hou S. Registry of pregnancy in dialysis patients. *American journal of kidney diseases: The official journal of the National Kidney Foundation.* 1998;31(5):766–773.

6. Malik GH, Al-Harbi A, Al-Mohaya S, Dohaimi H, Kechrid M, Shetaia MS, et al. Pregnancy in patients on dialysis – experience at a referral center. *The Journal of the Association of Physicians of India.* 2005;53:937–941.

7. Barua M, Hladunewich M, Keunen J, Pierratos A, McFarlane P, Sood M, et al. Successful pregnancies on nocturnal home hemodialysis. *Clinical journal of the American Society of Nephrology: CJASN.* 2008;3(2):392–396.

8. Shahir AK, Briggs N, Katsoulis J, Levidiotis V. An observational outcomes study from 1966–2008, examining pregnancy and neonatal outcomes from dialysed women using data from the ANZDATA registry. *Nephrology (Carlton, Vic).* 2013;18(4):276–284.

9. Piccoli GB, Minelli F, Versino E, Cabiddu G, Attini R, Vigotti FN, et al. Pregnancy in dialysis patients in the new millennium: A systematic review and meta-regression analysis correlating dialysis schedules and pregnancy outcomes. *Nephrology, dialysis, transplantation: Official publication of the European Dialysis and Transplant Association – European Renal Association.* 2015.

10. Piccoli GB, Conijn A, Consiglio V, Vasario E, Attini R, Deagostini MC, et al. Pregnancy in dialysis patients: Is the evidence strong enough to lead us to change our counseling policy? *Clinical journal of the American Society of Nephrology: CJASN.* 2010;5(1):62–71.

11. Lim VS, Henriquez C, Sievertsen G, Frohman LA. Ovarian function in chronic renal failure: Evidence suggesting hypothalamic anovulation. *Annals of internal medicine.* 1980;93(1):21–27.

12. Gomez F, de la Cueva R, Wauters JP, Lemarchand-Beraud T. Endocrine abnormalities in patients undergoing long-term hemodialysis: The role of prolactin. *The American journal of medicine.* 1980;68(4):522–530.

13. Mantouvalos H, Metallinos C, Makrygiannakis A, Gouskos A. Sex hormones in women on hemodialysis. *International journal of gynaecology and obstetrics: The official organ of the International Federation of Gynaecology and Obstetrics.* 1984;22(5):367–370.

14. Strippoli GF, Collaborative D, Sexual Dysfunction in Hemodialysis Working G, Vecchio M, Palmer S, De Berardis G, et al. Sexual dysfunction in women with ESRD requiring hemodialysis. *Clinical journal of the American Society of Nephrology: CJASN.* 2012;7(6):974–981.

15. Hou S. Conception and pregnancy in peritoneal dialysis patients. *Peritoneal dialysis international: Journal of the International Society for Peritoneal Dialysis.* 2001;21 Suppl. 3:S290–4.

16. Moranne O, Samouelian V, Lapeyre F, Pagniez D, Subtil D, Dequiedt P, et al. [Pregnancy and hemodialysis]. *Nephrologie.* 2004;25(7):287–292.

17. Tan LK, Kanagalingam D, Tan HK, Choong HL. Obstetric outcomes in women with end-stage renal failure requiring renal dialysis. *International journal of gynaecology and obstetrics: The official organ of the International Federation of Gynaecology and Obstetrics.* 2006;94(1):17–22.

18. Eroglu D, Lembet A, Ozdemir FN, Ergin T, Kazanci F, Kuscu E, et al. Pregnancy during hemodialysis: Perinatal outcome in our cases. *Transplantation proceedings.* 2004;36(1):53–55.

19. Haase M, Morgera S, Bamberg C, Halle H, Martini S, Hocher B, et al. A systematic approach to managing pregnant dialysis patients – the importance of an intensified haemodiafiltration protocol. *Nephrology, dialysis, transplantation: Official publication of the European Dialysis and Transplant Association – European Renal Association.* 2005;20(11):2537–2542.

20. Luders C, Castro MC, Titan SM, De Castro I, Elias RM, Abensur H, et al. Obstetric outcome in pregnant women on long-term dialysis: A case series. *American journal of kidney diseases: The official journal of the National Kidney Foundation.* 2010;56(1):77–85.

21. Hladunewich MA, Hou S, Odutayo A, Cornelis T, Pierratos A, Goldstein M, et al. Intensive hemodialysis associates with improved pregnancy outcomes: A Canadian and United States cohort comparison. *Journal of the American Society of Nephrology: JASN.* 2014;25(5):1103–1109.

22. Jesudason S, Grace BS, McDonald SP. Pregnancy outcomes according to dialysis commencing before or after conception in women with ESRD. *Clinical journal of the American Society of Nephrology: CJASN.* 2014;9(1):143–149.

23. Asamiya Y, Otsubo S, Matsuda Y, Kimata N, Kikuchi K, Miwa N, et al. The importance of low blood urea nitrogen levels in pregnant patients undergoing hemodialysis to optimize birth weight and gestational age. *Kidney international.* 2009;75(11):1217–1222.

24. Chou CY, Ting IW, Lin TH, Lee CN. Pregnancy in patients on chronic dialysis: A single center experience and combined analysis of reported results. *European journal of obstetrics, gynecology, and reproductive biology.* 2008;136(2):165–170.

25. Kioko EM, Shaw KM, Clarke AD, Warren DJ. Successful pregnancy in a diabetic patient treated with continuous ambulatory peritoneal dialysis. *Diabetes care.* 1983;6(3):298–300.

26. Bennett-Jones DN, Aber GM, Baker K. Successful pregnancy in a patient treated with continuous ambulatory peritoneal dialysis. *Nephrology, dialysis, transplantation: Official publication of the European Dialysis and Transplant Association – European Renal Association.* 1989;4(6):583–585.

27. Jakobi P, Ohel G, Szylman P, Levit A, Lewin M, Paldi E. Continuous ambulatory peritoneal dialysis as the primary approach in the management of severe renal insufficiency in pregnancy. *Obstetrics and gynecology.* 1992;79(5 [Pt 2]):808–810.

28. Gomez Vazquez JA, Martinez Calva IE, Mendiola Fernandez R, Escalera Leon V, Cardona M, Noyola H. Pregnancy in end-stage renal disease patients and treatment with peritoneal dialysis: Report of two cases. *Peritoneal dialysis international: Journal of the International Society for Peritoneal Dialysis.* 2007;27 (3):353–358.

29. Altay M, Akay H, Parpucu H, Duranay M, Oguz Y. A rare case: Full-term delivery in a lupus patient on CAPD. *Peritoneal dialysis international: Journal of the International Society for Peritoneal Dialysis.* 2007;27 (6):711–712.

30. Jefferys A, Wyburn K, Chow J, Cleland B, Hennessy A. Peritoneal dialysis in pregnancy: A case series. *Nephrology (Carlton, Vic).* 2008;13(5):380–383.

31. Okundaye I, Hou S. Management of pregnancy in women undergoing continuous ambulatory peritoneal dialysis. *Advances in peritoneal dialysis: Conference on Peritoneal Dialysis.* 1996;12:151–155.

32. Smith WT, Darbari S, Kwan M, C OR-G, Devita MV. Pregnancy in peritoneal dialysis: A case report and review of adequacy and outcomes. *International urology and nephrology.* 2005;37(1):145–151.

33. Chou CY, Ting IW, Hsieh FJ, Lee CN. Haemoperitoneum in a pregnant woman with peritoneal dialysis. *Nephrology, dialysis, transplantation: Official publication of the European Dialysis and Transplant Association – European Renal Association.* 2006;21(5):1454–1455.

34. Lew SQ. Persistent hemoperitoneum in a pregnant patient receiving peritoneal dialysis. *Peritoneal dialysis international: Journal of the International Society for Peritoneal Dialysis.* 2006;26 (1):108–110.

35. Gadallah MF, Ahmad B, Karubian F, Campese VM. Pregnancy in patients on chronic ambulatory peritoneal dialysis. *American journal of kidney diseases: The official journal of the National Kidney Foundation.* 1992;20(4):407–410.

36. Chao AS, Huang JY, Lien R, Kung FT, Chen PJ, Hsieh PC. Pregnancy in women who undergo long-term hemodialysis. *American journal of obstetrics and gynecology.* 2002;187(1):152–156.

37. Oosterhof H, Navis GJ, Go JG, Dassel AC, de Jong PE, Aarnoudse JG. Pregnancy in a patient on chronic haemodialysis: Fetal monitoring by Doppler velocimetry of the umbilical artery. *British journal of obstetrics and gynaecology.* 1993;100(12):1140–1141.

38. Malone FD, Craigo SD, Giatras I, Carlson J, Athanassiou A, D'Alton ME. Suggested ultrasound parameters for the assessment of fetal well-being during chronic hemodialysis. *Ultrasound in obstetrics & gynecology: The official journal of the International Society of Ultrasound in Obstetrics and Gynecology.* 1998;11(6):450–452.

39. Bamberg C, Diekmann F, Haase M, Budde K, Hocher B, Halle H, et al. Pregnancy on intensified hemodialysis: Fetal surveillance and perinatal outcome. *Fetal diagnosis and therapy.* 2007;22 (4):289–293.

40. Romero R, Espinoza J, Kusanovic JP, Gotsch F, Hassan S, Erez O, et al. The preterm parturition syndrome. *BJOG: An international journal of obstetrics and gynaecology.* 2006;113 Suppl. 3:17–42.

41. Brost BC, Newman RB, Hendricks SK, Droste S, Mathur RS. Effect of hemodialysis on serum progesterone level in pregnant women. *American journal of kidney diseases: The official journal of the National Kidney Foundation.* 1999;33(5):917–919.

42. Piccoli GB, Cabiddu G, Daidone G, Guzzo G, Maxia S, Ciniglio I, et al. The children of dialysis: Live-born babies from on-dialysis mothers in Italy – an epidemiological perspective comparing dialysis, kidney transplantation and the overall population. *Nephrology, dialysis, transplantation: Official publication of the European Dialysis and Transplant Association – European Renal Association.* 2014;29 (8):1578–1586.

43. Fahy BG, Gouzd VA, Atallah JN. Pregnancy tests with end-stage renal disease. *Journal of clinical anesthesia.* 2008;20(8):609–613.

44. Holley JL, Reddy SS. Pregnancy in dialysis patients: A review of outcomes, complications, and management. *Seminars in dialysis.* 2003;16 (5):384–388.

45. Batarse R, Steiger RM, Guest S. Peritoneal dialysis prescription during the third trimester of pregnancy. *Peritoneal dialysis international: Journal of the International Society for Peritoneal Dialysis.* 2014.

46. Hladunewich M, Hercz AE, Keunen J, Chan C, Pierratos A. Pregnancy in end stage renal disease. *Seminars in dialysis.* 2011;24(6):634–639.

47. Malek A, Sager R, Eckardt KU, Bauer C, Schneider H. Lack of transport of erythropoietin across the human placenta as studied by an in vitro perfusion system. *Pflugers Archiv: European journal of physiology.* 1994;427(1–2):157–161.

48. Bothwell TH. Iron requirements in pregnancy and strategies to meet them. *The American journal of clinical nutrition*. 2000;**72**(1 Suppl.):257S–64S.

49. Bates SM, Greer IA, Hirsh J, Ginsberg JS. Use of antithrombotic agents during pregnancy: The Seventh ACCP Conference on Antithrombotic and Thrombolytic Therapy. *Chest*. 2004;**126**(3 Suppl.): 627S–44S.

50. Lavainne F, Meffray E, Pepper RJ, Neel M, Delcroix C, Salama AD, et al. Heparin use during dialysis sessions induces an increase in the antiangiogenic factor soluble Flt1. *Nephrology, dialysis, transplantation: Official publication of the European Dialysis and Transplant Association – European Renal Association*. 2014;**29** (6):1225–1231.

51. Shenhav S, Gemer O, Sherman DJ, Peled R, Segal S. Midtrimester triple-test levels in women with chronic hypertension and altered renal function. *Prenatal diagnosis*. 2003;**23**(2):166–167.

52. Wittfooth S, Tertti R, Lepantalo M, Porela P, Qin QP, Tynjala J, et al. Studies on the effects of heparin products on pregnancy-associated plasma protein A. *Clinica chimica acta: International journal of clinical chemistry*. 2011;**412**(3–4):376–381.

53. Shulman LP, Briggs R, Phillips OP, Friedman SA, Sibai B. Renal hemodialysis and maternal serum triple analyte screening. *Fetal diagnosis and therapy*. 1998;**13** (1):26–28.

54. Tzitzikos G, Saridi M, Filippopoulou T, Makri A, Goulioti A, Stavropoulos T, et al. Measurement of tumor markers in chronic hemodialysis patients. *Saudi journal of kidney diseases and transplantation: An official publication of the Saudi Center for Organ Transplantation, Saudi Arabia*. 2010;**21**(1):50–53.

55. Khandelwal M. Vaginal progesterone in risk reduction of preterm birth in women with short cervix in the midtrimester of pregnancy. *International journal of women's health*. 2012;**4**:481–490.

56. Luciani G, Bossola M, Tazza L, Panocchia N, Liberatori M, De Carolis S, et al. Pregnancy during chronic hemodialysis: A single dialysis-unit experience with five cases. *Renal failure*. 2002;**24**(6):853–862.

Pregnancy and the Renal Transplant Recipient

Nadia Sarween, Martin Drage and Sue Carr

Introduction

The first successful birth in a renal transplant patient was in 1958, although it was not reported until 1963 [1]. Now the literature contains more than 14,000 reported pregnancies worldwide [2] and approximately 2 percent of women of childbearing age with a renal transplant will become pregnant [3].

Timing of Pregnancy

Fertility and the ability to conceive rapidly improve within a few months of successful renal transplantation [2, 4, 5]. In order to avoid pregnancy early post transplant, it is important that appropriate contraceptive advice is given to women before transplantation [2, 6–10].

Published guidelines [4, 11, 12] advise women to defer pregnancy for 12–24 months following a renal transplant (Box 11.1). Studies have reported favorable pregnancy outcomes 12 months post transplant [13] and the American Society of Transplantation guidelines state that in women with a stable renal transplant, who are at low risk of complications, pregnancy may be considered at 12 months (Box 11.2) [4]. The optimal timing of pregnancy is probably between 12 months and 5 years post transplant. However, some women who do not fulfill the recommendations regarding preferred timing of pregnancy will accidentally conceive or decide to conceive and then the situation has to be assessed on an individual basis. The safety of common drugs used in renal disease, including transplant recipients, are discussed in Chapter 7.

Effects of Pregnancy on the Renal Transplant Recipient

In normal pregnancy, the glomerular filtration rate (GFR) increases by approximately 50 percent owing to increased renal plasma flow (45 percent by nine weeks and 70 percent in mid-pregnancy) (see Chapter 1). This results in a fall in serum creatinine (SCr) by 45–70 μmol/l, which persists throughout normal pregnancy. In renal transplant patients, a similar increase in GFR has been reported during pregnancy, the magnitude of which is dependent upon prepregnancy renal function [14–16]. Fischer et al. reported the increase in GFR in pregnancy to be similar in both azathioprine- and ciclosporine-treated patients, although the prepregnancy SCr was lower in azathioprine-treated women [13].

Renal Function during and after Pregnancy

The UK Transplant Pregnancy Registry (UKTPR), US National Transplant Pregnancy Registry (NTPR), Australian and New Zealand registry (ANZDATA) and numerous single-center studies have investigated the effect of pregnancy on renal allograft function (Table 11.1) [13, 17–36].

In general, most [13, 18, 21, 23, 27, 35, 37–39] but not all [25, 28, 29, 40] studies report no significant deleterious effect of pregnancy on graft function. This is supported by a review published in 2012 summarizing international transplant registry and single-center data [12].

Bramham et al. used the UK Obstetric Surveillance System (UKOSS) to identify and follow up the outcome of 105 pregnancies in 101 women with renal transplants over a three-year period (2007–2009). The median SCr fell from 118 μmol/l prepregnancy to 104 μmol/l during the first and second trimesters and subsequently increased to 123 μmol/l in the third trimester. However, they reported that SCr did not fall in the second trimester in 49 percent of women and 38 percent of women had an increase in SCr of at least 20 percent during the pregnancy [38]. Stoumpos et al. recently reported outcomes in kidney transplant pregnancies over a 40-year period at a single center in Scotland (United Kingdom); a 27.5 percent rate of pregnancy-associated transplant dysfunction was observed [35].

BOX 11.1 Criteria for considering pregnancy in renal transplant recipients; MMF = mycophenolate mofetil; reproduced with permission from European Best Practice Guidelines Expert Group on Renal Transplantation [11]

1. Good general health for about two years after transplantation.
2. Good stable allograft function [serum creatinine < 177 µmol/l (2 mg/dl), preferably < 133 µmol/l (< 1.5 mg/dl)].
3. No recent episodes of acute rejection and no evidence of ongoing rejection.
4. Normal blood pressure or minimal antihypertensive regimen (only one drug).
5. Absence of or minimal proteinuria (< 0.50 g/day).
6. Normal allograft ultrasound (absence of pelvicalyceal distension).
7. Recommended immunosuppression:

   - prednisone < 15 mg/day
   - azathioprine ≤ 2 mg/day
   - ciclosporine or tacrolimus at therapeutic levels
   - MMF and sirolimus are contraindicated
   - MMF and sirolimus should be stopped six weeks before conception is attempted.

BOX 11.2 Criteria on which to determine the timing of pregnancy following renal transplant; American Society of Transplantation guidelines; reproduced with permission from McKay et al. [4]

Basis on which to determine timing of pregnancy:

- no rejection in the past year
- adequate and stable graft function (e.g. creatinine < 1.5 mg/dl but true GFR needs to be defined in prospective studies) or no or minimal proteinuria (level needs to be defined)
- no acute infections that might impact fetus
- maintenance immunosuppression at stable dosing

Special circumstances that impact recommendations:

- rejection within the first year (consider further graft assessment – biopsy and GFR)
- maternal age
- comorbid factors that may impact pregnancy and graft function
- established medical noncompliance

Pregnancies outside the guidelines need to be evaluated on a case-by-case basis. In general these considerations could be met at one year post-transplant based on individual circumstances.

Fewer studies have reported long-term renal transplant outcomes following pregnancy. Rahamimov et al. followed 39 women who became pregnant with a functioning allograft for 15 years and reported the long-term graft outcomes compared to three matched control patients. At 15 years, graft and patient survival were similar in both groups (72 percent and 85 percent in pregnant women versus 69 percent and 79 percent in the control group, respectively [28]). Stoumpos et al. also reported similar long-term patient and graft survival in kidney transplant recipients compared to a matched transplant control group [35].

Using data from the ANZDATA, Levidiotis et al. analyzed 40-year pregnancy-related outcomes of 381 women with renal allografts. One hundred twenty of these women were matched with 120 nulliparous women for various factors, including transplant date and prepregnancy renal function. There was no difference in 20-year graft or patient survival between the two groups [31].

Fischer et al. [13] also reported positive outcomes following 81 renal transplant pregnancies. There was no significant deterioration in renal function (mean Scr 115 µmol/l at conception and 119 µmol/l

Table 11.1 Studies on the effect of pregnancy on graft and patient survival

Study	Country	Time	Patients (pregnancies)	Patient survival	Graft survival	Hypertension (preeclampsia)
Rahamimov et al. [27]	Israel	1983–1998	39 (69)	84.8 percent (15y)	87 percent (2y)	44 percent (15 percent)
Thompson et al. [29]	United Kingdom	1976–2001	24 (48)		96.7 percent (3y)	77 percent (29 percent)
Miniero et al. [24]	Italy	1987–2002	96 (52 in kidney transplant)			16 percent onset 58.2 percent term
Yongwon et al. [48]	South Korea	Up to 2000	36 (47)			28 percent
Fischer et al. [13]	Germany		81 (81)	93.4 percent (10y)	62.5 percent (10y)	
Crowe et al. [18]	United Kingdom		29 (33)		0 percent (patients with creatinine > 200 µmol/l within two years)	
Salmela et al. [40]	Finland	1971–1991	22 (29)		69 percent (10y)	
Gutiérrez et al. [21]	Spain	1976–2004	35 (43)		87.5 percent (53 months)	64 percent (37.5 percent)
Keitel et al. [23]	Brazil	1977–2001	41 (44)			66 percent (20.4 percent)
Pour-Reza-Gholi et al. [26]	Iran	1984–2004	60 (74) (17.5 percent < one year post transplant)		No difference in 1-, 3-, 5- and 10-year graft survival pregnant patients versus controls	
Galdo et al. [20]	Chile	1982–2002	30 (37)		13.5 percent acute rejection	(19 percent)
Hooi et al. [22]	Malaysia	1984–2001	72 (46)	94 percent (10 y)	83 percent (10 y)	38 percent (15 percent)
Sibanda et al. [28]	United Kingdom	1994–2001	176 (193)	No different to controls (2y)		

Study	Country	Period	Number (controls)	Graft survival	Outcome	
Bramham et al. [38]	United Kingdom	2007–2009	101 (105)		94 percent (2y) no different to controls	(24 percent)
First et al. [39]	United States	1967–1990	18		2 percent acute rejection	
Levidiotis et al. [31]	Australia/NZ	1966–2005	381 (577) 120 were matched with controls		77.8 percent at 11–12 years	(27 percent)
Blume et al. [71]	Germany	1988–2010	34 (53)	92 percent (10y) 75 percent (20y)	No difference in 20-year graft survival in matched patients	(26.4 percent)
Rose et al. [33]	United States	1990–2010	729 (729)		Five-year all cause graft loss 36.6 percent	
Stoumpos et al. [35]	United Kingdom (Scotland)	1973–2013	89 (138)	95.5 percent (5 y)	At 10 years 54.2 percent (all cause) and 59.8 percent (death censored)	(14 percent)
				88.1 percent (10y)	No difference compared to matched controls	
				88.1 percent (20y) 27.5 percent pregnancy-associated graft dysfunction	No difference compared to matched controls	

postpartum) and no difference in graft survival at 10 years in female transplant recipients who became pregnant, or between women treated with azathioprine versus ciclosporine during pregnancy. Similarly, Crowe et al. [18] reported stable renal function during pregnancy and up to one year postpartum in 33 pregnancies. Keitel et al. [23], in a study from Brazil, reported no significant rise in Scr following pregnancy and no difference in long-term graft survival following pregnancy in 44 transplant recipients.

Piccoli et al., in an Italian multicenter study, have compared maternal and obstetric outcome in pregnant kidney transplant recipients to pregnancies in non-transplant chronic kidney disease (CKD) women [41]. Outcomes were split according to CKD-EPI stage. There was a higher incidence of CKD stage shift at delivery in the transplant CKD stage 1 group (31.6 percent) versus the CKD stage 1 cohort (6.7 percent). This difference was not observed in the more advanced stages of CKD.

However, some studies have reported less favorable outcomes. Rose et al. has recently, using Medicare data, reported rates of allograft failure from any cause including death at one, three and five years after pregnancy as 9.6 percent, 25.9 percent and 36.6 percent, respectively [33]. Of note this study was limited to women becoming pregnant within three years post transplantation and limited to first kidney transplant.

The UKTPR reported an increased SCr postpartum when the SCr was greater than 150 μmol/l before pregnancy [28]. Thompson et al. [29] performed a retrospective case note review and compared outcomes with registry data. It was evident that 20 percent of women experienced a decline in renal function that persisted up to six months postpartum. This effect was most marked in women with prepregnancy SCr level greater than 155 μmol/l. A lower eGFR, higher urine PCR and cadaveric versus live donation were reported by Stoumpos et al. to be associated with an increased risk of ≥20 percent loss of eGFR between prepregnancy and one year post delivery. [35].

Galdo et al. [20], in a single-center report of 37 renal transplant pregnancies in Chile, reported a significant decline in renal function from mean SCr 105 μmol/l at baseline to 127 μmol/l at delivery and 122 μmol/l at one year postpartum. In Brazil, Oliveira et al. [25] also found that 44 percent of women had a decline in renal function during pregnancy or postpartum.

A study from Iran reported outcomes for 74 pregnancies in recipients of living donor kidneys. Sixty-nine percent had no decline in renal function. Nine had significant deterioration in renal transplant function; however, 17.5 percent of pregnancies in this study were within 12 months of renal transplantation [26].

Rose et al. reported that pregnancy in the first year post transplantation was associated with an increased risk of all-cause allograft failure and death-censored graft loss [33]. Furthermore, pregnancy in the second year was also associated with an increased incidence of death-censored graft loss. Pregnancy in the third year was not associated with an increase in either outcome. This study suggests that the second year post transplant is also associated with an increased risk of allograft failure.

These studies indicate a considerable variation in renal transplant outcomes in different centers around the world. As a general rule, renal transplant patients with significantly impaired prepregnancy renal function *are* more likely to suffer a pregnancy-related decline in renal function. In a previous analysis of NTPR data, Armenti et al. [42] reported that all women with prepregnancy Scr above 177 μmol/l needed dialysis two years postpartum. Stratta et al. [36] concluded that renal prognosis following pregnancy was determined by prepregnancy graft and time post transplant. In summary, as of 2017, it is generally accepted that there is no need to alter optimistic counseling practices in women with good graft function.

Gestational Diabetes

Gestational diabetes (GDM) has been reported to be more prevalent in kidney transplant recipients in some [43–45] but not all studies [32]. A recent meta-analysis analyzed the outcome of 4,706 pregnancies in 3,570 kidney transplant recipients and the rate of GDM was 8 percent, which is double that found in the general US population. This may in part be explained by the use of prednisolone and tacrolimus in this group of patients.

Effects of Multiparity and Multiple Pregnancies

The European Dialysis and Transplant Association (EDTA) registry reported that 14 percent of 820 women had a second pregnancy following a successful first pregnancy between 1967 and 1990. Repeated pregnancy did not seem to adversely affect graft function provided that graft function was good at the onset of pregnancy [46].

The NTPR reported the outcome of multiple pregnancies (10 sets of twins, four sets of triplets) in 13 women from a cohort of 458 renal transplant recipients [43]. Five of the multiple pregnancies were conceived using assisted conception techniques. The pregnancies were complicated by hypertension in 77 percent of cases, preeclampsia in 29 percent and infection in 25 percent. Mean SCr at beginning or prepregnancy was on average 133 μmol/l with a rise to a mean of 150 μmol/l postpartum. In this group the mean gestational age was 33 weeks and birth weights were low at 1736 g. Seven of the 13 women were followed up, two of whom experienced reduced graft function and one of whom returned to dialysis.

Differential Diagnosis of Deteriorating Renal Function in Renal Transplant Patients

Renal transplant dysfunction may develop for many reasons during a pregnancy, and it is important to establish the underlying cause, which may be multifactorial. Table 11.2 lists the types of transplant dysfunction and their possible causes. Investigation of acute graft dysfunction in pregnancy may require the following investigations.

1. Biochemistry: urea and electrolytes, liver function tests and glucose.
   Lactate dehydrogenase (LDH) may be raised in a woman with hemolysis and may aid diagnosis of hemolytic anemia, elevated liver enzymes and low platelet count (HELLP) syndrome.
2. Full blood count, platelet count and a blood film to exclude schistocytes and microangiopathic hemolytic anemia.
3. Quantification of urinary protein excretion: 24-hour urine protein collection or protein/albumin creatinine ratio (PCR/ACR).
4. Ciclosporine or tacrolimus levels.
5. Urine culture to exclude infection.
6. Renal tract and allograft ultrasound scan: noting that urinary tract dilatation is a feature of normal pregnancy.
7. Renal transplant biopsy may be considered when acute rejection or recurrent or *de novo* glomerular disease is suspected. This should be performed after pre- and post-renal causes have been excluded and when clotting and platelet counts are normal (many patients will be receiving aspirin, which should be discontinued). An immunology screen (including antinuclear autoantibodies,

Table 11.2 Differential diagnosis of renal transplant dysfunction in pregnancy

Type of renal transplant dysfunction	Possible causes to consider
Pre-renal	Hypovolemia and/or hypotension due to vomiting, hemorrhage (postpartum or antepartum) or sepsis (often due to acute pyelonephritis)
	Vasoconstriction – especially associated with preeclampsia (may be exacerbated by ciclosporine)
Intrarenal transplant	Acute tubular necrosis due to prolonged pre-renal factors
	Microangiopathy – in preeclamptic syndromes, severe hypertension (or rarely *de novo* hemolytic uremic syndrome)
	Acute interstitial nephritis – diuretics, antibiotics
	Acute rejection
	Calcineurin inhibitor nephrotoxicity
	Viral infections – polyoma virus, cytomegalovirus infection
	Recurrent glomerular disease or *de novo* glomerulonephritis
Post-renal	Hydronephrosis of transplant kidney due to calculi, polyhydramniotic uterus or, rarely, exaggerated physiological dilatation of transplant kidney

dsDNA antibodies, complement levels C3 C4, antineutrophil cytoplasmic antibodies [ANCA] lupus anticoagulant and anticardiolipin antibodies) should be considered in suspected glomerular disease.

Risk of Acute Rejection

The immunological changes that occur in pregnancy may protect against acute rejection [2, 37]. Overall, the reported incidence of acute rejection during pregnancy is low and the consensus from the literature is that acute rejection rates in pregnancy are no higher than in nonpregnant patients. The incidence of acute rejection in published cohort studies range from 2 percent to 14.5 percent [27, 29, 34, 35, 37].

The American Society of Transplantation (AST) and the European Best Practice Guidelines (EBPG) Expert Group on Renal Transplantation guidelines recommend deferring pregnancy for 12–24 months to reduce the risk of acute rejection and other problems frequently associated with the early months following renal transplantation [4, 11].

Fluctuation in calcineurin inhibitor (CNI) levels during pregnancy may be an additional predisposing factor for acute rejection, as discussed in Chapter 7. Drug levels may fall and Fischer et al. [13] reported a 33 percent increase in dose requirement after 20 weeks of gestation. However, the authors found a sharp increase in levels postpartum and doses had to be reduced to avoid toxicity. Three out of six patients with biopsy-proven acute rejection during pregnancy in Stoumpos's study had sub-therapeutic tacrolimus levels prior to the rejection episodes [35]. Careful attention should thus be given to monitoring CNI levels during pregnancy and the puerperium.

Reviews of the treatment of acute rejection in pregnancy report treatment with corticosteroids is safe. However, there are limited data regarding the use of monoclonal antibodies, immobilized OKT3, antithymocyte globulin (ATG) or basiliximab or daclizumab. The AST guidelines support use of intravenous gammaglobulin, but ATG and rituximab should be avoided in pregnancy [2, 4, 11].

Hypertension

A systematic review and meta-analysis of 4,706 pregnancies in 3,570 renal transplant recipients from 2000 to 2010 reported 54.2 percent cases of hypertension and 27 percent cases of preeclampsia. The NTPR reported that 47–73 percent of renal transplant patients were hypertensive during pregnancy and other reports have endorsed this [2, 47].

The UKTPR reported 69 percent of renal transplant recipients were treated for hypertension pre-pregnancy and a further 8 percent were commenced on treatment during pregnancy [28]. Yongwon et al. [48] reported a lower incidence of hypertension (28 percent) in pregnant transplant patients, and an Italian study [24] reported hypertension in only 16 percent of pregnant transplant patients at booking, increasing to 58.2 percent at term. Bramham et al. reported 16 percent of women who were not previously taking antihypertensive medication were commenced on treatment during their pregnancy [38]. Several studies have reported the incidence of hypertension to be higher in ciclosporine-treated mothers (51.7 percent) [13, 47].

Registry reports and recent studies have indicated that the incidence of preeclampsia is between 15 percent and 58 percent in this group (Table 11.1). However, the diagnosis of preeclampsia can be difficult in renal transplant patients as blood pressure often rises in the second trimester and women with renal transplant often have preexisting proteinuria. Morken et al. has recently reported an increased risk of preeclampsia in pregnancies fathered by male patients following solid organ transplantation [49].

In high-risk populations aspirin has been shown to reduce the risk of preeclampsia [50]. In the UKOSS study only 30 percent of the pregnant women with renal transplants were on aspirin and no difference was found in rates of preeclampsia compared to those not on anti-platelet therapy [38].

Hypertension is an important determinant of pregnancy outcome in the renal transplant patient. Studies have reported an association with preterm delivery and the UKTPR found hypertension to be associated with poorer long-term graft survival in women with SCr above 150 µmol/l [2, 28].

Proteinuria

A pregnant renal transplant patient may have underlying chronic allograft nephropathy or recurrent glomerular disease associated with proteinuria in early pregnancy. Discontinuation of angiotensin-converting enzyme (ACE) inhibitor therapy before or at conception may also lead to a rise in baseline proteinuria. In general, renal transplant patients experience an increase in preexisting proteinuria during pregnancy, especially in the third trimester [15, 18, 29], which returns to baseline at three to six months. Forty percent of women with renal transplants developed 2–3 g proteinuria/day in the third trimester, even in the absence of superimposed preeclampsia [51]. Bramham's UK study reported that 13 percent of women had proteinuria at the start of pregnancy and 30 percent subsequently developed proteinuria, although none of these women were diagnosed with preeclampsia [38]. Thompson et al. [29] found an increase in proteinuria from 0.4 g/day prepregnancy to 1.37 g/day in the third trimester, which returned to baseline levels three to six months postpartum. Similarly, Crowe et al. [18] reported a rise in proteinuria from 0.45 g/day to 1.11 g/day at delivery, which returned to baseline at three months.

Obstetric Outcomes Following Pregnancy in Renal Transplant Recipients

While the NTPR and UKTPR have reported live birth rates of 75–80 percent in the renal transplant population, Gill et al. reported a much lower rate of 55.4 percent. He commented that the discrepancy may be due to the voluntary nature of registry reporting, which may underestimate early fetal losses [28, 43, 52]. However, a study using hospital episodes statistics (HES) data, which captures data submitted on a mandatory basis following a patient's discharge from hospital trusts in England, reported a live birth rate of more than 68 percent in pregnant renal transplant recipients [45].

In Deshpande's meta-analysis the reported live birth rate was 73.3 percent, which is similar to that reported in more recent studies [35, 2]. The miscarriage rate was 14 percent, which was lower than that of the US general population (17.1 percent). Although chances of successful delivery in renal transplant recipients were high, there was a higher risk of obstetric complications, including preeclampsia (27 percent), gestational diabetes (8 percent), delivery by caesarean section (56.9 percent), preterm birth (45.6 percent) and lower birth weight (2,420g versus US mean 3,298g) [44]. These findings are also supported by analysis of English HES data. As compared to the general population, the rate of delivery by caesarean section and pregnancy complications, including intrauterine grown restriction, gestational diabetes and postpartum infections, were increased in the renal transplant cohort. There was also a possibility that early pregnancy losses may be increased in this group [45].

Registry data show that good renal function and normal or well-controlled blood pressure are the most important factors for a favorable obstetric outcome. A review of the obstetric outcomes in 7,110 pregnancies between 1961 and 2000 concluded that SCr below 125 µmol/l was an important prognostic factor (Table 11.3) [3]. In addition, the UKOSS study identified more than one previous kidney transplant or a diastolic BP > 90 mmHg in the second and third trimesters as additional predictive factors for poor pregnancy outcome [38]. Stoumpos et al., in their single-center study of 138 pregnancies, reported lower eGFR and a higher urine PCR at conception as independent predictors of poor obstetric outcome (pregnancy loss, stillbirth, neonatal mortality, birth < 32 weeks and/or fetal congenital anomalies) [35].

Deshpande reported more favorable pregnancy outcomes in studies with lower maternal age and a higher rate of obstetric complications with shorter intervals between transplantation and pregnancy [44].

Perinatal Mortality

In the 1980s in the United States, perinatal mortality was 3 percent in the renal transplant population and 1.3 percent in the general population [37]. Ten years later this had improved and was reported to be 2.8 percent in renal transplant patients and 0.58 percent

Table 11.3 Influence of renal allograft function on pregnancy outcome; reproduced with permission from Davison and Bailey [3]

Serum creatinine	Complicated pregnancy	Successful outcome	Long-term obstetric problems
≤ 125 µmol/l (1.4 mg/dl)	30 percent	9 percent	7 percent
≥ 125 µmol/l (1.4 mg/dl)	82 percent	75 percent	27 percent

Estimates are based on data from 7,110 pregnancies in 5,370 women (1961–2000) that attained at least 28 weeks of gestation.

Table 11.4 Studies on fetal outcomes in kidney transplant recipients

Study	Miscarriage (%)	Therapeutic termination of pregnancy (%)	Stillbirth (%)	Neonatal death (%)	Live birth (%)
UK Transplant Pregnancy Registry 1994–2001 [28]	11	6	1.6	2	79 (and one infant died before three months)
Armenti et al. [17]	12–24	1–8	1–3	1–2	76
Rahamimov et al. [27]	20			55	
Thompson et al. [29]				6	69
Miniero et al. [24]	29			68	
Yongwon et al. [48]	4	18			
Gutiérrez et al. [21]	21	23			65.6
Keitel et al. [23]	14	23	3.2 fetal death		61.4
Pour-Reza-Gholi et al. [26]	24	9.5		43.2	
Cruz Lemini et al. [19]		15 abortions			84
Galdo et al. [20]	19				
Hooi et al. [22]					63
Oliveira et al [25]	17.3	4.5	2.5	1	73.8
NTPR [73]	(9 percent loss or termination)			91	
Bramham et al. [37]	24.5	13.2	0		
Blume et al. [71]			1.9	1.1	60
Gill et al. [52]		3.813 (1966–2005)	2 (1966–2005)		76 (1966–2005)
		5 (1996–2005)	0.5 (1996–2005)		83 (1996–2005)
Levidiotis et al. [31]	9 percent		1.5		55.4
Stoumpos et al. [35]	16.7	5.8	1.4	2,	73.9
	2.2 ectopic births			2.2 congenital anomalies	
Sarween et al. [45]	17.5	13.2	≤3.2		68.8

in the general US population [53]. Studies of transplant pregnancies worldwide have reported live birth rates of between 43.2 percent and 84 percent (Table 11.4).

Using NTPR data Armenti et al. reported a lower live birth rate in tacrolimus-treated women compared with ciclosporine-treated women [54]. However, the pregnancies reported may have occurred at the time when tacrolimus therapy was mainly used in women with highest immunological risk and as rescue therapy following acute rejection.

Preterm Birth

Rates of preterm birth in renal transplant recipients are high, particularly in women with hypertension [28]. The incidence of preterm birth is increased by the high incidence of urinary tract infection in renal transplant patients [14, 37], the effects of CNIs [2, 13, 47] and the increased incidence of preeclampsia in these women. The timing of delivery is often influenced by the medical and obstetric team and may be hastened by the presence of severe hypertension, deteriorating graft function or fetal growth restriction. The incidence of preterm birth ranges from 26 percent to 60 percent in reported studies. The average gestational age is 35–37 weeks (Table 11.5).

Sibanda et al. reported a 50 percent incidence of preterm birth in renal transplant patients compared with 7 percent in the general population. Women

Table 11.5 Studies on obstetric outcomes for kidney transplant recipients

Study	Preterm birth before 37 weeks (mean gestation)	Low birth weight less than 2,500 g (mean weight)	Lower segment caesarean section
Sibanda et al. [28]	50 percent (35.6 weeks)	54 percent (2,316 g)	64 percent
Armenti et al. [17]	52–54 percent (35–36 weeks)	46–50 percent (2,378–2,493 g)	46–55 percent
Rahamimov et al. [27]	60 percent	52 percent	
Thompson et al. [29]	56 percent (34.9 weeks)	41 percent, associated creatinine > 133 µmol/l	59 percent
Miniero et al. [24]	42 percent (36.1 weeks)		91 percent
Yongwon et al. [48]	25.5 percent (36.9 weeks)	40 percent (2,260 g)	34 percent
Gutiérrez et al. [21]	29 percent	33 percent	46 percent
Keitel et al. [23]	36.4 percent	(2,195 g)	
Cruz Lemini et al. [19]	37 weeks	19 percent	
Galdo et al. [20]	56 percent (30 weeks)	(2,463 g)	55 percent
Hooi et al. [22]	35 percent		37 percent
Oliveira et al. [25]	38.4 percent	30 percent	61.5 percent
Bramham et al. [37]	52 percent (36 weeks)	48 percent	64 percent
NTPR [73]	52 percent		
Gill et al. [52]	32.7 percent		50.6 percent
Blume et al. [71]	50 percent	Median: 2,290g mean: 2,194 g	75 percent
Piccoli et al. [41]	46.2 percent (CKD-EPI stage 1), 60.8 percent (stage 2), 68.3 percent (stage 3)	SGA <10th centile 16.0 percent (stage 1; 810g), 16 percent (stage 2,610g), 25 percent (stage 3–5,672g)	73.1 percent (stage 1), 76.5 percent (stage 2), 86 percent (stage 3–5)
Stoumpos et al. [35]	61 percent	45.1 percent	78.4 percent
Yi-ping et al. [36]	53.3 percent	40 percent <10th centile (2,208.8)	60 percent

with hypertension and SCr above 150 µmol/l were at particularly high risk of preterm birth [28]. Bramham et al. also found a higher rate of both premature and very premature (< 32 weeks) delivery compared to a comparison cohort (52 percent versus 8 percent and 9 percent versus 2 percent, respectively) [38]. Piccoli et al. reported preterm and early preterm delivery was linked to a higher pre-pregnancy CKD stage (2–5 versus 1) and the presence of hypertension, but not with transplant versus non-transplant CKD patient [41].

Fetal Growth

Infants of transplant recipients frequently have lower birth weight. Recent studies have reported the incidence of low birth weight babies to be 19–54 percent (average 42 percent) and very low birth weight babies (less than 1,500 g) to be 11–17.8 percent [29, 47, 55].

In addition to the effects of preterm birth, several authors have reported an association between ciclosporine use and low birth weight infants. The NTPR reported significantly lower birth weights in infants of ciclosporine-treated mothers compared with women receiving alternative immunosuppressive regimens (2,250 g versus 2,505 g) [11, 42, 47]. Some studies have reported an association between low birth weight and hypertension and impaired renal function (SCr above 130 µmol/l) [28].

Delivery

Caesarean section should only be performed for obstetric indications such as preterm births, preeclampsia and deteriorating renal function. The incidence of caesarean section has varied in the literature from 34 percent in South Korea [48] to 91 percent in an Italian study [24] (Table 11.5). Sibanda et al. reported that 83 percent of preterm infants were born by caesarean section compared with only 5 percent by spontaneous delivery [28]. In Bramham's study 64 percent of the cohort had caesarean sections, with the most common indication before onset of labor being concern about fetal well-being (23 percent), previous caesarean section (19 percent) and deteriorating renal function (16 percent) [38]. Surgical aspects relating to delivery are discussed in what follows.

An Italian multicenter study reported increased rates of delivery by caesarean section in all groups of renal transplant recipients regardless of CKD stage; 73.1 percent (stage 1), 76.5 percent (stage 2) and 86 percent (stage 3–5) [41]. An increase in caesarean section rates when compared to the non-transplant cohort was only observed in the stage 1 group and not in more advanced stages of CKD.

Simultaneous Pancreas-Kidney Transplant Recipients

Successful pregnancies following simultaneous pancreas-kidney transplants have been reported. The NTPR reported higher rates of preeclampsia, preterm delivery, low birth weight, infection, acute rejection and graft loss in later years compared to kidney transplant recipients [17]. Pregnancies in these women should be managed as high risk, delivery planned in transplant centers with early involvement of the transplant surgical team.

The Effect of Live Kidney Donation on Subsequent Pregnancies

Garg et al. recently published the results of a retrospective Canadian cohort study looking at pregnancy outcomes of 85 living kidney donors matched with 510 healthy non-donors from the general population [56]. Gestational hypertension or preeclampsia was more common among the donors compared to the control group (11 percent versus 5 percent). Importantly, there was no difference in other adverse maternal/fetal outcome between the two groups. Other previous studies have reported similar findings and thus women of childbearing age wishing to act as live donors should be counseled appropriately and

managed as "high risk" for developing hypertensive disorders in any future pregnancies.

Outcomes in Children of Renal Transplant Patients

Children of transplant recipients are frequently born preterm, suffer fetal growth restriction and are of low birth weight (Table 11.6) [53, 57–59]. This leads to an increased risk of developmental and neurodevelopmental problems in later life. It is important that women understand the implications and risks facing a small and/or preterm baby and this should be addressed when advice is given before pregnancy or in early pregnancy.

Children of transplant patients are exposed to immunosuppressive and other medications in pregnancy, which may affect their long-term outcomes. Concerns regarding late effects of exposure to CNIs in utero were originally raised by Tendron-Franzin et al. [60] following experiments in an animal model.

Immunological Risks

The long-term effects of in utero exposure to immunosuppressive agents are unknown. Some authors have hypothesized that immunological abnormalities may be induced in the fetus [2, 37]. In animal studies, administration of CNIs during pregnancy resulted in abnormal T cell development and had a profound effect on the fetal immune system. Data in humans are limited, but one study showed children of immunosuppressed women had low B cell numbers and another reduced T and B cells at birth, which normalized in a few months [61, 62]. One case report of a child with multiple autoimmune problems [63] raised concerns regarding the induction of autoimmune disease in later life, but subsequent reports have shown no increased incidence above the general population [2]. The response of neonates to routine childhood vaccinations may alter following exposure to ciclosporine in utero and may be better delayed until after six months of age [61].

Effects on Fetal Renal Development

Cochat et al. reported that children exposed to immunosuppressants in utero may be at theoretical risk of renal impairment due to fetal growth restriction (associated with reduced nephron number and oligomeganephronia) and fetal nephrotoxicity [64].

Table 11.6 Neurodevelopment of children exposed to immunosuppressive agents in utero

Study	Number of children	Immunosuppressive drugs	Follow-up	Outcome
Willis et al. [58]	48 (56 percent preterm)		5.2 years	
Stanley et al. [59]	175 (4 months to 12 years; 71 at school)	Ciclosporine	4 months to 12 years	Mean gestation 34 weeks: 16 percent developmental delays (mean gestation < 33 weeks: 48 percent developmental delays, especially language)
				14 percent needed educational support versus 11 percent US public schools
				1.7 percent major disabilities
Sgro et al. [53]	44		3 months to 11 years	Three developmental or learning disabilities
Coscia et al. [43]	249	Ciclosporine	Mean follow-up 9.2 years	5.2 percent attention deficit hyperactivity disorder (6–7 percent general population)
				4 percent neurocognitive defects
				4 percent structural malformations
Nulman et al. [57]	39 (15 singleton, 24 multiple pregnancy)	Ciclosporine (18 concomitant azathioprine)	8 years	No difference in neurocognitive or behavioral measures (IQ, visuomotor skills, behavioral measures) associated with exposure to ciclosporine or azathioprine Prematurity (13/39 children born before 37 weeks) associated with poorer neurocognitive and behavioral outcomes.

Preliminary data in children do not support the hypothesis, however [2].

Pediatric Neurodevelopment

A small number of studies have reported outcomes in the offspring of renal transplant recipients (Table 11.6) [43, 53, 57–60, 66]. A study of 20 children (age 3–13 years) exposed to ciclosporine and azathioprine in pregnancy identified no differences in global, verbal or performance IQ or in language skills compared with controls [57].

McKay and Josephson highlighted the outcome of several studies that reported that small numbers of children suffered from sensorineural deafness and behavioral disorders [2]. Nulman et al. reported on the neurodevelopment of 39 children who were exposed to ciclosporine during gestation compared to matched unexposed children [57]. There was no association between in utero exposure to ciclosporine and long-term neurocognitive or behavioral development in children of renal transplant mothers. However, the higher rate of prematurity in children of renal transplant mothers was associated with poorer neurodevelopmental outcomes. As the number of babies born to transplant recipients grows, it is important to collect further prospective data on the outcome of children in the longer term.

Fertility Issues in Renal Transplant Patients

Fertility rapidly improves in patients with advanced CKD following successful renal transplantation. There are limited data on how fertility rates in transplant recipients compare with the general population, however. Medicare claim reports from 1990 to 2003 estimated a pregnancy rate of 3.3 percent in women of childbearing age in the first three years following renal transplantation compared with > 10 percent in the general population [52]. In a study of 63 female renal transplants, 68.1 percent had a regular menstrual cycle, and this was more likely in women who had been transplanted for longer. Ovulation was present in 59.5 percent of these women, compared to 70 percent in a control group, all of whom had regular cycles (p > 0.05) [66]. Increased levels of estrogen and similar serum FSH, LH and prolactin concentrations were observed in the transplant group. The authors concluded that although menstrual function greatly improved following a renal transplant, it was not fully restored to normal.

Contraception

There is a high reported rate of therapeutic termination of pregnancy within the renal transplant population (1–23 percent) in published studies (Table 11.4). It is therefore very important that women are given appropriate contraceptive advice prior to or immediately following transplantation [2, 7]. Approximately 50 percent of pregnancies in transplant patients are unplanned and 93.8 percent of these women were not using any specific contraception [6, 7, 23]. Both reversible and irreversible methods of contraception can be considered, but the approach has to be tailored to the needs of the individual woman or couple. Comprehensive details of options are discussed in Chapter 3.

Assisted Reproduction

The use of assisted reproductive technology has increased and such treatments may be sought by renal transplant patients who have difficulty conceiving naturally. The rate of infertility is similar to that in the general population (10.4 percent) [7].

Techniques include ovulation induction, *in vitro* fertilization and embryo transfer. There are case reports of successful treatment of male infertility using intracytoplasmic sperm injection for male renal transplant recipients with infertility [66] and successful *in vitro* fertilization in female transplant recipients [67–69]. Ethical issues regarding fertility treatment in women with organ transplants are discussed in previous reviews [70] and Chapter 4.

Preparation of Renal Transplant Patients for Pregnancy

Prepregnancy, antenatal and postpartum care of the renal transplant patient is a complex situation requiring multidisciplinary team care. The renal transplant patient may also have other comorbid conditions that need consideration and management both prepregnancy and during pregnancy. A simple checklist for the care of the renal transplant patients in the clinic is given in Box 11.3.

In 2014 the UK NHS-BT recommended that all rhesus-negative women of childbearing age receiving a kidney transplant from a rhesus-positive donor are administered Anti-RhD immunoglobulin in order to prevent sensitization.

Anatomical Considerations of Kidney Transplantation and Pregnancy

Most kidneys are placed in the extra-peritoneal plane in the iliac fossa. Depending on the side of donor kidney used, the renal pelvis of the transplanted kidney can be anterior or posterior. The renal artery is generally anastomosed on to the external iliac artery, though it may be placed onto the common iliac artery. Around 10 percent of transplanted kidneys have accessory arteries, so multiple vessels may be present. Sometimes, the internal iliac artery can be used to supply one of the accessory vessels. If the kidney is from a living donor, the vessels are very short. With deceased donor kidneys the vessels can be relatively long, with the kidney transplant lying some way from the iliac vessels. The ureter of the transplant kidney is then directly joined to the bladder laterally or anteriorly. Transplanted tissue is very immunogenic and often causes an inflammatory response in the recipient. The ureter can therefore be adherent to the anterior abdominal wall. For example, when performing a

BOX 11.3 Checklist for the care of pregnant renal transplant patients

1. **Prepregnancy or early pregnancy (if no opportunity prepregnancy)**
    *   Rubella vaccination pre-transplant and confirm antibody status
    *   Stop smoking
    *   Folic acid
    *   Discuss medicines in pregnancy:
        –   Medicines that are contraindicated in pregnancy, e.g. statins, ACE inhibitors, angiotensin II receptor blockers (ARBs), mycophenolate mofetil. Plan when to stop and how to convert to a safer alternative if required
        –   Medications that need to be modified in pregnancy including antihypertensives. Discuss safety of drugs and convert to methyldopa, labetalol or calcium channel blocker
        –   Consider other medication carefully. Stop bisphosphonates
    *   Advise about monitoring of calcineurin inhibitor (CNI) levels
    *   Advise about prevention of urinary tract infections. Plan monthly midstream urine (MSU) sample and consider prophylaxis
    *   Advise about other conditions: diabetes, systemic lupus erythematosus (SLE), implications in pregnancy, including testing for anti-Ro, anti-La, check anticardiolipin antibodies and lupus anticoagulant
    *   Consider aspirin prophylaxis
    *   In patients with proteinuria discuss thromboembolic risk associated with increasing proteinuria and need for prophylaxis
    *   Advise about genetic issues: polycystic kidney disease or chronic pyelonephritis. Baby will need an ultrasound scan (record in maternal notes)
    *   Discuss Down syndrome testing
2. **Antenatal**
    *   Monitor blood pressure
    *   Monitor CNI levels
    *   Monthly MSU
    *   Monitor proteinuria
    *   Monitor renal function
3. **Later pregnancy**
    *   Fetal growth monitoring
    *   Continue monitoring blood pressure, blood count, biochemistry, protein excretion, urate, platelets
    *   CNI levels
    *   MSU
    *   At 26–28 weeks, consider glucose tolerance test for women treated with tacrolimus
4. **Postpartum**
    *   Careful monitoring of fluid balance
    *   Monitoring of CNI levels to avoid nephrotoxicity
    *   Advise about breastfeeding and medications – balance between maternal and child factors
    *   Restore ACE inhibitor or ARB medication when breastfeeding permits
    *   Consider childhood vaccinations
    *   Arrange ultrasound scan for children of parents with vesicoureteric reflux
    *   Organize ongoing nephrology follow-up appointments
    *   Continue low-molecular-weight heparin in heavily proteinuric subjects for up to six weeks

caesarean section, the transplant ureter is at risk of damage.

If a patient is transplanted as a small child, the kidney can be placed directly onto the aorta and inferior vena cava. The ureter is often midline and should be placed on the posterior bladder wall, though sometimes if the bladder is small it is placed anteriorly. Great care must be taken to preserve the ureter if the patient goes on to have a caesarean section and liaison with transplant surgical colleagues is recommended.

One of the complications of kidney transplantation is the formation of a lymphocele. During a transplant many lymphatic vessels are divided – both around the donor renal artery and along the iliac vessels. This can result in a chronic collection of fluid called a lymphocele. If this compromises kidney function, it is surgically treated. However, in many patients it can be asymptomatic, resulting in a chronic collection of fluid near the kidney. Eventually this is reabsorbed, but it is important to be aware of a pre-existing lymphocele if surgery is planned in pregnancy.

Transplant Hydronephrosis in Pregnancy

Mild hydronephrosis, up to 1.6cm, is relatively common in the denervated transplant kidney, and if the creatinine is at baseline warrants no further treatment or investigation. If there is hydronephrosis, there is an increased risk of upper tract infection due to reflux. The transplant ureter is likely to lie directly on the uterus and is therefore at risk of compression. Serum creatinine levels should be measured and if there is a significant increase, then an ultrasound scan must be performed. If the ultrasound scan is normal, then other possible causes of renal dysfunction need to be investigated.

If hydronephrosis is present, the pregnancy is the likely cause, but differential diagnoses need to be considered such as a renal calculus, fibrosis, post-transplant lymphoproliferative disorder, rejection and viral infection. Drainage of the hydronephrosis can be achieved with insertion of a percutaneous nephrostomy tube. Insertion of a retrograde ureteric stent might be considered in early pregnancy, but is more challenging in more established stages. These interventions are likely to be needed for the rest of the pregnancy, so should be considered only when simple measures fail.

Pregnancy and Pancreas Transplantation

There are three categories of pancreas transplantation. The most common is a simultaneous pancreas and kidney (SPK) transplant for patients with type 1 or 2 diabetes and kidney failure. The second category is a pancreas after kidney (PAK) transplant for patients with diabetes who already have a functioning kidney transplant. The third category is a pancreas transplant alone (PTA) reserved for diabetics with good kidney function, but who have the life-threatening condition of hypoglycemia unawareness. The pancreas is placed on the right side of the abdomen. Commonly, the pancreas is anastomosed to the right common iliac artery and directly to the inferior vena cava. Most surgeons will place the head of the pancreas and duodenum upward, and the tail of the pancreas down in the pelvis. As well as producing insulin, the pancreas also produces digestive enzymes. These are drained by joining the attached transplant duodenum to the recipient's small bowel. To monitor pancreas function throughout pregnancy, a baseline serum amylase and HbA1c should be measured. The serum amylase should be monitored regularly. As the pancreas lies in the pelvis, there is the theoretical possibility that a growing uterus can compress the pancreas and cause an acute pancreatitis. If this is diagnosed, then the patient must be transferred to a transplant center. Transplant pancreatitis is a potentially serious condition that needs to be managed by an expert multidisciplinary team.

Planning Delivery in a Pregnant Transplant Patient

Careful planning of the mode of delivery is essential for the well-being of the mother and child. In most cases, vaginal delivery is thought to be the preferred option [4]. Damage to the transplant is rare at vaginal delivery and more likely during caesarean section. The main risk to the transplant during delivery is surgical damage to the kidney parenchyma or to the transplant ureter at the time of caesarean section. Damage to the kidney or ureter at the time of caesarean section is likely to be underreported. Following a number of case reports [72], it is estimated that the risk of transplant damage at the time of caesarean section is in the order of 1 percent. Women should be offered assessment at around 30 weeks' gestation by an obstetrician and a transplant surgeon. A decision should be made for a vaginal delivery or a planned caesarean section. A decision has also to be made whether the planned labor is in a local non-transplant center, or whether, from 36 weeks' gestation, the patient should be transferred to a center with transplant surgeons present to assist the obstetricians if necessary. A detailed plan for a caesarean section must be made for all pregnant women with a transplant. If there is any concern about the proximity of the transplant kidney or ureter, then the incision through the abdominal wall should be vertical and midline. If the transplant patient has had multiple previous transplants or is a recipient of a kidney and pancreas, then it is reasonable for a transplant surgeon to be present at the time of a caesarean section.

References

1. Murray JE, Reid DE, Harrison JH, Merrill JP. Successful pregnancies after human renal transplantation. *The New England journal of medicine*. 1963;**269**:341–343.

2. McKay DB, Josephson MA. Pregnancy in recipients of solid organs – effects on mother and child. *The New England journal of medicine*. 2006;**354**(12):1281–1293.

3. Davison JM, Bailey DJ. Pregnancy following renal transplantation. *J Obstet Gynaecol Res*. 2003;**29**(4):227–233.

4. McKay DB, Josephson MA, Armenti VT, August P, Coscia LA, Davis CL, et al. Reproduction and transplantation: Report on the AST Consensus Conference on Reproductive Issues and Transplantation. *Am J Transplant*. 2005;**5**(7):1592–1599.

5. Hou S. Pregnancy in renal transplant recipients. *Adv Chronic Kidney Dis*. 2013;**20**(3):253–259.

6. Lessan-Pezeshki M. Pregnancy after renal transplantation: Points to consider. *Nephrol Dial Transplant*. 2002;**17**(5):703–707.

7. Lessan-Pezeshki M, Ghazizadeh S, Khatami MR, Mahdavi M, Razeghi E, Seifi S, et al. Fertility and contraceptive issues after kidney transplantation in women. *Transplant Proc*. 2004;**36**(5):1405–1406.

8. Josephson MA, McKay DB. Women and transplantation: Fertility, sexuality, pregnancy, contraception. *Adv Chronic Kidney Dis*. 2013;**20**(5):433–440.

9. Ramhendar T, Byrne P. Contraception for renal transplant recipients in the Republic of Ireland: A review. *Ir J Med Sci*. 2013;**182**(3):315–317.

10. French VA, Davis JS, Sayles HS, Wu SS. Contraception and fertility awareness among women with solid organ transplants. *Obstetrics and gynecology*. 2013;**122**(4):809–814.

11. European best practice guidelines for renal transplantation. Section IV: Long-term management of the transplant recipient. IV.10. Pregnancy in renal transplant recipients. *Nephrol Dial Transplant*. 2002;**17** Suppl. 4:50–55.

12. Richman K, Gohh R. Pregnancy after renal transplantation: A review of registry and single-center practices and outcomes. *Nephrol Dial Transplant*. 2012;**27**(9):3428–3434.

13. Fischer T, Neumayer HH, Fischer R, Barenbrock M, Schobel HP, Lattrell BC, et al. Effect of pregnancy on long-term kidney function in renal transplant recipients treated with ciclosporine and with azathioprine. *Am J Transplant*. 2005;**5**(11):2732–2739.

14. Davison JM. Renal disorders in pregnancy. *Curr Opin Obstet Gynecol*. 2001;**13**(2):109–114.

15. Davison JM. The effect of pregnancy on kidney function in renal allograft recipients. *Kidney Int*. 1985;**27**(1):74–79.

16. Hou S, Firanek C. Management of the pregnant dialysis patient. *Adv Ren Replace Ther*. 1998;**5**(1):24–30.

17. Armenti VT, Radomski JS, Moritz MJ, Gaughan WJ, Hecker WP, Lavelanet A, et al. Report from the National Transplantation Pregnancy Registry (NTPR): Outcomes of pregnancy after transplantation. *Clin Transpl*. 2004:103–114.

18. Crowe AV, Rustom R, Gradden C, Sells RA, Bakran A, Bone JM, et al. Pregnancy does not adversely affect renal transplant function. *QJM*. 1999;**92**(11):631–635.

19. Cruz Lemini MC, Ibarguengoitia Ochoa F, Villanueva Gonzalez MA. Perinatal outcome following renal transplantation. *Int J Gynaecol Obstet*. 2007;**96**(2):76–79.

20. Galdo T, Gonzalez F, Espinoza M, Quintero N, Espinoza O, Herrera S, et al. Impact of pregnancy on the function of transplanted kidneys. *Transplant Proc*. 2005;**37**(3):1577–1579.

21. Gutierrez MJ, Acebedo-Ribo M, Garcia-Donaire JA, Manzanera MJ, Molina A, Gonzalez E, et al. Pregnancy in renal transplant recipients. *Transplant Proc*. 2005;**37**(9):3721–3722.

22. Hooi LS, Rozina G, Shaariah MY, Teo SM, Tan CH, Bavanandan S, et al. Pregnancy in patients with renal transplants in Malaysia. *Med J Malaysia*. 2003;**58**(1):27–36.

23. Keitel E, Bruno RM, Duarte M, Santos AF, Bittar AE, Bianco PD, et al. Pregnancy outcome after renal transplantation. *Transplant Proc*. 2004;**36**(4):870–871.

24. Miniero R, Tardivo I, Curtoni ES, Bresadola F, Calconi G, Cavallari A, et al. Outcome of pregnancy after organ transplantation: A retrospective survey in Italy. *Transpl Int*. 2005;**17**(11):724–729.

25. Oliveira LG, Sass N, Sato JL, Ozaki KS, Medina Pestana JO. Pregnancy after renal transplantation – a five-yr

single-center experience. *Clin Transplant*. 2007;**21** (3):301–304.

26. Pour-Reza-Gholi F, Nafar M, Farrokhi F, Entezari A, Taha N, Firouzan A, et al. Pregnancy in kidney transplant recipients. *Transplant Proc*. 2005;**37** (7):3090–3092.

27. Rahamimov R, Ben-Haroush A, Wittenberg C, Mor E, Lustig S, Gafter U, et al. Pregnancy in renal transplant recipients: Long-term effect on patient and graft survival. A single-center experience. *Transplantation*. 2006;**81**(5):660–664.

28. Sibanda N, Briggs JD, Davison JM, Johnson RJ, Rudge CJ. Pregnancy after organ transplantation: A report from the UK Transplant pregnancy registry. *Transplantation*. 2007;**83**(10):1301–1307.

29. Thompson BC, Kingdon EJ, Tuck SM, Fernando ON, Sweny P. Pregnancy in renal transplant recipients: The Royal Free Hospital experience. *QJM*. 2003;**96** (11):837–844.

30. Yildirim Y, Uslu A. Pregnancy in patients with previous successful renal transplantation. *Int J Gynaecol Obstet*. 2005;**90**(3):198–202.

31. Levidiotis V, Chang S, McDonald S. Pregnancy and maternal outcomes among kidney transplant recipients. *J Am Soc Nephrol*. 2009;**20**(11):2433–2440.

32. Stratta P, Canavese C, Giacchino F, Mesiano P, Quaglia M, Rossetti M. Pregnancy in kidney transplantation: satisfactory outcomes and harsh realities. *J Nephrol*. 2003;**16**(6):792–806.

33. Rose C, Gill J, Zalunardo N, Johnston O, Mehrotra A, Gill JS. Timing of pregnancy after kidney transplantation and risk of allograft failure. *American journal of transplantation: Official journal of the American Society of Transplantation and the American Society of Transplant Surgeons*. 2016;**16**(8):2360–2367.

34. Kwek JL, Tey V, Yang L, Kanagalingam D, Kee T. Renal and obstetric outcomes in pregnancy after kidney transplantation: Twelve-year experience in a Singapore transplant center. *The journal of obstetrics and gynaecology research*. 2015;**41**(9):1337–1344.

35. Stoumpos S, McNeill SH, Gorrie M, Mark PB, Brennand JE, Geddes CC, et al. Obstetric and long-term kidney outcomes in renal transplant recipients: A 40-yr single-center study. *Clinical transplantation*. 2016;**30**(6):673–681.

36. Li YP, Shih JC, Lin SY, Lee CN. Pregnancy outcomes after kidney transplantation-A single-center experience in Taiwan. *Taiwan J Obstet Gynecol*. 2016;**55**(3):314–318.

37. Stratta P, Canavese C, Giacchino F, Mesiano P, Quaglia M, Rossetti M. Pregnancy in kidney transplantation: Satisfactory outcomes and harsh realities. *J Nephrol*. 2003;**16**(6):792–806.

38. Bramham K, Nelson-Piercy C, Gao H, Pierce M, Bush N, Spark P, et al. Pregnancy in renal transplant recipients: A UK national cohort study. *Clinical journal of the American Society of Nephrology: CJASN*. 2013;**8**(2):290–298.

39. First MR, Combs CA, Weiskittel P, Miodovnik M. Lack of effect of pregnancy on renal allograft survival or function. *Transplantation*. 1995;**59**(4):472–476.

40. Salmela KT, Kyllonen LE, Holmberg C, Gronhagen-Riska C. Impaired renal function after pregnancy in renal transplant recipients. *Transplantation*. 1993;**56** (6):1372–1375.

41. Piccoli GB, Cabiddu G, Attini R, Gerbino M, Todeschini P, Perrino ML, et al. Outcomes of pregnancies after kidney transplantation: Lessons learned from CKD. A comparison of transplanted, nontransplanted chronic kidney disease patients and low-risk pregnancies: a multicenter nationwide analysis. *Transplantation*. 2017.

42. Armenti VT, McGrory CH, Cater JR, Radomski JS, Moritz MJ. Pregnancy outcomes in female renal transplant recipients. *Transplant Proc*. 1998;**30** (5):1732–1734.

43. Coscia LA, Constantinescu S, Moritz MJ, Frank A, Ramirez CB, Maley WL, et al. Report from the National Transplantation Pregnancy Registry (NTPR): Outcomes of pregnancy after transplantation. *Clin Transpl*. 2009:103–122.

44. Deshpande NA, James NT, Kucirka LM, Boyarsky BJ, Garonzik-Wang JM, Montgomery RA, et al. Pregnancy outcomes in kidney transplant recipients: A systematic review and meta-analysis. *American journal of transplantation: Official journal of the American Society of Transplantation and the American Society of Transplant Surgeons*. 2011;**11**(11):2388–2404.

45. Sarween N, Hughes S, Evison F, Day C, Knox E, Lipkin G. SO012 Pregnancy outcomes in renal transplant recipients in England over 15 years. *Nephrology Dialysis Transplantation*. 2016;**31**(Suppl. 1):i6.

46. Ehrich JH, Loirat C, Davison JM, Rizzoni G, Wittkop B, Selwood NH, et al. Repeated successful pregnancies after kidney transplantation in 102 women (Report by the EDTA Registry). *Nephrol Dial Transplant*. 1996;**11** (7):1314–1317.

47. Armenti VT, Ahlswede KM, Ahlswede BA, Jarrell BE, Moritz MJ, Burke JF. National Transplantation Pregnancy Registry – outcomes of 154 pregnancies in ciclosporine-treated female kidney transplant recipients. *Transplantation*. 1994;**57**(4):502–506.

48. Yongwon PJC, Younghan K, Changee L, Hyungmin C, Taeyoon K. 360 pregnancy outcome in renal transplant recipients: The experience of a single center in Korea. *Am J Obstet Gynecol* 2001;**185**(Suppl. 6:S180).

49. Morken NH, Diaz-Garcia C, Reisaeter AV, Foss A, Leivestad T, Geiran O, et al. Obstetric and neonatal

outcome of pregnancies fathered by males on immunosuppression after solid organ transplantation. *American journal of transplantation: Official journal of the American Society of Transplantation and the American Society of Transplant Surgeons.* 2015;**15**(6):1666–1673.

50. Duley L, Henderson-Smart DJ, Meher S, King JF. Antiplatelet agents for preventing pre-eclampsia and its complications. *The Cochrane database of systematic reviews.* 2007(2):CD004659.

51. Davison JM. Pregnancy in renal allograft recipients: Problems, prognosis and practicalities. *Baillieres Clin Obstet Gynaecol.* 1994;**8**(2):501–525.

52. Gill JS, Zalunardo N, Rose C, Tonelli M. The pregnancy rate and live birth rate in kidney transplant recipients. *American journal of transplantation: Official journal of the American Society of Transplantation and the American Society of Transplant Surgeons.* 2009;**9**(7):1541–1549.

53. Sgro MD, Barozzino T, Mirghani HM, Sermer M, Moscato L, Akoury H, et al. Pregnancy outcome post renal transplantation. *Teratology.* 2002;**65**(1):5–9.

54. Armenti VT, Radomski JS, Moritz MJ, Gaughan WJ, Philips LZ, McGrory CH, et al. Report from the National Transplantation Pregnancy Registry (NTPR): Outcomes of pregnancy after transplantation. *Clin Transpl.* 2002:121–130.

55. Penny JA, Halligan AWF, Shennan AH, Lambert PC, Jones DR, de Swiet M, et al. Automated, ambulatory, or conventional blood pressure measurement in pregnancy: Which is the better predictor of severe hypertension? *American journal of obstetrics and gynecology.* 1998;**178**(3):521–526.

56. Garg AX, Nevis IF, McArthur E, Sontrop JM, Koval JJ, Lam NN, et al. Gestational hypertension and preeclampsia in living kidney donors. *The New England journal of medicine.* 2014.

57. Nulman I, Sgro M, Barrera M, Chitayat D, Cairney J, Koren G. Long-term neurodevelopment of children exposed in utero to ciclosporin after maternal renal transplant. *Paediatr Drugs.* 2010;**12**(2):113–122.

58. Willis FR, Findlay CA, Gorrie MJ, Watson MA, Wilkinson AG, Beattie TJ. Children of renal transplant recipient mothers. *J Paediatr Child Health.* 2000;**36**(3):230–235.

59. Stanley CW, Gottlieb R, Zager R, Eisenberg J, Richmond R, Moritz MJ, et al. Developmental well-being in offspring of women receiving ciclosporine post-renal transplant. *Transplant Proc.* 1999;**31**(1–2):241–242.

60. Tendron-Franzin A, Gouyon JB, Guignard JP, Decramer S, Justrabo E, Gilbert T, et al. Long-term effects of in utero exposure to cyclosporin A on renal function in the rabbit. *J Am Soc Nephrol.* 2004;**15**(10):2687–2693.

61. Di Paolo S, Schena A, Morrone LF, Manfredi G, Stallone G, Derosa C, et al. Immunologic evaluation during the first year of life of infants born to ciclosporine-treated female kidney transplant recipients: Analysis of lymphocyte subpopulations and immunoglobulin serum levels. *Transplantation.* 2000;**69**(10):2049–2054.

62. Pilarski LM, Yacyshyn BR, Lazarovits AI. Analysis of peripheral blood lymphocyte populations and immune function from children exposed to ciclosporine or to azathioprine in utero. *Transplantation.* 1994;**57**(1):133–144.

63. Scott JR, Branch DW, Holman J. Autoimmune and pregnancy complications in the daughter of a kidney transplant patient. *Transplantation.* 2002;**73**(5):815–816.

64. Cochat P, Decramer S, Robert-Gnansia E, Duborg L, Audra P. Renal outcome of children exposed to ciclosporine in utero *Transplantation proceedings.* 2004; 36(Suppl 2S): S208–10.

65. Sifontis NM, Coscia LA, Constantinescu S, Lavelanet AF, Moritz MJ, Armenti VT. Pregnancy outcomes in solid organ transplant recipients with exposure to mycophenolate mofetil or sirolimus. *Transplantation.* 2006;**82**(12):1698–1702.

66. Pietrzak B, Cyganek A, Jabiry-Zieniewicz Z, Bobrowska K, Durlik M, Paczek L, et al. Function of the ovaries in female kidney transplant recipients. *Transplantation proceedings.* 2006;**38**(1):180–183.

67. Berkkanoglu M, Bulut H, Coetzee K, Ozgur K. Intracytoplasmic sperm injection in male renal transplant recipients. *Middle East Fertility Society Journal.* 2015;**20**(2):127–130.

68. Norrman E, Bergh C, Wennerholm UB. Pregnancy outcome and long-term follow-up after in vitro fertilization in women with renal transplantation. *Hum Reprod.* 2015;**30**(1):205–213.

69. Pietrzak B, Mazanowska N, Kociszewska-Najman B, et al. Successful Pregnancy Outcome after In Vitro Fertilization in a Kidney Graft Recipient: A Case Report and Literature Review. *Ann Transplant.* 2015;**20**:338–341.

70. Ross LF. Ethical considerations related to pregnancy in transplant recipients. *N Engl J Med.* 2006;**354**(12):1313–6.

71. Blume C, Sensoy A, Gross MM, Guenter HH, Haller H, Manns MP, et al. A comparison of the outcome of pregnancies after liver and kidney transplantation. *Transplantation.* 2013;**95**(1):222–227.

72. Shrestha BM, Throssell D, McKane W, Raftery AT. Injury to a transplanted kidney during caesarean section: a case report. *Exp Clin Transplant.* 2007;5(1):618–20.

73. *National Transplant Pregnancy Registry: 2011 annual report.* Philadelphia, PA: Thomas Jefferson University, 2012.

Chapter 12

Comorbid Conditions Affecting Pregnancy in Renal Transplant Patients

Sue Carr, Nadia Sarween and Joyce Popoola

Many renal transplant patients have coexisting comorbid conditions that could influence the outcome of a pregnancy. It is essential that each comorbid condition is recognized and a management plan made for these factors at every stage of pregnancy – from the time of preconception counseling to postpartum care. An overall integrated management plan for the pregnancy can then be developed and followed by the patient and the multidisciplinary team. Some of the more common comorbid conditions found in renal transplant patients are considered in what follows.

Hypertension

A high proportion of renal transplant recipients are hypertensive before pregnancy (47–73 percent) [1]. A further 25 percent will become hypertensive during pregnancy and indeed, in the later stages of pregnancy, superimposed preeclampsia develops in 15–37 percent [2] (see Chapter 9).

Infections in Pregnancy

Urinary Tract Infections

Normal pregnancy-related changes in the urinary tract (diminished bladder tone and physiological dilatation of ureter and renal pelvis) predispose all women to urinary tract infection (UTI) in pregnancy. The overall incidence of UTI is approximately 8 percent [3].

The risk of UTI in pregnancy is increased further in renal transplant patients owing to a number of factors:

- surgical factors, such as transplant surgery or re-implantation of ureters
- preexisting urological abnormalities, such as bladder problems, calculi or reflux to native or transplant kidney
- underlying renal disease, such as reflux nephropathy

- immunosuppression
- comorbid diseases, such as diabetes.

The common pathogens include *Escherichia coli*, *Enterobacter, Klebsiella, Pseudomonas* and *Proteus* [3].

UTI in pregnancy, including asymptomatic bacteriuria, has been associated with an increased risk of adverse pregnancy outcomes, including preterm birth, low birth weight and perinatal mortality in most but not all studies [3–6].

In a transplant patient, it is important to ensure that immunosuppression is optimized and that diabetes, when present, is well controlled to reduce risk of infection.

Asymptomatic Bacteriuria

As part of routine antenatal care, all women are screened for the presence of asymptomatic bacteriuria (ASB). In normal pregnancy, ASB affects 2–10 percent of women and 30 percent will develop a symptomatic UTI if left untreated [6]. Antibiotic treatment should be prescribed, which will reduce the risk of symptomatic infections by up to 70 percent. Furthermore, effective treatment of ASB during pregnancy has been shown to reduce the incidence of preterm delivery and low birth weight [4, 5]. Commonly used antibiotics in renal transplant patients during pregnancy include cephalexin, amoxicillin and trimethoprim (avoid in early pregnancy) (see Chapter 7). A Cochrane review recommends that treatment courses are guided by urine cultures and sensitivities and continued for at least seven days [6].

It is important to perform a follow-up urine culture. The European Best Practice Guidelines (EBPG) recommendation is that all renal transplant patients should have a monthly midstream urine sample sent to screen for ASB and additional samples sent if symptoms develop [7].

EBPG recommends two weeks of antibiotic treatment for ASB and prophylactic antibiotics for the remainder of the pregnancy following treatment of ASB.

Symptomatic Urinary Tract Infection

In renal transplant patients, the reported incidence of UTI varies from 19 percent to 42 percent in recent studies [8–11]. Thompson et al. reported UTI in 26 percent [8] of renal transplant pregnancies, Galdo et al. 13.5 percent [9], Oliveira et al. 42.3 percent [10] and Hooi et al. 13 percent [11].

In general, a pregnant renal transplant recipient with UTI should receive 7–10 days of antibiotic therapy [3], depending on local antibiotic policies. A systematic review from the Cochrane database concluded that there were insufficient data to recommend a superior or specific drug regimen for treatment of symptomatic UTI during pregnancy [12]. Pregnant renal transplant patients with a UTI in pregnancy should be considered for prophylactic antibiotic therapy for the remainder of the pregnancy with low-dose cephalexin, amoxicillin or trimethoprim (depending on stage of pregnancy and sensitivities) at night. Women receiving antibiotic prophylaxis for UTI pre-pregnancy should continue on an appropriate antibiotic through the pregnancy.

Pyelonephritis

The incidence of acute pyelonephritis in normal pregnancy is 1–2 percent and up to 40 percent in women with untreated bacteriuria in pregnancy. In a transplant patient, acute pyelonephritis can develop in either the native or transplanted kidney and, in view of the immunosuppressed state, the symptoms and signs may be masked or altered. It is important to be alert to this possible diagnosis and to reduce the risk by monthly urinary screening and prompt treatment of urinary tract sepsis during pregnancy. Intravenous antibiotic therapy should be started promptly while awaiting specific urine culture and sensitivity results that will further guide management. It is recommended that antimicrobial treatment is continued for a minimum of 10 days and up to 21 days to reduce the risk of recurrence of infection [7].

Other Bacterial Infections

Listeria Monocytogenes

Pregnant women are at risk of developing Listeria, but this risk is increased by the use of immunosuppression.

The condition may present with flu-like symptoms and gastroenteritis, but though rare, it may cause congenital infection and lead to preterm delivery, stillbirths, miscarriages, neonatal sepsis/meningitis and congenital anomalies. In pregnancy women are advised to avoid potentially contaminated foods [13].

Group B Streptococcus (GBS)

Streptococcus agalactiae is part of the normal vaginal flora in up to 30 percent of pregnant women The updated CDC guidelines recommend universal prenatal screening for vaginal and rectal GBS colonization of all pregnant women at 35–37 weeks' gestation such that if positive penicillin can be given intrapartum [14].

Whooping Cough (Bordetella Pertussis)

Reduced uptake of the vaccine has led to an increased incidence in the condition, particularly among infants. Vaccination is recommended in women between 28–38 weeks of pregnancy. There is no contraindication to whooping cough vaccination in the renal transplant patient.

Viral Infections

Cytomegalovirus

Following renal transplantation, patients are potentially at risk of cytomegalovirus (CMV) infection or reactivation. At the time of transplantation, all transplant recipients and donor kidneys are tested for evidence of previous CMV infection. The presence of detectable immunoglobulin G (IgG) anti-CMV antibodies in the plasma indicates a previous CMV infection and is present in more than two-thirds of donors and recipients prior to transplantation. A CMV-negative transplant recipient can be at risk of CMV infection from a CMV-positive transplant kidney and CMV-positive transplant recipients can be subject to reactivation of CMV virus or re-infection, usually related to high levels of immunosuppression. The risk of CMV infection is highest in the first year following renal transplantation. CMV-negative recipients of CMV-positive kidneys and CMV-positive recipients of CMV-positive kidneys who have been significantly immunosuppressed will receive prophylaxis against CMV infection using ganciclovir or valganciclovir [15]. Based upon the IMPACT study some centers have adopted prolonged valganciclovir prophylaxis (200 days) [16] and late-onset CMV infection may become more common.

If pregnancy occurs during the first 12 months following transplant, when the risk of acute rejection and immunosuppression levels are still quite high, CMV infection may occur. However, continuation of valganciclovir is not recommended due to reports of fetotoxicity and teratogenicity in animal studies, although no human cases are reported. In general, when patients delay pregnancy by 12–24 months, post-transplant CMV is unlikely to be a problem as the risk of acute rejection and the immunosuppressive drug levels are generally lower.

In the fetus, approximately 90 percent of congenital infections are asymptomatic and affected children can present in later life with impaired psychomotor development and hearing, neurological, eye or dental abnormalities. In symptomatic congenital CMV, infants can develop splenomegaly, jaundice and a petechial rash. In the more severe form of the disease, cytomegalovirus inclusion disease, there can be multi-organ involvement with microcephaly, motor disability, chorioretinitis, cerebral calcifications, lethargy, respiratory distress and seizures.

When CMV infection is suspected, samples should be sent urgently from mother's serum and where appropriate the amniotic fluid for detection and quantification of CMV DNA using quantitative polymerase chain reaction (PCR). If infection is confirmed, treatment should be considered with appropriate counseling.

Rubella

Women with chronic kidney disease who may become pregnant should be vaccinated against rubella infection before renal transplant. The vaccine is a live vaccine and cannot be administered to an immunosuppressed patient.

Varicella Zoster

Women of childbearing age should be considered for vaccination against this virus to prevent chicken pox known to be particularly life threatening in adults and those on immunosuppression. Shingles occurs as a result of reactivation of the virus usually in the elderly or immunosuppressed. The vaccination, however, needs to be given prior to transplantation as it is a live attenuated virus.

Hepatitis C

The prevalence of hepatitis C virus (HCV) infection has increased in dialysis patients and hence there are an increasing number of HCV-positive patients who receive a renal transplant.

In pregnancy, vertical transmission of the HCV virus occurs in 5–10 percent of pregnancies of HCV RNA-positive mothers and is related to the viral load. The incidence of vertical transmission is also increased in the presence of human immunodeficiency virus. Pregnancy should be planned at a time of minimal viral load to reduce the risk of vertical transmission to the fetus. In non-transplant HCV-positive pregnancies, the outcome is usually good. And there appears to be no evidence of increased fetal malformation.

It is important that HCV infection is diagnosed early in infants of mothers who are HCV-positive using HCV DNA PCR as HCV antibodies are passively transferred from the mother. There is no evidence of transmission of HCV by breastfeeding. There have been few reports of pregnancy in HCV-positive renal transplant patients. Ventura et al. [17] reported three cases of pregnancy in HCV-positive renal transplant patients without chronic liver disease. In these three cases there was no evidence of progression of liver disease during follow-up two years postpartum.

Many patients with hepatitis C are treated with ribavirin, which is contraindicated in pregnancy because of teratogenicity in animal studies. There are several new agents emerging, including direct-acting antivirals that combine NS5A (Nonstructural protein 5A) inhibition and a nucleotide analog polymerase inhibitor, which are also contraindicated during pregnancy.

It is advised that effective contraception be used during oral administration and for six months after treatment in women and in men [18]. Interferon is generally avoided in renal transplant patients.

Hepatitis B

The presence of hepatitis B virus (HBV) infection is increasing in the dialysis population and increasingly HBV-positive patients without evidence of liver disease on a FibroScan/liver biopsy are considered for renal transplantation. Some patients may acquire HBV following renal transplantation. Patients who are HBV DNA-positive require antiviral therapy following transplantation, which may need to be continued long term.

Renal transplant patients with HBV infection have reduced survival and are at increased risk of graft loss. Outcomes are improving with improvements in antiviral therapies. Lamivudine should be avoided in the first trimester of pregnancy, likewise tenofovir and entecavir. Tenofovir is used later in pregnancy to reduce viral load in those with high viral titers. In general, pregnancy is uneventful in women who are hepatitis B carriers and exacerbation of disease during pregnancy is uncommon. The most significant risk is of vertical transmission to the infant during delivery, which can occur in up to 80 percent of cases. The administration of HBV immunoglobulin and vaccination is effective in reducing infection in the infant. Infants born to HBSAg-positive mothers should be given hepatitis B Immunoglobulin within 12 hours of birth and HBV vaccine at another site within 48 hours followed by a booster injection at one and six months. It is important that close liaison takes place between hepatologists, renal physicians, virologists and obstetricians when managing pregnancy in a renal transplant patient with hepatitis B or C positivity.

Herpes Simplex

Persistent viral infections can occur in renal transplant patients, including herpes simplex infection. Infection within the first 20 weeks of gestation can be associated with an increased risk of miscarriage. The majority of infections occur in the second (30 percent) and third (40 percent) trimesters, but provided there is seroconversion prior to delivery there is no increased incidence of neonatal mortality [19]. A child can be infected with herpes simplex virus (HSV) as a result of spread due to contact at the time of birth. The risk of transmission and subsequent neonatal herpes can be reduced by caesarean delivery in women with positive HSV cervical cultures. Aciclovir is safe in pregnancy. Clinically insignificant amounts of aciclovir are secreted into breast milk.

Human Immunodeficiency Virus

Historically, patients with HIV were considered unsuitable candidates for transplantation; however, there is declining morbidity among patients with HIV infection. Additionally, there is now several years' experience of transplanting this group that includes multicenter cohort studies mainly from the United States [20]. Where recipients are appropriately selected, outcomes for patients and grafts are similar to transplantation in the older population > 65 years. Clearly as more experience is gained in this area, female recipients may well consider conception similar to the general population with HIV. Care in pregnancy requires a multidisciplinary team that would include HIV specialists, transplant specialists, obstetricians, immunologists, pharmacists, psychologists, social workers and specialist nurses. Awareness of drug interactions (antiretrovirals and immunosuppressants), potential for increased risk of rejection, increased monitoring, reduced graft survival and implications around conception is important.

Toxoplasmosis

Congenital toxoplasmosis has been reported following reactivation in an immunosuppressed mother. The majority of infants with congenital toxoplasmosis (70–90 percent) are asymptomatic at birth but have a high risk of developing subsequent abnormalities, especially chorioretinitis with potential visual impairment, if adequate treatment is not given. Symptomatic infants may present the classic triad of chorioretinitis, hydrocephalus and intracranial calcification, although other manifestations may include fever, rash, hepatosplenomegaly, microcephaly, seizures, jaundice, thrombocytopenia and sometimes lymphadenopathy. In addition, neurodevelopmental delay, deafness, seizures and spasticity can be seen in a minority of untreated children.

This condition can be diagnosed pre- or postnatally using serology or PCR testing. Treatment is generally reported to improve prognosis in affected infants and is usually spiramycin (a macrolide antibiotic), pyrimethamine or sulfadiazine (unlicensed) [21]. These agents may interact with immunosuppressive drugs and some are renally excreted: specific advice should be sought from a pharmacist and infectious disease specialist. There is also a risk of developing urolithiasis and subsequent acute kidney injury with agents such as sulfadiazines.

Hematological Abnormalities

Anemia

In normal pregnancy the red cell mass increases under the control of erythropoietin (EPO) but, because the relative increase in plasma volume is greater, hemodilution occurs and there is a decrease in hemoglobin concentration. As a result of this a renal transplant patient may become anemic as well as iron deficient or may have anemia related to chronic renal impairment. Women with impaired transplant function may be receiving treatment with EPO before pregnancy or require this treatment during pregnancy if renal transplant function has deteriorated. It is important to exclude other causes of anemia, including vitamin deficiencies, bleeding and hemolysis in an anemic renal transplant patient. The frequency of anemia in renal transplant patients is quoted as 65–85 percent [22].

Anemia if untreated can cause both fetal and maternal morbidity. In the fetus, anemia can lead to an increased risk of infections and is associated with growth restriction and preterm birth [23, 24]. In the mother, cardiovascular symptoms may develop, including breathlessness and delayed wound healing and infection. Parenteral iron may be required in women with renal transplants who are unable to tolerate oral iron supplements or who are receiving EPO therapy. A published Cochrane review [25] concluded that intravenous iron enhanced hematological response compared with oral iron and there are now further trials to support this [23] (see Chapter 7). In general, for a pregnant transplant patient similar to the general population, the aim is to maintain the hemoglobin level at around 110 g/L in the first trimester and 105g/L in the second and third trimesters. If hemoglobin falls below this level, the following investigations should be considered starting with the sample and in discussion with a hematologist in relation to the more complex tests:

- Full blood count and red cell indices
- Blood film
- Serum ferritin, Vitamin B12, Folate
- Serum iron (Fe) and total iron binding capacity (TIBC)
- C-reactive protein (to exclude inflammation)
- Hemolysis screen
- Zinc protoporphyrin level, transferrin saturation ratio
- Soluble transferrin receptor (sTIR)
- Parvovirus infection test
- Trial of iron therapy
- Bone marrow iron

Anemia in pregnancy may be exacerbated by anemia of chronic kidney disease (CKD) owing to transplant dysfunction (the aforementioned additional factors excluded). Magee et al. [29] found that serum EPO levels were inappropriately low and rate of erythropoiesis low in transplant patients in a study comparing 30 transplant patients with 30 normal pregnant controls. Hou [30] suggested EPO should be started if hematocrit falls below 30 percent and the dose titrated to maintain hemoglobin at 100–120 g/L.

There are several reports of the safe use of EPO in renal transplant pregnancies [30–32]. Goshorn and Yuell [31] reported successful use of darbepoetin-alpha in a woman with impaired renal function (serum creatinine 203 µmol/l) and hemoglobin 75 g/L at 28 weeks of gestation. EPO does not appear to cross the placenta and has not been reported to be teratogenic, but it has been associated with increases in blood pressure, which needs careful monitoring [32]. Experimental studies have shown direct vasoconstriction following administration of recombinant human EPO (rHuEPO) on placental blood vessel rings [33]. EPO does not appear to cross the placenta because of its large molecular size. EPO is found in both breast milk and colostrum and appears to have a beneficial effect on the development of the infant's gastrointestinal system. It also interacts with other growth factors to optimize development and increase the rate of certain cell migration [34].

EPO is not known to have a direct effect on fertility; however, it increases energy levels and sexual function and regulates menstrual cycles. This is possibly by normalizing prolactin levels, thereby increasing the chance of pregnancy [35].

EPO can be used safely in pregnancy, and in certain instances replacement of hematinics such as iron are inadequate and correction of anemia can only be brought about by replacement of EPO or a blood transfusion [36].

Blood transfusions should be avoided in pregnancies and in transplant recipients and only used where essential such as acute significant blood loss associated with postpartum hemorrhage, placenta previa or abruptio placenta.

Post-transplant Erythrocytosis

Post-transplant erythrocytosis (PTE) or polycythemia is defined as a hematocrit of more than 51 percent and occurs in up to 20 percent of transplant patients, usually within the first two years of transplantation. The etiology of PTE remains uncertain, but it may be due to an over-secretion of EPO by native kidneys, the transplanted kidney or the liver. Erythrocytosis, if untreated, is associated with increased incidence of vascular and thromboembolic disorders. This condition is often treated with angiotensin converting enzymes (ACE) inhibitors or ARBs, which are contraindicated in pregnancy. Pregnant transplant patients known to have PTE need regular monitoring of the hemocrit and assessment of thromboembolic risk. If hemocrit rises significantly, venesection could be considered.

Hemoglobinopathies

Long-term morbidity and mortality has improved significantly in sickle cell patients and other hereditary hemoglobinopathies like Thalassemia such that they are living well into adulthood. Individuals with these conditions require additional genetic counseling during their workup in order to ensure they are aware of the inheritance pattern and that their partners have undergone screening. There is an increased incidence of deep vein thrombosis, pulmonary embolism, obstetric complications, pneumonia, sepsis and postpartum infection. Less common are acute kidney injury, cerebrovascular disorder, respiratory distress syndrome, eclampsia, postpartum hemorrhage, preterm birth and ventilation [37]. In addition they are more likely to require transfusions, ideally exchange transfusions to avoid iron overload, particularly as the transfusion requirements increase as pregnancy progresses. Erythropoietin can also be employed, but response is usually inadequate to preclude the need for transfusions. The addition of a transplant means enhanced potential complications and there is an increased risk of deterioration in graft function, thereby impacting overall graft survival. Management of such cases requires the multispecialist input of transplant specialist, obstetrician, and specialist hematologist.

Thromboembolic Risk

Renal transplant patients often have proteinuria during pregnancy (which may increase following discontinuation of an ACE inhibitor or ARB) or other comorbid factors or clotting abnormalities that may increase their thromboembolic risk. In this situation a pregnant renal transplant patient may be prescribed

prophylaxis with low-molecular-weight heparin (or unfractionated heparin depending on their renal function) (see Chapter 5).

Hyperlipidemia

An increasing number of renal transplant recipients are treated with statin therapy for hypercholesterolemia and to reduce the risk of coronary events, stroke and cardiovascular morbidity following renal transplantation. It is not clear, however, whether transplantation confers an additional risk. Some immunosuppressant agents such as calcineurin inhibitors, mTOR inhibitors and steroids lead to an increase in lipid levels. Pregnancy is associated with an increase in lipid levels (mainly triglycerides). This change is most marked in the third trimester. Profound increases in triglyceride levels can lead to pancreatitis.

None of the widely used lipid lowering agents (statins, fibrates or ezetimibe) is used routinely in pregnancy. Animal studies have suggested that statins are teratogenic and case reports in humans reported central nervous system and limb defects in newborns exposed to statins in utero [38]. The highly lipophilic statins such as atorvastatin and simvastatin reach concentrations in the fetal circulation that are similar to maternal levels. These agents are contraindicated in pregnancy. Pravastatin is more hydrophilic and to date has not been associated with abnormal pregnancy outcomes. These drugs should be discontinued before conception. Fibrates may be used in cases of extreme hypertriglyceridemia.

Skeletal Problems

Preexisting bone problems are a common consideration in the pregnant renal transplant patient.

Seventy-seven percent of renal transplant patients have abnormal parathyroid hormone concentrations [39], owing to chronic renal impairment following renal transplantation or because of incomplete resolution of pre-transplant hyperparathyroidism. In addition, some patients may have had a previous parathyroidectomy.

Severe primary hyperparathyroidism is associated with poor pregnancy outcome, with increased neonatal death (31 percent) and hypocalcemia (19 percent) [40]. In a single case report of a renal transplant patient with mild tertiary hyperparathyroidism (adjusted calcium 2.74 mmol/l, parathyroid hormone

Table 12.1 Management of skeletal problems in pregnant renal transplant patients

	Usual treatment	Treatment during pregnancy
Secondary hyperparathyroidism	Phosphate binders	Continue calcium carbonate
		Discontinue sevelamer or lanthanum
	Alfacalcidol	Continue alfacalcidol
Tertiary hyperparathyroidism	Parathyroidectomy	In very severe cases consider surgery in second trimester [39]
		Monitor calcium levels closely in pregnancy
	Cinacalcet	Discontinue cinacalcet
Previous parathyroidectomy	Alfacalcidol	Continue alfacalcidol
	Calcium supplements	Continue calcium supplements
Osteoporosis	Calcium supplements	Continue calcium supplements and vitamin D?
	Bisphosphonates	Discontinue bisphosphonates
Osteopenia	Calcium supplements	Continue calcium supplements and vitamin D?

14 pmol/l), serum calcium level remained stable during pregnancy despite deterioration in renal function. The infant developed mild neonatal hypocalcemia, requiring treatment with intravenous calcium gluconate. It is important that infants of mothers with hyperparathyroidism are monitored for clinical signs of hypocalcemia (irritability, jerking, grimacing and convulsions) and that serum calcium levels are checked regularly following delivery.

Renal transplant patients may be prescribed numerous medications for the management of skeletal problems, including calcium supplements, alfacalcidol, phosphate binders, bisphosphonates and, more recently, cinacalcet. The use of these agents must be carefully considered before and during pregnancy (Table 12.1). Calcium supplements and alfacalcidol are safe in pregnancy and should be continued. Some phosphate binders are safe, including calcium carbonate-based binders, but the newer phosphate binders, including sevelamer and lanthanum carbonate, should be avoided in pregnancy, although there is little evidence at present and each case must be assessed individually.

As a result of steroid therapy pre and/or post transplantation, some young women who have had a transplant may have osteoporosis or osteopenia. Bisphosphonates used in the treatment and prevention of osteoporosis act to inhibit bone resorption. Due to their small molecular weight, bisphosphonates are known to cross the placenta, but very little is known about their safety in pregnancy. Early information was conflicting with some reports from animal studies indicating accumulation in fetal bones and possible maternal hypocalcemia in late pregnancy. One report in humans found no adverse effect of bisphosphonates on the human fetus [41], which was endorsed by Onroy et al. [42] reporting no adverse effects on pregnancy outcome when alendronate was taken prepregnancy or in early pregnancy in 24 pregnancies. Reports of women who have had bone scintigraphy with ^{99m}Tc-methylene diphosphonate showed radionuclide uptake by both placenta and fetus [43].

There may be an association with fetal skeletal anomalies, reduced gestational age and hypocalcemia in infants; the first two, however, may be related to other comorbidities in mothers. Animal models demonstrate anomalies in both mother and fetus such as embryolethality, general underdevelopment, marked skeletal retardation of fetus (increased diaphyseal bone trabeculae, decreased diaphyseal length, small fetal weight and abnormal tooth growth). It is noteworthy that these changes are at doses much higher than those used clinically [44].

The safety of these agents in pregnancy is an area that requires more research. In general, bisphosphonates should be discontinued at least six months to a year if possible prepregnancy, particularly for the older formulations such as pamidronate and alendronate, which have a long half-life, or as soon as pregnancy is suspected.

Careful consideration should be given before these agents are prescribed to women of childbearing age. In situations where a bisphosphonate is thought to be essential, there may be a case for using one of the new-generation bisphosphonates, which have a much shorter half-life.

Other Comorbid Diseases

Diabetes

A renal transplant patient may have end-stage renal disease due to diabetic nephropathy or may have developed new-onset diabetes after transplant (NODAT). In addition, transplant patients receiving steroids and tacrolimus are at increased risk of gestational diabetes (3–12 percent) [1]. Therefore, glucose tolerance testing may be warranted during pregnancy in tacrolimus / steroid-treated patients (see Chapter 15).

There are several additional issues to consider in a diabetic renal transplant recipient who is pregnant. The risks of preterm delivery and preeclampsia are increased by both diabetes and renal transplantation. Intrauterine growth restriction is less common in diabetic pregnancies as macrosomia is more common particularly in those with preexisting or poorly controlled diabetes. Patients with diabetic nephropathy affecting the transplanted kidney may have significant proteinuria during pregnancy (especially if ACE inhibitors and ARBs have been discontinued at conception) and present an increased thromboembolic risk during pregnancy as previously described. In addition, edema and severe nephrotic syndrome may require diuretic treatment during pregnancy.

Those with gestational diabetes are ideally treated with lifestyle changes, diet and exercise only, but some may require treatment with insulin and/or oral hypoglycemic agents during pregnancy. Alpha-glucosidase inhibitors (acrabase) are contraindicated in pregnancy. Sulphonyureas and biguanides, particularly metformin, have been used in South Africa and Australasia for more than three decades. Metformin had been in use particularly in Australasia prior to formal clinical trials [45]. Data generated from clinical trials suggest that benefit outweighs potential risk to the mother, fetus and breastfeeding infant [46–49]. Use of biguanides may help in women struggling with weight gain. As a result of the clearer understanding of the pathophysiology of diabetes several new agents have been developed such as incretin-based therapies (glucagons like therapies), SGLT2 inhibitors (gliflozins), glucokinase inhibitor, dipeptidyl peptidase 4 (DDP-4) and thioglitazones. In the absence of adequate pregnancy data on these agents they should be avoided in pregnancy and ideally stopped three months prior to conception. In the pregnant diabetic renal transplant patient, it is very important to maintain close liaison between specialist renal and diabetic obstetric teams throughout the pregnancy.

Systemic Lupus Erythematosus

One to two percent of patients on the renal transplant waiting list have lupus nephritis as a cause of end-stage renal disease. The success of renal transplantation in this group is comparable to that of other recipient groups. Systemic lupus erythematosus (SLE) is a disease that frequently affects young women and pregnancy is often a consideration for this group of renal transplant recipients. The transplant patient with an underlying diagnosis of SLE can face several additional problems during pregnancy, including recurrent miscarriages (see Chapter 14). A further consideration in this group is the potential presence of lupus anticoagulant and anticardiolipin antibody in some patients, which further increases the risk of fetal loss. Such patients may require prophylactic low-molecular-weight heparin therapy during pregnancy and aspirin. The presence of anti-Ro and anti-La antibodies leads to an increased risk of fetal cardiac problems. In this situation there is a risk of congenital heart block. SLE is associated with increased risk of preterm delivery and preeclampsia. Infants require monitoring for neonatal lupus, which includes a rash and thrombocytopenia, as well as congenital heart block.

Post-transplant Malignancy

Renal transplant patients are at increased risk of malignancy compared with the general population. In particular, the risks of skin cancers, lymphomas and in situ carcinomas, including carcinoma of the cervix, are increased.

Cervical Neoplasia

Several authors have reported increased incidence of cervical neoplasia in renal transplant recipients [50–52]. Kasiske et al. reported the incidence of cervical cancer to be increased five-fold [52]. However, Halpert et al. [50] reported a 17-fold increase and Ozsaran et al. [51] reported a 75 percent incidence in heavily immunosuppressed kidney transplant recipients.

Table 12.2 Management plan for pregnant renal transplant patients with additional comorbidities

Comorbidity	Prepregnancy	First trimester	Second trimester	Third trimester	Postpartum
General antenatal care in renal transplant patients	Confirm rubella antibody status. Hb electrophoresis. Advice regarding stopping smoking. Folic acid.	Folic acid. Discuss Down syndrome testing options. GTT in high-risk cases. Commence Aspirin 75mg od	Consider GTT in tacrolimus/steroid-treated patients at 24–28 weeks if indicated. Fetal USS monitoring	Consider steroid cover in labor. Fetal USS monitoring	
Renal transplant	Discuss implications of pregnancy on: • graft function • BP • proteinuria • risk of preeclampsia • obstetric risks. Immunosuppression: review current regimen and discuss/plan modification or conversion to alternative drugs, e.g. azathioprine. Review other medications, e.g. statins, diuretics, ACE inhibitors.	Discuss prepregnancy issues if not seen before conception. Monitor BP. Monitor CNI levels. Monitor proteinuria. Monitor renal function. Advise regarding genetic issues: polycystic kidney disease or chronic pyelonephritis (baby will need a USS) (record in maternal notes). Review other medications, e.g. statins, diuretics, ACE inhibitors.	Monitor BP. Monitor CNI levels. Monthly MSU. Monitor proteinuria. Monitor renal function.	Monitor BP. Monitor CNI levels. Monthly MSU. Monitor proteinuria. Monitor renal function. Discuss mode of delivery, review transplant operation note/discuss with transplant surgeon.	Monitor CNI levels. Monitor renal function. Arrange transplant OPD follow-up.
Recurrent UTIs	Discuss increased risk of UTIs and implications in pregnancy. Optimize immunosuppression and diabetic control. Advise regarding prevention of UTI. Plan monthly MSU and consider appropriate prophylaxis.	Monthly MSU. Treat infections promptly. Consider antibiotic prophylaxis if recurrent UTI. May require further investigation if additional pathology suspected clinically – USS.	Monthly MSU. Treat infections promptly. Consider antibiotic prophylaxis if recurrent UTI. May require further investigation if additional pathology suspected clinically – USS.	Monthly MSU. Treat infections promptly. Consider antibiotic prophylaxis if recurrent UTI. May require further investigation if additional pathology suspected clinically – USS.	Continue prophylaxis if previously prescribed. In mothers with chronic pyelonephritis and vesicoureteric reflux liaise with pediatricians regarding renal USS for the child.

Bone disease	Discuss and review current medication. Stop bisphosphonates and consider/convert phosphate binders.	Monitor bone biochemistry.	Monitor bone biochemistry.	Monitor bone biochemistry.	Monitor neonatal calcium levels if mother has marked hyperparathyroidism. Recommence the most suitable treatment for mother (depending on infant feeding). Avoid bisphosphonates if mother is planning further pregnancies.
Hypertension	Discuss implications of hypertension and safety of drugs in pregnancy. Plan conversion to alternative BP agents if required. Discuss risk of preeclampsia and consider aspirin prophylaxis.	Stop ACE inhibitors and ARBs, Convert other agents to methyldopa, labetalol or calcium channel blocker. Stop diuretics unless strong clinical indication to continue.	Monitor BP and titrate medication.	Monitor BP and titrate medication.	Monitor BP. Depending on infant feeding, restart ACE inhibitors and ARBs, change methyldopa, labetalol to alternative antihypertensive agents.
Proteinuria	Discuss implications of proteinuria, possible thromboembolic risks and edema.	Assess thromboembolic risk. Assess need for LMWH prophylaxis.	Monitor proteinuria. Assess thromboembolic risk. Assess need for LMWH prophylaxis.	Monitor proteinuria. Assess thromboembolic risk. Assess need for LMWH prophylaxis.	Continue LMWH prophylaxis for up to six weeks postpartum. Consider degree of proteinuria, mode of delivery, other risk factors for thrombosis. Restart ACE inhibitors and/or ARBs.
Diabetes	Discuss risk in pregnancy and management plan. Increased risk of preeclampsia	Arrange liaison/combined follow-up with diabetes antenatal team. Monitor proteinuria. Monitor diabetes.	Monitor proteinuria. Monitor diabetes.	Monitor proteinuria. Monitor diabetes.	Monitor diabetes. Recommence ACE inhibitors and/or ARBs
SLE	Discuss risks in pregnancy and increased risk of	Check and monitor lupus serology.	Fetal heart scanning/monitoring in Ro and La	Fetal heart scanning/monitoring in Ro and La	Review LMWH duration and whether there is

Table 12.2 (cont.)

Comorbidity	Prepregnancy	First trimester	Second trimester	Third trimester	Postpartum
	preeclampsia. Check anticardiolipin antibodies, lupus anticoagulant. Check anti Ro and La antibodies.	Consider need for LMWH in antiphospholipid antibody-positive women. Plan fetal heart monitoring in Ro and La antibody-positive women.	antibody-positive women.	antibody-positive women.	a need to continue longer term. Depends on other factors: proteinuria, delivery, other risk factors, etc.
Anemia	In women with CKD (T) discuss possibility of anemia requiring iron therapy and/or EPO. Check hematinics.	Monitor Hb: if < 11 g/dl consider Fe and or EPO on an individual patient basis.	Monitor Hb: if < 11 g/dl consider Fe and or EPO on an individual patient basis. Check hematinics.	Monitor Hb: if < 11 g/dl consider Fe and or EPO on an individual patient basis. Check hematinics	Decide re continuation or discontinuation of therapy.

ACE = angiotensin-converting enzyme; ARB = angiotensin II receptor blocker; BP = blood pressure; CKD = chronic kidney disease; CNI = calcineurin inhibitor; EPO = erythropoietin; GTT = glucose tolerance test; Hb = hemoglobin; LMWH = low-molecular-weight heparin; MSU = midstream urine; OPD = outpatients department; SLE = systemic lupus erythematosus; USS = ultrasound scan; UTI = urinary tract infection

The diagnosis of precancerous changes in the cervix was associated with an increased risk of preterm birth in an Australian study of 17,633 women between 1982 and 2000. The risk was increased in treated and untreated women compared with the general population [53]. In view of the increased risk it is important that renal transplant patients undergo annual cervical screening to detect early disease [52], which can then be treated prepregnancy. The use of HPV vaccination may also confer some benefit [54, 55], but as an additive measure and not as a replacement for regular, timely screening [56].

Abnormal smears should be followed by colposcopy, but biopsies should be deferred until the second trimester to minimize the risk of pregnancy loss. If the diagnosis is made during pregnancy, definitive management with ablation or excision should be delayed until postpartum. More aggressive lesions including carcinoma in situ may require more definitive management during pregnancy.

References

1. Deshpande NA, James NT, Kucirka LM, Boyarsky BJ, Garonzik-Wang JM, Montgomery RA, et al. Pregnancy outcomes in kidney transplant recipients: A systematic review and meta-analysis. *American journal of transplantation: Official journal of the American Society of Transplantation and the American Society of Transplant Surgeons.* 2011;**11**(11):2388–2404.

2. McKay DB, Josephson MA. Pregnancy in recipients of solid organs – effects on mother and child. *The New England journal of medicine.* 2006;**354**(12):1281–1293.

3. McCormick T, Ashe RG, Kearney PM. Urinary tract infection in pregnancy. *The Obstetrician & Gynaecologist.* 2008;**10**(3):156–162.

4. Harris RE. The significance of eradication of bacteriuria during pregnancy. *Obstetrics and gynecology.* 1979;**53**(1):71–73.

5. Romero R, Oyarzun E, Mazor M, Sirtori M, Hobbins JC, Bracken M. Meta-analysis of the relationship between asymptomatic bacteriuria and preterm delivery/low birth weight. *Obstetrics and gynecology.* 1989;**73**(4):576–582.

6. Smaill F, Vazquez JC. Antibiotics for asymptomatic bacteriuria in pregnancy. *The Cochrane database of systematic reviews.* 2007;(2):CD000490.

7. European Best Practice Guidelines for Renal Transplantation. Section IV: Long-term management of the transplant recipient. IV.10. Pregnancy in renal transplant recipients. *Nephrol Dial Transplant.* 2002;**17** Suppl. 4:50–55.

8. Thompson BC, Kingdon EJ, Tuck SM, Fernando ON, Sweny P. Pregnancy in renal transplant recipients: The Royal Free Hospital experience. *QJM.* 2003;**96**(11):837–844.

9. Galdo T, Gonzalez F, Espinoza M, Quintero N, Espinoza O, Herrera S, et al. Impact of pregnancy on the function of transplanted kidneys. *Transplant Proc.* 2005;**37**(3):1577–1579.

10. Oliveira LG, Sass N, Sato JL, Ozaki KS, Medina Pestana JO. Pregnancy after renal transplantation – a five-yr single-center experience. *Clin Transplant.* 2007;**21**(3):301–304.

11. Hooi LS, Rozina G, Shaariah MY, Teo SM, Tan CH, Bavanandan S, et al. Pregnancy in patients with renal transplants in Malaysia. *Med J Malaysia.* 2003;**58**(1):27–36.

12. Vazquez JC, Villar J. Treatments for symptomatic urinary tract infections during pregnancy. *Cochrane Database Syst Rev.* 2000;(3):CD002256.

13. Stamm AM, Dismukes WE, Simmons BP, Cobbs CG, Elliott A, Budrich P, et al. Listeriosis in renal transplant recipients: Report of an outbreak and review of 102 cases. *Reviews of infectious diseases.* 1982;**4**(3):665–682.

14. Verani JR, McGee L, Schrag SJ, Division of Bacterial Diseases NCfI, Respiratory Diseases CfDC, Prevention. Prevention of perinatal group B streptococcal disease – revised guidelines from CDC, 2010. *MMWR recommendations and reports: Morbidity and mortality weekly report Recommendations and reports/Centers for Disease Control.* 2010;**59**(RR-10):1–36.

15. Andrews PA, Emery VC, Newstead C. Summary of the British Transplantation Society guidelines for the prevention and management of CMV disease after solid organ transplantation. *Transplantation.* 2011;**92**(11):1181–1187.

16. Humar A, Limaye AP, Blumberg EA, Hauser IA, Vincenti F, Jardine AG, et al. Extended valganciclovir prophylaxis in D+/R- kidney transplant recipients is associated with long-term reduction in cytomegalovirus disease: Two-year results of the IMPACT study. *Transplantation.* 2010;**90**(12):1427–1431.

17. Ventura AM, Imperiali N, Dominguez-Gil B, del Prado Sierra M, Munoz MA, Andres A, et al. Successful pregnancies in female kidney-transplant recipients with hepatitis C virus infection. *Transplantation proceedings.* 2003;**35**(3):1078–1080.

18. [bnf.org/bnf]. JFCBNFLBMAaRPSoGB.

19. Brown ZA, Selke S, Zeh J, Kopelman J, Maslow A, Ashley RL, et al. The acquisition of herpes simplex virus during pregnancy. *The New England journal of medicine.* 1997;**337**(8):509–515.

20. Harbell J, Terrault NA, Stock P. Solid organ transplants in HIV-infected patients. *Current HIV/AIDS reports.* 2013;**10**(3):217–225.

21. Diaz F, Collazos J, Mayo J, Martinez E. Sulfadiazine-induced multiple urolithiasis and acute renal failure in a patient with AIDS and Toxoplasma encephalitis. *The Annals of pharmacotherapy.* 1996;**30**(1):41–42.

22. Coyne DW BDAitRTRUwuc.

23. Breymann C. Treatment of iron deficiency anaemia in pregnancy and postpartum with special focus on intravenous iron sucrose complex. *Journal of the Medical Association of Thailand = Chotmaihet thangphaet.* 2005;**88** Suppl. 2:S108–S109.

24. Sifakis S, Angelakis E, Vardaki E, Koumantaki Y, Matalliotakis I, Koumantakis E. Erythropoietin in the treatment of iron deficiency anemia during pregnancy. *Gynecologic and obstetric investigation.* 2001;**51**(3):150–156.

25. Reveiz L, Gyte GM, Cuervo LG, Casasbuenas A. Treatments for iron-deficiency anaemia in pregnancy. *The Cochrane database of systematic reviews.* 2011(**10**): CD003094.

26. Perewusnyk G, Huch R, Huch A, Breymann C. Parenteral iron therapy in obstetrics: 8 years experience with iron-sucrose complex. *The British journal of nutrition.* 2002;**88**(1):3–10.

27. Pavord S, Myers B, Robinson S, Allard S, Strong J, Oppenheimer C, et al. UK guidelines on the management of iron deficiency in pregnancy. *British journal of haematology.* 2012;**156**(5):588–600.

28. Breymann C, von Seefried B, Stahel M, Geisser P, Canclini C. Milk iron content in breast-feeding mothers after administration of intravenous iron sucrose complex. *Journal of perinatal medicine.* 2007;**35**(2):115–118.

29. Magee LA, von Dadelszen P, Darley J, Beguin Y. Erythropoiesis and renal transplant pregnancy. *Clinical transplantation.* 2000;**14**(2):127–135.

30. Thorp M, Pulliam J. Use of recombinant erythropoietin in a pregnant renal transplant recipient. *American journal of nephrology.* 1998;**18**(5):448–451.

31. Goshorn J, Youell TD. Darbepoetin alfa treatment for post-renal transplantation anemia during pregnancy. *American journal of kidney diseases: The official journal of the National Kidney Foundation.* 2005;**46**(5):e81–6.

32. Kashiwagi M, Breymann C, Huch R, Huch A. Hypertension in a pregnancy with renal anemia after recombinant human erythropoietin (rhEPO) therapy.

Archives of gynecology and obstetrics. 2002;**267**(1):54–56.

33. Resch BE, Gaspar R, Sonkodi S, Falkay G. Vasoactive effects of erythropoietin on human placental blood vessels in vitro. *American journal of obstetrics and gynecology.* 2003;**188**(4):993–996.

34. Juul SE, Joyce AE, Zhao Y, Ledbetter DJ. Why is erythropoietin present in human milk? Studies of erythropoietin receptors on enterocytes of human and rat neonates. *Pediatric research.* 1999;**46**(3):263–268.

35. Schaefer RM, Kokot F, Wernze H, Geiger H, Heidland A. Improved sexual function in hemodialysis patients on recombinant erythropoietin: A possible role for prolactin. *Clinical nephrology.* 1989;**31**(1):1–5.

36. Krafft A, Bencaiova G, Breymann C. Selective use of recombinant human erythropoietin in pregnant patients with severe anemia or nonresponsive to iron sucrose alone. *Fetal diagnosis and therapy.* 2009;**25**(2):239–245.

37. Boulet SL, Okoroh EM, Azonobi I, Grant A, Craig Hooper W. Sickle cell disease in pregnancy: Maternal complications in a Medicaid-enrolled population. *Maternal and child health journal.* 2013;**17**(2):200–207.

38. Edison RJ, Muenke M. Central nervous system and limb anomalies in case reports of first-trimester statin exposure. *The New England journal of medicine.* 2004;**350**(15):1579–1582.

39. Morton A, Dalzell F, Isbel N, Prado T. Pregnancy outcome in a renal transplant recipient with residual mild tertiary hyperparathyroidism. *BJOG: An international journal of obstetrics and gynaecology.* 2005;**112**(1):124–125.

40. Schnatz PF, Curry SL. Primary hyperparathyroidism in pregnancy: Evidence-based management. *Obstetrical & gynecological survey.* 2002;**57**(6):365–376.

41. Rutgers-Verhage AR, deVries TW, Torringa MJ. No effects of bisphosphonates on the human fetus. *Birth defects research Part A, Clinical and molecular teratology.* 2003;**67**(3):203–204.

42. Ornoy A, Wajnberg R, Diav-Citrin O. The outcome of pregnancy following pre-pregnancy or early pregnancy alendronate treatment. *Reproductive toxicology.* 2006;**22**(4):578–579.

43. McKenzie AF, Budd RS, Yang C, Shapiro B, Hicks RJ. Technetium-99 m-methylene diphosphonate uptake in the fetal skeleton at 30 weeks gestation. *Journal of nuclear medicine: Official publication, Society of Nuclear Medicine.* 1994;**35**(8):1338–1341.

44. Stathopoulos IP, Liakou CG, Katsalira A, Trovas G, Lyritis GG, Papaioannou NA, et al. The use of bisphosphonates in women prior to or during pregnancy and lactation. *Hormones.* 2011;**10**(4):280–291.

45. Kyle PM. Drugs and the fetus. *Current opinion in obstetrics & gynecology.* 2006;**18**(2):93–99.

46. Gutzin SJ, Kozer E, Magee LA, Feig DS, Koren G. The safety of oral hypoglycemic agents in the first trimester of pregnancy: A meta-analysis. *The Canadian journal of clinical pharmacology = Journal canadien de pharmacologie clinique.* 2003;**10**(4):179–183.

47. Gilbert C, Valois M, Koren G. Pregnancy outcome after first-trimester exposure to metformin: A meta-analysis. *Fertility and sterility.* 2006;**86**(3):658–663.

48. Ekpebegh CO, Coetzee EJ, van der Merwe L, Levitt NS. A 10-year retrospective analysis of pregnancy outcome in pregestational Type 2 diabetes: comparison of insulin and oral glucose-lowering agents. *Diabetic medicine: A journal of the British Diabetic Association.* 2007;**24**(3):253–258.

49. Rowan JA, Hague WM, Gao W, Battin MR, Moore MP, Mi GTI. Metformin versus insulin for the treatment of gestational diabetes. *The New England journal of medicine.* 2008;**358**(19):2003–2015.

50. Halpert R, Fruchter RG, Sedlis A, Butt K, Boyce JG, Sillman FH. Human papillomavirus and lower genital neoplasia in renal transplant patients. *Obstetrics and gynecology.* 1986;**68**(2):251–258.

51. Ozsaran AA, Ates T, Dikmen Y, Zeytinoglu A, Terek C, Erhan Y, et al. Evaluation of the risk of cervical intraepithelial neoplasia and human papilloma virus infection in renal transplant patients receiving immunosuppressive therapy. *European journal of gynaecological oncology.* 1999;**20**(2):127–130.

52. Kasiske BL, Snyder JJ, Gilbertson DT, Wang C. Cancer after kidney transplantation in the United States. *American journal of transplantation: Official journal of the American Society of Transplantation and the American Society of Transplant Surgeons.* 2004;**4**(6):905–913.

53. Bruinsma F, Lumley J, Tan J, Quinn M. Precancerous changes in the cervix and risk of subsequent preterm birth. *BJOG: An international journal of obstetrics and gynaecology.* 2007;**114**(1):70–80.

54. Markowitz LE, Hariri S, Lin C, Dunne EF, Steinau M, McQuillan G, et al. Reduction in human papillomavirus (HPV) prevalence among young women following HPV vaccine introduction in the United States, National Health and Nutrition Examination Surveys, 2003–2010. *The Journal of infectious diseases.* 2013;**208**(3):385–393.

55. Kahn JA. HPV vaccination for the prevention of cervical intraepithelial neoplasia. *The New England journal of medicine.* 2009;**361**(3):271–278.

56. Tomljenovic L, Spinosa JP, Shaw CA. Human papillomavirus (HPV) vaccines as an option for preventing cervical malignancies: (How) effective and safe? *Current pharmaceutical design.* 2013;**19**(8):1466–1487.

Chapter 13

Reflux Nephropathy in Pregnancy

Nigel Brunskill

Vesicoureteric Reflux and Reflux Nephropathy – Epidemiology, Pathogenesis and Clinical Features

One third of all anomalies detected by routine fetal ultrasonography are congenital abnormalities of the kidney and urinary tract (CAKUT) [1, 2]. The spectrum of abnormalities seen in individuals with CAKUT is wide and includes ureteric abnormalities (e.g. vesicoureteric reflux [VUR], megaureter and ureterovesical junction obstruction) and kidney abnormalities (e.g. aplastic kidneys, multicystic dysplasic kidneys, hydronephrosis and duplex kidney). CAKUT are observed more frequently in the offspring of women with conditions such as obesity [3] or diabetes mellitus [3, 4] in the first 20 weeks of pregnancy.

In clinical practice, VUR is the most common manifestation of CAKUT with an incidence in the general population of at least 0.4 percent to 1.8 percent [5–7]. Primary VUR results in the retrograde passage of urine from the bladder through the ureter into the upper urinary tract. In the majority, VUR resolves with time and is most often manifest in childhood [8]. There is now clear recognition that this has a familial component. Early segregation analysis pointed to a single dominant gene [9], but more recent evidence points to a polygenic genetically heterogeneous trait with multiple candidate genes affecting males and females equally [10–14].

Reflux nephropathy is a term that describes coarse unilateral or bilateral renal scarring often found in association with VUR, an appearance previously known as *chronic pyelonephritis*. However, only a proportion of children with VUR subsequently develops reflux nephropathy. Under the age of eight years 26 percent of children diagnosed with VUR have renal scars, whereas in children older than eight years, 47 percent have renal scars at the time of diagnosis of VUR [15]. Reflux nephropathy is the most common cause of end-stage renal disease (ESRD) in children and accounts for 10 percent of all ESRD [16].

In the majority of affected children, the focal scars characteristic of reflux nephropathy develop early in childhood, usually in the setting of severe intra-renal reflux and urinary infection. Some children with VUR, particularly boys, demonstrate small, smooth kidneys at birth with histological evidence of renal dysplasia in addition to VUR [8]. Hypertension is common [17] and progressive renal impairment toward ESRD occurs predominantly in those with gross VUR with severe bilateral scarring. The bulk of the initiating injury occurs in early childhood and ESRD may develop thereafter despite the resolution of VUR and in the absence of infection [18].

Some individuals with VUR and reflux nephropathy are detected through screening programs in the context of a family history. The commonest clinical presentation of VUR and reflux nephropathy, however, is a complicated urinary tract infection (UTI). The finding of hypertension, proteinuria and/or renal impairment in children and adults may also lead to the subsequent discovery of reflux nephropathy.

Reflux Nephropathy in Pregnancy

Some asymptomatic and otherwise healthy women with reflux nephropathy may present in pregnancy largely because the antenatal care setting often provides the first opportunity for blood pressure monitoring, urine dipstick analysis and the detection of urinary infection in affected women. Renal scarring and impaired renal function may be detected during subsequent investigation of these abnormal findings. There are several reasons why a maternal diagnosis of reflux nephropathy may impact the outcome of a pregnancy.

Reflux Nephropathy and Urinary Sepsis in Pregnancy

Urinary tract infections are one of the commonest health problems during normal pregnancy, complicating 8 percent of pregnancies [19, 20], and women with VUR are at particularly increased risk. Although patients with VUR and reflux nephropathy are prone to urine infection, the reasons are not fully understood. With the combination of physiological dilatation of the urinary tract in pregnancy and severe VUR, urinary stasis certainly plays a part [18].

Given that it is generally accepted that urine infection may hasten renal scar formation, such infections in pregnancy merit treatment on this basis alone. The occurrence of symptomatic UTI in pregnancy is associated with increased risk of preterm rupture of membranes, preterm birth and low birth weight in addition to serious maternal complications such as septic shock [21]. Asymptomatic bacteriuria in pregnancy may be accompanied by similar complications, although this remains controversial [22]. Nonetheless, current consensus suggests that both asymptomatic bacteriuria and UTI in pregnancy should be promptly treated with antibiotics to prevent obstetric and maternal complications [21, 22]. In the presence of reflux nephropathy, screening for bacteriuria should be performed regularly. No studies have assessed the optimum timing for such surveillance, although at least once in each trimester has been suggested [18]. If bacteriuria or UTI are detected, eradication should be achieved using appropriate antibiotics. If urinary infection is recurrent, prophylactic antibiotics should be considered.

Effect of Reflux Nephropathy on Obstetric and Maternal Outcomes in Pregnancy

How renal disease impacts pregnancy outcomes has been an issue of interest and debate for 30 years. Based on a number of predominantly retrospective studies, it is currently believed that for pregnancy in the presence of renal disease: i) outcomes are largely dependent on renal function such that if renal functional loss is less than 50 percent, then pregnancy is likely to be successful; ii) complications such as preeclampsia and preterm birth are increased; iii) poorly controlled hypertension predicts a worse outcome; iv) the presence of heavy proteinuria is accompanied by increased risks; and v) renal impairment associated with systemic diseases such as lupus and scleroderma carries a worse prognosis [23–31] (see Chapters 2 and 5).

Several authors have specifically studied the outcome of pregnancies complicated by reflux nephropathy and the results have sometimes been controversial. The series of Katz and colleagues (32) included 26 (out of 121) pregnancies in women with renal biopsy proven interstitial nephritis likely due to reflux nephropathy, with serum creatinine (SCr) levels ≤1.4 mg/dL (≤125 μmol/L). The course of pregnancy and the underlying renal disease in these women did not appear different from those with other pathologies.

In 1986 the Australian group of Becker and colleagues [33] reported in pregnancy outcomes in six women with reflux nephropathy, diagnosed according to typical radiological features, who formed part of a subgroup of 20 women with "moderate" renal failure (serum creatinine [SCr] 200–400 μmol/L) among a larger cohort of 184 female patients with reflux nephropathy under long-term follow-up. Pregnancy was associated with rapid loss of renal function in all six, with four women requiring dialysis within two years of delivery. Two babies of mothers with reflux did not survive. The authors suggested that women with reflux nephropathy contemplating pregnancy should be specifically warned of the risk of ESRD. However, in the French series of 245 pregnancies in 99 patients with reflux nephropathy reported by Jungers and colleagues [34, 35, 26] in 1986, 1987 and 1997, pregnancy outcomes were more favorable, and rapidly decreasing renal function was seen only in two hypertensive patients with SCr > 200μmol/L, but not in the majority with better-preserved renal function.

Updating the Australian experience in 1997, El-Khatib and colleagues [37] presented data from 345 pregnancies in 137 women with unequivocal reflux nephropathy and/or VUR. More than 50 percent of these pregnancies were complicated. Twenty-six percent of women developed UTI with 6 percent developing acute pyelonephritis. The rate of fetal loss of 18 percent in those with SCr > 110 μmol/L was significantly greater than that of 8 percent in those with SCr < 110 μmol/L at conception. Maternal complications such as preeclampsia were greater in the presence of bilateral renal scarring, but persistent VUR had no impact on any pregnancy outcomes. Overall therefore in this study, the risk of maternal and obstetric complications was predominantly related to the degree of underlying renal impairment and severity of renal scarring.

Jungers and colleagues [38] updated their French series by reporting outcomes in a cohort of 375 pregnancies in 158 women with reflux nephropathy seen over a period of 30 years up to 1994. The diagnosis of reflux nephropathy was carefully established using standard radiological investigations, and in 113 women, the presence or absence of persisting VUR was determined by micturating cystourethrography. In this latter group, persistent reflux was present in 43 percent. Interestingly, the diagnosis of reflux nephropathy was unknown in 56 percent of these women prior to their first pregnancy, and was only revealed after investigation of UTI, proteinuria, hypertension and/or renal impairment. The most common complication was UTI in 22 percent of pregnancies, and UTI was more common and severe in those with persistent VUR, but UTI did not appear to have substantial deleterious effects on fetal outcomes. The authors suggested that prospective mothers with VUR and recurrent UTI, particularly pyelonephritis, should consider prophylactic ureteric re-implantation. Maternal renal function deterioration was observed in 87 percent of women with SCr > 110 μmol/L pre-pregnancy compared to only 1.2 percent of those with SCr < 110 μmol/L before pregnancy. Live births occurred in 92 percent of pregnancies where preconception SCr was < 110 μmol/L, but in only 63 percent of pregnancies with preconception SCr was > 110 μmol/L. Fetal loss was much more common in hypertensive mothers. Taking the 30-year cohort as a whole, outcomes generally seemed to show evidence of significant improvement over time and were better when management of pregnancy was intensified and carefully coordinated between obstetricians and nephrologists. Taken together, the literature suggests that in women with VUR, the presence of renal scarring is the key determinant of the risk of gestational hypertension, preeclampsia and other morbidity in pregnancy [39].

Recently, Roihuvuo-Leskinen and colleagues reported a Finnish case series of 175 deliveries in 87 women with VUR definitively diagnosed in childhood. Urinary tract infections were common and seen in around a third of women. Taken together, maternal complications were observed in 64 percent of women in pregnancy, and were significantly more common in those with renal scars. Fetal complications such as preterm birth, low birth weight and poor intrauterine growth were less common and observed in 13 percent of women. However, in this study, renal scars were not associated with increased fetal complications [40].

Some studies have suggested that outcomes in pregnancies complicated by glomerular diseases may be less favorable than those complicated by reflux nephropathy [23, 25, 26]. These comparisons are seriously limited by small numbers of women in such studies.

Screening for VUR

Infants born to mothers with VUR may inherit the condition. If the maternal diagnosis is apparent during pregnancy, the antenatal ultrasound may be used to detect characteristic changes of reflux nephropathy in the fetus [18, 41]. Failing this, the offspring of patients with either known VUR or a first-degree relative with VUR should be investigated as soon as possible after birth [18]. In the past, some interest has been shown in screening for bacteriuria in schoolchildren as a potential indicator of underlying VUR, but this is no longer regarded as a practical or useful undertaking [42].

Conclusion

Reflux nephropathy is relatively common in pregnancy. However, while there are particular problems relating to UTI in pregnancies with reflux nephropathy, these can be adequately treated with standard antibiotics (see Chapter 7). There is no justification for prospective mothers to undergo micturating cystourethrography with a view to prophylactic ureteral re-implantation prior to pregnancy. Overall outcomes of pregnancies with reflux nephropathy appear to be related predominantly to the degree of underlying renal impairment and presence of hypertension rather than the underlying renal disease per se. Women with reflux nephropathy should be screened regularly for urinary infection in pregnancy and treated promptly should it occur. The offspring of the women should be screened for VUR.

References

1. Noia G, Masini L, De Santis M and Caruso A. The impact of invasive procedures on prognostic, diagnostic and therapeutic aspects of urinary tract anomalies. In *Neonatal nephrology in progress*, edited by Cataldi L, Fanos V, Simeoni U. Lecce, Italy, Agora, 1996, pp. 67–84.

2. Pope JCI, Brock JW, III, Adams MC, Stephens FD and Ichikawa I. How they begin and how they end: Classic and new theories for the development and deterioration of congenital anomalies of the kidney and urinary tract, CAKUT. *J Am Soc Nephrol* **10**, 2018–2028, 1999.

3. Hsu CW, Yamamoto KT, Henry RK, De Roos AJ and Flynn JT. Prenatal risk factors for childhood CKD. *J Am Soc Nephrol* **25**, 2105–2111, 2014.

4. Dart AB, Ruth CA, Sellers EA, Au W and Dean HJ. Maternal diabetes mellitus and congenital anomalies of the kidney and urinary tract (CAKUT) in the child. *Am J Kid Dis* S0272-6386(14)01527-3. doi: 10.1053/j.ajkd.2014.11.017. 2015. [Epub ahead of print]

5. Kincaid-Smith P and Becker G. Reflux nephropathy and chronic atrophic pyelonephritis: A review. *J Infect Dis* **138**, 774–780, 1978.

6. Bailey R. Vesicoureteric reflux in healthy infants and children. In *Reflux nephropathy*, edited by Hodson J and Kincaid-Smith P Masson, New York, 1979, pp. 59–61.

7. Sargent MA. What is the normal prevalence of vesicoureteral reflux? *Pediatr Radiol* **30**, 587–593, 2000.

8. Dillon MJ and Goonasekera CD. Reflux nephropathy. *J Am Soc Nephrol* **9**, 2377–2383, 1998.

9. Chapman CJ, Bailey RR, Janus ED, Abbott GD and Lynn KL. Vesicoureteric reflux: Segregation analysis. *Am J Med Genet* **20**, 577–584, 1985.

10. Feather SA, Malcolm S, Woolf AS, Wright V, Blaydon D, Reid CJ, Flinter FA, Proesmans W, Devriendt K, Carter J, Warwicker P, Goodship TH and Goodship JA. Primary, nonsyndromic vesicoureteric reflux and its nephropathy is genetically heterogeneous, with a locus on chromosome 1. *Am J Hum Genet* **66**, 1420–1425, 2000.

11. Mak RH and Kuo HJ. Primary ureteral reflux: Emerging insights from molecular and genetic studies. *Curr Opin Pediatr* **15**, 181–185, 2003.

12. Woolf AS, Price KL, Scambler PJ and Winyard PJD. Evolving concepts in human renal dysplasia. *J Am Soc Nephrol* **15**, 998–1007, 2004.

13. Murawski IJ and Gupta IR. Vesicoureteric reflux and renal malformations: A developmental problem. *Clinical Genetics* **69**: 105–117, 2006.

14. Lu W, Van Eerde AM, Fan X, Quintero-Rivera F, Kulkarni S, Ferguson H, Kim HG, Fan Y, Xi Q, Li QG, Sanlaville D, Andrews W, Sundaresan V, Bi W, Yan J, Giltay JC, Wijmenga C, de Jong TP, Feather SA, Woolf AS, Rao Y, Lupski JR, Eccles MR, Quade BJ, Gusella JF, Morton CC and Maas RL. Disruption of ROBO2 is associated with urinary tract anomalies and confers risk of vesicoureteral reflux. *Am J Hum Genet* **80**, 616–632, 2007.

15. Smellie J, Edwards D, Hunter N, Normand IC and Prescod N. Vesico-ureteric reflux and renal scarring. *Kidney Int Suppl* **4**: S65-72, 1975.

16. Bailey R. Vesicoureteric reflux and reflux nephropathy. In *Diseases of the kidney*, edited by Schrier RW GG. Boston, MA: Little Brown, 1988, pp. 747–783.

17. Goonasekera CDA and Dillon MJ. Hypertension in reflux nephropathy. *BJU International* **83**, 1–12, 1999.

18. Lynn K. Vesicoureteral reflux and reflux nephropathy. In *Comprehensive clinical nephrology*, edited by Feehally J, Floege J and Johnson RJ. Elsevier Health Sciences, 2007, p. 691–702.

19. Lucas MJ CF. Urinary infection in pregnancy. *Clin Obstet Gynecol* **36**, 855–868, 1993.

20. Mikhail MS AA. Lower urinary tract dysfunction in pregnancy: A review. *Obstet Gynecol Surv* **50**, 675–683, 1995.

21. Vazquez JC and Villar J. Treatments for symptomatic urinary tract infections during pregnancy. *Cochrane Database of Systematic Reviews* Article number CD002256: 2003.

22. Smaill F and Vazquez JC. Antibiotics for asymptomatic bacteriuria in pregnancy. *Cochrane Database of Systematic Reviews* Article number CD000490: 2007.

23. Imbasciati E and Ponticelli C. Pregnancy and renal disease: Predictors for fetal and maternal outcome. *Am J Nephrol* **11**, 353–362, 1991.

24. Jones DC and Hayslett JP. Outcome of pregnancy in women with moderate or severe renal insufficiency. *N Engl J Med* **335**, 226–232, 1996.

25. Jungers P and Chauveau D. Pregnancy in renal disease. *Kidney Int* **52**, 871–885, 1997.

26. Jungers P, Chauveau D, Choukroun G, Moynot A, Skhiri H, Houillier P, Forget D and Grunfeld JP. Pregnancy in women with impaired renal function. *Clin Nephrol* **47**, 281–288, 1997.

27. Davison JM. Renal disorders in pregnancy. *Curr Opin Obstet Gynecol* **13**, 109–114, 2001.

28. Fischer MJ, Lehnerz SD, Hebert JR and Parikh CR. Kidney disease is an independent risk factor for adverse fetal and maternal outcomes in pregnancy. *Am J Kidney Dis* **43**, 415–423, 2004.

29. Franceschini N, Savitz DA, Kaufman JS and Thorp JM. Maternal urine albumin excretion and pregnancy outcome. *Am J Kidney Dis* **45**, 1010–1018, 2005.

30. Imbasciati E, Gregorini G, Cabiddu G, Gammaro L, Ambroso G, Del Giudice A and Ravani P. Pregnancy in CKD stages 3 to 5: Fetal and maternal outcomes. *Am J Kidney Dis* **49**, 753–762, 2007.

31. Lindheimer MD and Davison JM. Pregnancy and CKD: Any progress? *Am J Kidney Dis* **49**, 729–731, 2007.

32. Katz AI, Davison JM, Hayslett JP, Singson E and Lindheimer MD. Pregnancy in women with kidney disease. *Kidney Int* **18**, 192–206, 1980.

33. Becker GJ, Ihle BU, Fairley KF, Bastos M and Kincaid-Smith P. Effect of pregnancy on moderate renal failure

in reflux nephropathy. *Br Med J (Clin Res Ed)* **292**, 796–798, 1986.

34. Jungers P, Forget D, Henry-Amar M, Albouze G, Fournier P, Vischer U, Droz D, Noel LH and Grunfeld JP. Chronic kidney disease and pregnancy. *Adv Nephrol Necker Hosp* **15**, 103–141, 1986.

35. Jungers P, Forget D, Houillier P, Henry-Amar M and Grunfeld JP. Pregnancy in IgA nephropathy, reflux nephropathy, and focal glomerular sclerosis. *Am J Kidney Dis* **9**, 334–338, 1987.

36. Jungers P, Houillier P and Forget D. Reflux nephropathy and pregnancy. *Baillieres Clin Obstet Gynaecol* **1**, 955–969, 1987.

37. El-Khatib M, Packham DK, Becker GJ and Kincaid-Smith P. Pregnancy-related complications in women with reflux nephropathy. *Clin Nephrol* **41**, 50–55, 1994.

38. Jungers P, Houllier P, Chaveau D, Choukroun G, Moynot A, Skhiri H, Labrunie M, Descamps-Latscha B and Grunfeld J-P. Pregnancy in women with reflux nephropathy. *Kidney Int* **50**, 593–609 1996.

39. Hollowell JG. Outcome of pregnancy in women with a history of vesico-ureteric reflux. *BJUI* **102**, 780–784, 2008.

40. Roihuvuo-Leskinen H-M, Vainio MI, Niskanen KM and Lahdes-Vasama TT. Pregnancies in women with childhood vesicoureteral reflux. *Acta Obstet Gynecol Scand* **94**, 847–851, 2015.

41. Blumenthal I. Vesicoureteric reflux and urinary tract infection in children. *Postgrad Med J* **82**, 31035, 2006.

42. Hansson S, Martinell J, Stokland E and Jodal U. The natural history of bacteriuria in childhood. *Inf Dis Clin North Am* **11**, 499–512, 1997.

Lupus and Vasculitis in Pregnancy

Liz Lightstone

Introduction

Lupus is a disease of women of childbearing age and so it is common to encounter women with lupus who wish to become pregnant or are pregnant. Lupus nephritis affects up to 60 percent or more of women with lupus and imposes increased risks to the mother and fetus. The treatments for lupus, especially for lupus nephritis, can impair fertility, and some are teratogenic. Women with lupus may have antibodies associated with miscarriage and poor placentation or antibodies that can cause neonatal lupus syndromes. Prepregnancy counseling is essential to ensure women are aware of the risks of pregnancy to them and their baby, to know the best timing for pregnancy and to ensure they are on safe medications. Vasculitis, which can affect large and small vessels, less commonly presents in women of childbearing age, and the literature surrounding management is much sparser. However, many of the same principles apply – planning, timing and correct medications. In both conditions, the health professionals caring for these women in pregnancy need to be able to recognize a disease flare and also to judge whether the women is having a disease flare and/or superimposed preeclampsia – a true clinical challenge, especially in women with lupus nephritis. This chapter focuses on women with lupus nephritis and those with vasculitis affecting the kidneys – most commonly the small-vessel vasculitidies – Granulomatous polyangiitis (GPA – formerly known as Wegener's granulomatosis) and microscopic polyangiitis (MPA) – and rarely the large vessel Takayasu vasculitis. For recent reviews, see references [1–6].

Lupus and Lupus Nephritis

Diagnosis

The diagnosis of lupus has recently been revised by the Systemic Lupus International Collaborating Clinics (SLICC) group. A patient can be classified as having lupus if they have four of the clinical and immunologic criteria used in the SLICC classification criteria, including at least one clinical criterion and one immunologic criterion, or if they have biopsy-proven nephritis compatible with SLE in the presence of anti-nuclear antibodies (ANAs) or anti-double stranded DNA antibodies (dsDNA) [7]. This is not always easy even in the nonpregnant woman, but new-onset rash or arthralgias may not initially be appreciated as part of systemic disease in pregnancy. Because of the close relationship, not fully understood, between hormonal state and lupus presentation and flares, it is not uncommon for patients to present for the first time during pregnancy. The combination of rash, arthralgias (overt arthritis is rare), unusual fatigue, and/or pleurisy and/or pericarditis, with or without proteinuria and/or hematuria should raise suspicion. Lupus has protean manifestations and clinicians need to be alert to the possibility in a woman with persisting and unexplained symptoms. Of course pregnancy can be associated with unusual fatigue, rashes, aches and pains, and pleuritic pain should raise the possibility of a pulmonary embolus before the diagnosis of lupus is addressed. Blood tests can be very useful in this setting.

Blood Tests

Patients with lupus tend to be penic – anemic, lymphopenic, often neutropenic and thrombocytopenic. If they have marked proteinuria they may be hypoalbuminemic – however, remember that a normal albumin for pregnancy is significantly lower than in the nonpregnant state. Serology is probably the most useful marker. Since pregnancy is essentially an acute phase response, serum complement should be normal or raised. A falling complement in the normal range might start to raise suspicion of active lupus and a low complement should definitely. In patients with lupus, C4 is often persistently low, but C3 falls with more active disease. ANA are very nonspecific, but the finding of anti dsDNA and/or anti Sm or anti RNP antibodies would confirm the diagnosis. The combination of rising anti dsDNA antibodies and falling complement should raise serious concern about impending flare.

Renal Function

Most women with lupus have apparently normal renal function with a serum creatinine within the normal range but their estimated glomerular filtration rate (eGFR) may well be reduced. The key signs of a renal flare are increasing proteinuria and hematuria on renal dip and a rise in creatinine, though it is very possible to have active lupus nephritis, especially class V, without any change in renal function.

Principles of Treatment

Lupus nephritis is usually diagnosed on the basis of renal biopsy – classification is based on glomerular findings, and if there is endocapillary, proliferation will be considered as either class III (if fewer than 50 percent of glomeruli involved) or class IV (if more than 50 percent involved); if there is membranous change, it is class V, which can be present with class III or IV. While proliferative lupus nephritis (class III/IV) is generally considered as having a worse long-term prognosis than class V, both forms can be associated with significant nephrotic syndrome, hypertension and impaired renal function. Women with additional antiphospholipid antibodies can have a superimposed vasculopathy/thrombotic microangiopathy. Outside of pregnancy lupus nephritis is generally treated with an induction regimen followed by maintenance immunosuppression. Induction regimens generally include steroids with either mycophenolate mofetil (MMF) or cyclophosphamide (CyP) – both drugs absolutely contraindicated in pregnancy (see Chapter 7). Clinical trial data suggest that for those who respond to induction, MMF is the more effective agent for maintenance therapy [8]. However, in Caucasians at least, azathioprine (safe in pregnancy) is a reasonable maintenance drug [9]. All patients with lupus should be on the immunomodulatory drug hydroxychloroquine (HCQ), which is good for extra-renal symptoms such as alopecia and arthralgias, as well as reducing the risk of clots, infections and flares. Since lupus and lupus nephritis can relapse and remit, long-term treatment is required. Herein lies one of the many challenges of ensuring safe pregnancies for women with lupus nephritis.

Prepregnancy Planning

Planning is crucial for a successful outcome. The key determinants of success of pregnancies in women with lupus and with lupus nephritis have recently been clarified in two large prospective studies [10–12]. These include having quiescent disease, especially nephritis, at the time of conception and ideally for at least six months prior; the absence of hypertension; not being lupus anticoagulant positive; and being on HCQ. For women with lupus nephritis, it is imperative they understand that their disease needs to be treated and then they can plan for pregnancy. This should be addressed very early on in management of women with acute lupus nephritis (see Chapter 2).

Cyclophosphamide can cause ovarian failure. The risk is dose- and age-related such that a dose over greater than 10g in a woman over 30 years is almost invariably associated with amenorrhea, which may be permanent [13]. The Eurolupus regimen of cyclophosphamide (using 6 x 500mg doses every two weeks) should be the standard regimen and the dose of 3g is rarely associated with infertility [14]. Indeed a recent study has shown anti-mullerian hormone levels are well preserved in women receiving one Eurolupus course [15]. That said, many women have more than one course of treatment and may be at risk of premature menopause. If there are any doubts about fertility, it is worth early referral to a specialist for assessment. Importantly, it is worth considering doing this while the woman is on treatment for her lupus nephritis so there is minimal delay once her nephritis is quiescent. During treatment with cyclophosphamide, many centers use ovarian protection with GnRH agonists, but the validity of this has recently been questioned. Egg collection may be considered to preserve fertility options in women with lupus [16]. The problem with egg collection is that the hormones required to stimulate egg production may well exacerbate already active disease and hence be contraindicated.

The issues with fertility highlight the challenges of advising on correct timing to conceive. It is very clear that active lupus nephritis at the time of conception is associated with worse maternal and fetal outcomes [10, 17]. Current advice is that disease should be quiescent for six months prior to conception. However, many women with lupus nephritis are in their mid- to late 30s – hence the need to ensure that everything is in place – medicines management, fertility investigations and so forth – for as soon as it is safe to try to conceive. We often recommend a renal biopsy to ensure that residual proteinuria is not associated with active disease.

Medications need to be optimized prior to conception. Women with lupus nephritis are often on multiple medications – immunosuppressants, prophylactic medications to protect them from the side effects of treatment or to reduce long-term cardiovascular risk. For an overview of the risks and safety of regularly used medications, see Chapter 7 and reference [18]. Steroids, azathioprine and hydroxychloroquine can and should all be continued. Hydroxychloroquine should be advised for all pregnant women with lupus. It has been shown to reduce disease activity with no adverse effects on the baby and withdrawal leads to an increased risk of lupus flare [19–22]. If a woman is in a stable remission on these maintenance medications, generally they should not be weaned off prior to pregnancy lest she flares and is set back another year or so. Mycophenolate mofetil, cyclophosphamide and methotrexate are all teratogenic and must be stopped at least three months prior to conception. Most women do not just stop their immunosuppression but need to convert to azathioprine for maintenance. There is good evidence this is a safe strategy [23], though flares may be more common once switched, which will delay the time to advising that it is safe to conceive. Establishing a woman on the correct dose and monitoring her response will usually require at least three months. Specifics about immunosuppressants are discussed in Chapter 7. Rituximab is used increasingly, especially for refractory lupus nephritis – it crosses the placenta and will deplete fetal B cells. The current recommendation is to wait at least a year from treatment to conception. However, there is also a school of thought that it may be a strategy to prevent relapse (perhaps more in women with vasculitis than lupus) if given not long before pregnancy. If the baby is delivered at term, its B cells are likely to have recovered. However, there are no long-term data on the impact of such a perturbation of immune cell development.

Hypertension is an adverse prognostic factor for all pregnancies, and women with lupus nephritis are very likely to have significant hypertension. It is critical to optimize blood pressure control prepregnancy. Depending on her residual proteinuria, the woman needs to be advised on whether to continue ACE inhibitors(ACEi) or angiotensin receptor blockers (ARB) until pregnancy is confirmed (to offer renoprotection) or to switch e.g. to labetalol or nifedipine. There is a growing consensus that the risk of congenital abnormalities is probably lower than previously attributed to first-trimester exposure [24]. However, ACEi and ARB diminish proteinuria nonspecifically, and for women with lupus and prior lupus nephritis, there is a strong argument to stop their ACEi or ARB at the prepregnancy planning stage to define the level of proteinuria off the medications. If it is significant, the woman can be advised to have a renal biopsy to ensure no active nephritis has been unmasked.

Prepregnancy biopsy – as alluded to in the discussion about ACEI/ARB cessation, knowing that the lupus nephritis is quiescent is important prognostically. It is our practice to advise a renal biopsy prior to switching e.g. from maintenance MMF to azathioprine, particularly if the woman has persistent low-level proteinuria.

How to Advise on Impact of Lupus on Maternal and Fetal Outcomes?

Ideally, prepregnancy, a woman with lupus nephritis needs to be aware of the risks to her and to her baby. A systematic review of 37 studies from 1980 to 2009, evaluating data from 2,751 pregnancies in 1,842 women with lupus was published in 2010 [17]. It is important to remember this covers a very long time period during which care of high-risk pregnancies improved hugely, neonatal care strengthened and treatment of lupus underwent considerable change. However, overall the systematic review showed that pregnancies in women with lupus were complicated by a lupus flare in 25.6 percent, hypertension in 16.3 percent, lupus nephritis in 16.1 percent, preeclampsia in 7.6 percent and eclampsia, stroke or death in 1 percent. Unsuccessful pregnancies occurred in 23.4 percent and of those that progressed, 34.9 percent were delivered at < 37 weeks' gestation, stillbirth was seen in 3.6 percent, neonatal death in 2.5 percent and intrauterine growth restriction (IUGR) in 12.7 percent. These rates are higher than in the general population of women. Importantly, active nephritis was significantly associated with maternal hypertension ($p < 0.001$) and premature birth ($p = 0.02$). A history of nephritis was also associated with hypertension ($p < 0.001$) and preeclampsia ($p = 0.017$). Hence, even if lupus nephritis is in remission, it is important to counsel women they are at increased risk of adverse pregnancy outcomes and need to be managed as high risk even if really well. Women with positive antiphospholipid antibodies were found to have a higher risk of hypertension (p = 0.029) and having a premature birth (p = 0.004).

A very recent meta-analysis comparing women with and without systemic lupus confirms the high impact on maternal and fetal outcomes following pregnancy and stresses the need for special care to be offered before and during pregnancy to women with lupus [25]. The study reported on 11 studies with a total of 529,788 women included. They showed the risk for having a caesarean section was significantly higher in the women with lupus (RR: 1.85, 95 percent CI: 1.63–2.10; P = 0.00001). Women with lupus were also more likely to have preeclampsia and hypertension (RR: 1.91, 95 percent CI: 1.44–2.53; P = 0.00001 and RR: 1.99, 95 percent CI: 1.54–2.56; P = 0.00001 respectively). Spontaneous abortion, thromboembolic disease and postpartum infection were also significantly higher among the women with lupus (RR: 1.51, 95 percent CI: 1.26–1.82; P = 0.0001, RR: 11.29, 95 percent CI: 6.05–21.07; P = 0.00001 and RR: 4.35, 95 percent CI: 2.69–7.03; P = 0.00001, respectively). Women without lupus were more likely to have a live birth (RR: 1.38, 95 percent CI: 1.14–1.67; P = 0.001), while women with lupus were much more likely to have premature deliveries and small-for-gestational-age (SGA) babies (RR: 3.05, 95 percent CI: 2.56–3.63; P = 0.00001 and RR: 1.69, 95 percent CI: 1.53–1.88; P = 0.00001, respectively). Babies born to mothers with lupus were significantly more likely to require a neonatal intensive care unit and, perhaps most worryingly, have congenital defects (RR: 2.76, 95 percent CI: 2.27–3.35; P = 0.00001) and (RR: 2.63, 95 percent CI: 1.93–3.58; P = 0.00001), respectively.

There has now been an excellent prospective cohort study published – the PROMISSE study [10], which importantly defines not only a high-risk group of women with lupus, but also a low-risk one. The study followed a cohort of 385 patients (49 percent non-Hispanic white, 31 percent with prior lupus nephritis) with lupus. They excluded women with active severe disease – specifically relevant to women with lupus nephritis, they excluded those with a protein-to-creatinine ratio > 1,000mg/g (equivalent to about 1g/ 24 hours), creatinine greater than 1.2mg/dl (> 106μmol/l), prednisolone dose > 20mg/day and multifetal pregnancy. This means that the cohort comprised women who, if they had had lupus nephritis, likely had quiescent disease. They used "hard" endpoints to define adverse pregnancy outcomes (APOs): fetal or neonatal death; birth before 36 weeks due to placental insufficiency, hypertension or preeclampsia (i.e. not just because the obstetrician was "concerned" should deliver earlier); and SGA neonate (birth weight below the fifth percentile). Importantly, the women were largely followed in lupus centers and had optimal care. A high proportion were taking hydroxychloroquine. While APOs occurred in 19.0 percent (95 percent CI, 15.2 percent to 23.2 percent) of pregnancies, the corollary is that 81 percent of pregnancies had a good outcome – this is a very important message for women with mild or quiescent disease to hear. The rates of APO were lower than seen in the systematic review cited earlier. Fetal death occurred in 4 percent, neonatal death occurred in 1 percent, preterm delivery occurred in 9 percent and SGA neonate occurred in 10 percent. Severe flares in the second and third trimesters were infrequent – occurring in 2.5 percent and 3.0 percent, respectively. Baseline predictors of APOs included presence of lupus anticoagulant (LAC) (odds ratio [OR], 8.32 [CI, 3.59 to 19.26]), antihypertensive use (OR, 7.05 [CI, 3.05 to 16.31]), Physician Global Assessment (PGA) score greater than 1 (OR, 4.02 [CI, 1.84 to 8.82]), and low platelet count (OR, 1.33 [CI, 1.09 to 1.63] per decrease of 50×10^9 cells/L). These data are very relevant to women with lupus nephritis as many will be on maintenance antihypertensives, though for some more for proteinuria control than blood pressure control. Non-Hispanic white race was protective (OR, 0.45 [CI, 0.24 to 0.84]). Perhaps unsurprisingly, maternal flares, higher disease activity and smaller increases in C3 level later in pregnancy also predicted APOs. Again, important to stress to women in prepregnancy planning, among women without baseline risk factors, the APO rate was 7.8 percent – hence the need to control disease prior to pregnancy. The less-good news for women with lupus nephritis is that for women who either were LAC-positive or were LAC-negative but non-white or Hispanic and using antihypertensives, the APO rate was 58.0 percent and fetal or neonatal mortality was 22.0 percent. Lupus nephritis is more common and more severe in nonwhite patients, so will be overrepresented among those with higher risk factors for APOs. While this study remains very important, it was not focused on women with lupus nephritis.

However, it does support the view that for women who become pregnant with inactive or stable mild/moderate SLE, severe flares are infrequent during pregnancy and, in the absence of specific risk factors such as LAC positivity, outcomes are favorable.

Moroni and colleagues have published a further series of pregnancies in women with lupus nephritis [26]. The study prospectively followed 71 pregnancies in 61 Italian women between 2006 and 2013, so it was very much a modern era study. All women had received prepregnancy counseling. At the time of conception, 78.9 percent were in complete renal remission and 21.1 percent had mild active lupus nephritis. Flares (very loosely defined by a relatively small rise in proteinuria) occurred in 19.7 percent (n = 14) and all responded to treatment. Flares were predicted by low C3 (consistent with the PROMISSE data), and high anti-dsDNA antibodies. Interestingly, there was no increased risk of flares with prior lupus nephritis or clinical activity at baseline. The rate of preeclampsia was 8.4 percent (n-6), surprisingly similar to the 7.6 percent reported in Smyth's systematic review. Hemolysis elevated liver enzymes, low platelets (HELLP) syndrome was seen in two patients, and both preeclampsia and HELLP were predicted by prior lupus nephritis or longer disease duration or hypertension.

In the Moroni study, they also assessed fetal outcomes [12]. Fetal loss was seen in 6/71 pregnancies (8.4 percent) and was predicted by baseline hypertension, being LAC-positive, having anticardiolipin IgG antibodies or anti-β2 IgG antibodies and by being triple positive for antiphospholipid antibodies. Preterm delivery was common and predicted by high baseline SLE Disease Activity Index (SLEDAI), proteinuria, history of renal flares, hypertension and active lupus nephritis. Odds for preterm delivery increased by 60 percent for each unit increase in SLEDAI and by 15 percent for each increase in proteinuria by 1 g per day. The rate of fetal loss was considered reasonably low and mostly associated with the presence of antiphospholipid antibodies. Prematurity was common and largely predicted by lupus activity and lupus nephritis at baseline. Importantly, while having an SGA baby was not uncommon (16.4 percent), the probability was highly significantly reduced by 85 percent in those women taking hydroxychloroquine (p = 0.023).

What these recent studies highlight are the messages to share with women with lupus prior to conception and indeed from early on in their treatment for the lupus itself. The disease needs to be quiescent, the medications need to be safe and ideally pregnancy needs to be achieved when renal function is normal, proteinuria is minimal and hypertension is well controlled. All women should be screened at baseline for lupus anticoagulant and if positive, counseled that they are at much higher risk for adverse pregnancy outcomes.

During Pregnancy

There are three key aspects to care during pregnancy for women with lupus nephritis.

a) Monitoring of women with prior lupus or lupus nephritis

b) Diagnosing those with *de novo* lupus nephritis or a flare of lupus nephritis

c) Treatment of *de novo* lupus nephritis or flares

Monitoring

Women with lupus or prior lupus nephritis ideally will have had prepregnancy counseling and know to book early to facilitate accurate dating and early assessment of disease activity, and to ensure optimization of medications and baseline bloods. Even if a woman has had prepregnancy counseling, it is worth early review to ensure she knows to continue taking hydroxychloroquine, has started aspirin (75mg od) if not already on it, to continue folic acid (throughout pregnancy if also on azathioprine), that she is on appropriate antihypertensives and has stopped any inappropriate medications.

Lupus activity is monitored by checking for symptoms and signs of a lupus flare as well as by regular measurement of serology and urine dip. Guidelines suggest monthly monitoring of specific lupus serology in addition to monitoring full blood count, renal profile and serum albumin. Lupus serology should include serum complement and anti-dsDNA antibodies. If presenting for the first time, it is critical to test for the presence of lupus anticoagulant, antiphospholipid antibodies and anti-Ro antibodies as these confer specific risks for the pregnancy and fetus, respectively. Urine should be dipped at each visit to evaluate new-onset hematuria and proteinuria. If proteinuria is detected it should be quantified with a protein-to-creatinine ratio.

All women with lupus or lupus nephritis should be advised to have low-dose aspirin through to 36 weeks' gestation to reduce the risk of preeclampsia. Women with antiphospholipid syndrome (with confirmed thromboembolic event, or adverse obstetric outcome – excluding recurrent early fetal loss) should receive low-molecular-weight heparin (LMWH) in pregnancy and for six weeks postpartum. Similarly, women with significant proteinuria (the level that is considered significant is debated but certainly if greater than 2g per day and serum albumin falling), regardless of lupus anticoagulant, should be given prophylactic LMWH. Dose should be adjusted for the mother's weight and renal function.

During pregnancy, recent data have suggested early measurement of angiogenic factors can predict those women destined to have adverse pregnancy outcomes as defined by the PROMISSE study [10, 27, 28]. They showed that having soluble Flt1 (sFlt1) in the highest quartile vs the lowest quartile between weeks 12–15 of gestation gave an OR of 17.3 for predicting severe adverse pregnancy outcomes (95 percent CI, 3.5–84.8); positive predictive value 61 percent, negative predictive value 93 percent. From weeks 16–19 of gestation, the combination of sFlt1 and PlGF were most predictive of severe adverse pregnancy outcomes, with the greatest risk conferred if PlGF was in the lowest quartile (< 70.3pg/ml) and sFlt1 in the highest quartile (> 1,872pg/ml); OR 31.1; (95 percent CI, 8.0–121.9); PPV, 58 percent, NPV, 95 percent. In this subgroup, if lupus anticoagulant was positive or a history of hypertension was also present, the severe adverse pregnancy outcome rate was a staggering 94 percent (95 percent CI, 70–99.8 percent). In contrast, among those women with the PlGF > 70.3pg/ml and sFlt1 < 1,872pg/ml, the rate of severe adverse pregnancy outcomes was only 4.6 percent (95 percent CI, 2.1–8.6 percent). While these factors are not yet being routinely measured through pregnancy, they could give really useful guidance about continuing with a pregnancy in a woman presenting with severe lupus in early pregnancy.

Women with anti-Ro or anti-La antibodies should have the fetal heart rate checked every two weeks from 18 weeks. Fetal echocardiography is often offered at 17–18 weeks' gestation to screen for cardiac abnormalities. Fetal echocardiography is recommended where there is any suspicion of fetal dysrhythmia or myocarditis [1].

All women with lupus and/or prior lupus nephritis should be seen at least monthly through pregnancy to ensure optimal blood pressure control, no evidence of flare and good fetal growth.

Fetal Monitoring in Pregnancy

This is a somewhat contentious issue. There is little debate that the fetus of a woman with lupus is more prone to being growth restricted and regular ultrasounds for fetal growth are recommended. However, the recent EULAR recommendations [1] are very specific about detailed fetal surveillance: "Women with SLE and/or APS should undergo supplementary fetal surveillance with Doppler ultrasonography and biometric parameters, particularly in the third trimester to screen for placental insufficiency and small for gestational age fetuses." However, there is much less agreement among fetal medicine experts about what constitutes evidence of placental insufficiency and when to intervene. We routinely offer growth scans for women with lupus nephritis (prior or current) from 24 or 28 weeks' gestation.

Flares of Lupus Nephritis in Pregnancy

Diagnosing a flare of lupus nephritis in pregnancy presents significant challenges. If a woman with known lupus, especially prior lupus nephritis, develops new-onset proteinuria with or without microscopic hematuria, with or without a rise in creatinine, then it is very likely she is having a flare of lupus nephritis. Serology may help confirm (falling complement, rising dsDNA) as may extra-renal symptoms – however, these are not required to make the diagnosis. Outside of pregnancy a woman with this constellation of findings would undoubtedly be offered a renal biopsy. This is safe to do in early pregnancy (probably up to 20 weeks' gestation and some do later [29–31]). However, if the diagnosis is already known and she has had prior lupus nephritis, then it may not be an absolute requirement. The need is greater in women presenting for the first time in pregnancy as the differential diagnosis is much wider and systemic lupus can occur in the presence of different renal disease. The key factors to weigh up are the risk of bleeding versus the benefit of an accurate diagnosis. The problem with bleeding is not that there is necessarily an increased risk of bleeding, but if the woman bleeds, she cannot be anticoagulated – and she may require anticoagulation more than she requires the biopsy, especially if nephrotic and LAC-positive. The downside of no biopsy is flying blind with potentially harmful treatment without a confirmed tissue diagnosis.

Later in pregnancy the main question is whether new-onset proteinuria is due to preeclampsia or nephritis or both. Renal biopsy should not be undertaken late in pregnancy and the judgment until recently has rested on the constellation of clinical findings (e.g. clear extra-renal manifestations of a lupus flare such as rash, arthralgias) and serology. However, many of the clinical features of lupus are common to both preeclampsia and lupus and relatively nonspecific. Patients with preeclampsia can also develop anemia and thrombocytopenia, as well as nephrotic syndrome. A rising dsDNA antibody titer and falling complement make lupus nephritis more likely but not a certainty, and of course the two can coincide. More recently, angiogenic factors, particularly a low and falling PlGF, have been shown to predict the need for delivery due to preeclampsia within 14 days in women with chronic kidney disease, some of whom in the study had lupus [32]. While these tests are not yet generally in routine clinical use they are likely to become more widely used.

The differential between a flare of lupus nephritis and preeclampsia can present a real dilemma particularly around 26–30 weeks' gestation. If it is a flare of lupus nephritis at this stage of gestation, the correct thing to do is to treat, monitor carefully and only expedite delivery if the flare worsens or if preeclampsia supervenes. However, if it is preeclampsia, then early delivery is likely to be required. Clearly the impact for the mother and baby is immense, and this highlights the need for these women to be cared for by an expert multidisciplinary team with at a minimum an obstetrician and an obstetric physician, but ideally in conjunction with a nephrologist or rheumatologist with specific expertise.

Treating Lupus Nephritis Flares in Pregnancy

Treatment of lupus nephritis in pregnancy should always be done in conjunction with a nephrologist or rheumatologist expert in the management of the disease. In early pregnancy it is appropriate to discuss the option of therapeutic abortion, treating the lupus nephritis optimally and planning for pregnancy at a later stage. However, many women choose not to take this route and later in pregnancy it is not an option. The selection of drugs that can be used to treat active lupus nephritis in pregnancy is more limited as mycophenolate and cyclophosphamide – standardly used for induction therapy – are contraindicated absolutely in the first trimester and

probably well into the second trimester. The mainstays of treatment are steroids and azathioprine. While some recommendations suggest starting with steroids alone, there is no evidence this approach works outside of pregnancy [33], so this should not be the approach during pregnancy. For acute lupus nephritis, it is appropriate to pulse with intravenous methyl prednisolone e.g. three doses of 500mg intravenous methyl prednisolone. This should get rapid control of systemic and renal inflammation. Larger doses are not needed (see for instance [34, 35]). Oral prednisolone should be started at 0.5mg/kg (maximum dose 60mg) (with proton pump inhibitor cover, as well as bone protection) [36]. However, where possible, dose and duration of steroids should be kept to a minimum due to the short-term significantly increased risks of maternal hypertension and gestational diabetes, as well as preeclampsia (though of course this might reflect the underlying disease state). The impact of steroids on mood should not be underestimated – while frank steroid-induced psychosis is infrequent, given the combination of acute illness and concerns regarding their babies, women treated with high-dose steroids should be warned of possible mood changes, including hypomania and severe depression.

The main steroid sparing agent to treat lupus nephritis in pregnancy is azathioprine. The mother's thiopurine methyl transferase (TPMT) should be ascertained to guide start dose and maximum dose. The maximum dose regardless should be 2mg/kg to minimize fetal immunosuppression and cytopenias. Women should have their full blood count and liver function monitored regularly while on azathioprine. Recent data have suggested tacrolimus, a calcineurin inhibitor, could be an effective treatment for lupus nephritis in pregnancy [37, 38]. Both azathioprine and tacrolimus are steroid sparing and tapering of steroids as rapidly as tolerated is to be encouraged. Tacrolimus and steroids are both diabetogenic, so women must be screened for gestational diabetes. Tacrolimus levels need to be monitored with a target range of around 5–8ng/l. Bound levels of tacrolimus fall quite markedly in pregnancy and quite high doses might be required though free levels (not routinely measured) may well remain stable or increase. If toxicity is suspected (tremor, unexplained rise in creatinine), then the dose should be reduced.

In the face of severe systemic lupus or severe lupus nephritis, alternative or additional therapeutic options include intravenous immunoglobulin (IVIg) and plasma exchange. IVIg does increase thrombotic risk, but is of value for thrombocytopenia and as an adjunctive therapy, especially when there is concomitant infection precluding increasing immunosuppression. There have been case series and reports to support its safety in pregnancy [39–41]. Plasma exchange requires (generally) central venous access and so is an invasive procedure with concomitant risk of infection from central line. However, for refractory lupus nephritis and severe antiphospholipid syndrome with poor obstetric outcomes there have been some reports of success [42].

While not generally recommended, in order to prolong a pregnancy complicated by severe lupus nephritis, it is possible to use cyclophosphamide in the third trimester of pregnancy [43]. There are almost no data supporting the use of mycophenolate mofetil in the third trimester, but the logic to be applied would be the same – the danger from teratogenicity has passed by this stage and the main risks to the fetus are those of immunosuppression and cytopenias. This logic was applied in a recently reported complex case [41].

Breastfeeding

Women should be encouraged to breastfeed and there are data to support them doing so while taking azathioprine and tacrolimus [44,45]. As yet breastfeeding while taking mycophenolate mofetil has not been recommended.

Vasculitis

Systemic vasculitides are classified according to the smallest vessel involved. The ones most likely to be encountered in pregnant women that can impact kidney function are a) the large vessel Takayasu arteritis and b) the small vessel ANCA associated vasculitides – granulomatous polyangiitis (GPA, formerly known as Wegener's granulomatosis) and microscopic polyangiitis (MPA). Takayasu via inflammatory changes leads to stenosis of affected vessels. Renal artery involvement is common and can lead to severe hypertension and renal impairment if the stenosis is complete. GPA and MPA are characterized by the presence of anti-neutrophil cytoplasmic antibodies (ANCA) – the ANCA in GPA are typically directed against proteinase 3 (anti PR3) and in MPA against myeloperoxidase (anti MPO).

Diagnosis

Takayasu arteritis is rare but classically affects women of childbearing age. It is challenging to diagnose as systemic symptoms may be very nonspecific (e.g. malaise, fever) and distinguishing between active disease (inflammation) and damage (often presenting as stenotic vessels long after the inflammation has subsided) is challenging. Patients are often diagnosed late but can present with hypertension (due to renal artery stenosis), ischemic limbs or gut and strokes depending on which arteries are involved. Imaging is central to diagnosis and includes MRA, ultrasound, PET-CT and formal angiography [46, 47].

Granulomatous polyangiitis (GPA) and microscopic polyangiitis (MPA) classically affect older people, but GPA in particular can present in women of childbearing age. Both can cause constitutional symptoms, arthralgias, vasculitic rashes, pulmonary hemorrhage and necrotizing glomerulonephritis (often with just blood and small amounts of proteinuria on dipstick). GPA can also cause upper airway disease, including subglottic stenosis, deafness, sinus symptoms, nasal crusting and bridge collapse and pulmonary granulomas and cavitations. MPA can be associated with neuropathies.

Blood Tests

In contrast to lupus, vasculitis is generally associated with an acute phase response, so women may well have a raised CRP, anemia, high white count, high platelets, high alkaline phosphatase and low serum albumin. Patients are rarely nephrotic on presentation. Takayasu arteritis is rarely associated with a positive ANCA. In GPA and MPA, patients are usually ANCA positive, but not always, and less likely if limited e.g. to renal disease only or upper airway disease only.

Renal Function

Patients with Takayasu arteritis may lose renal function due to significant renal artery stenosis, but often develop collateral circulation, which leads to preservation of eGFR unless both kidneys are severely affected. In contrast, the classical focal necrotizing glomerulonephritis associated with GPA and MPA can lead to rapid loss of renal function – the so-called rapidly progressive glomerulonephritis (RPGN). RPGN is a medical emergency requiring prompt diagnosis and intervention if renal function is not to be permanently lost.

Principles of Treatment

As with lupus, treatment is focused on induction of remission and maintenance of remission. Takayasu arteritis is challenging because defining when remission has occurred is very difficult, as highlighted by the recent data using anti-interleukin 6 (IL-6). Anti-IL -6 treatment led to normalization of all the measurable inflammatory markers e.g. CRP, but new lesions were still seen in some patients on detailed imaging [46]. Prednisolone remains the cornerstone of treatment for Takayasu arteritis, but most would advocate steroid sparing with e.g. azathioprine, or anti-TNF inhibitors.

The treatment of acute RPGN or other organ-threatening disease in GPA and MPA has changed in recent years. Steroids are used, whereas cyclophosphamide was the standard of care in addition to steroids for induction; however, there are now strong data supporting the use of rituximab especially in those with a flare from remission rather than *de novo* disease [48]. Milder small-vessel vasculitis, especially non-renal disease, can be treated with methotrexate or mycophenolate mofetil. Maintenance treatment with steroids and azathioprine for at least two years from remission (especially in GPA which is more likely to relapse) is recommended, though recent data showed far few relapses in those maintained on prednisolone and intermittent low doses of rituximab versus those maintained on prednisolone and azathioprine [49].

Prepregnancy Planning

All patients with vasculitis should be under specialist care before and during pregnancy – as with lupus the route to success is collaborative care by an expert multidisciplinary team. Similarly, fertility needs to be considered in women who have been exposed to cyclophosphamide (see earlier).

Medications need to be reviewed prepregnancy. Prednisolone, azathioprine, MMF, methotrexate and cyclophosphamide have all been discussed. Use of TNF inhibitors is common for Takayasu arteritis. The commonly used ones are IgG1 antibodies, which are actively transported by the placenta and cord blood levels will exceed those in the mother if given in the third trimester. The advice varies but is largely based on the half-life of the inhibitors – thus infliximab should probably be stopped no later than 18–19 weeks of gestation, adalimumab six to eight weeks before delivery if disease active, and by the end of the second trimester if quiescent; Etanercept should be stopped by 30–32 weeks [50–52]. There is no evidence of these drugs causing congenital abnormalities, but exposed babies are substantially immunosuppressed and should not have live vaccines for at least five months post exposure. Rituximab also crosses the placenta and it is advised to avoid exposure for a year before conception. However, it is very effective at preventing flares of small-vessel vasculitis and there is a growing school of thought that it might be the ideal drug to give soon before pregnancy or in early pregnancy to avoid vasculitic flares during pregnancy, which are considerably more of a risk for the women and her fetus.

How to Advise on Impact of Vasculitis on Maternal and Fetal Outcomes?

The generality holds that it is much safer to get pregnant with quiescent disease than active disease. There are far fewer data to draw inferences from in vasculitis than lupus as the frequency of pregnancy in women with vasculitis is much lower.

Takayasu Arteritis

Four recent studies (reviewed in [47]) from four different countries (France, Brazil, India and Turkey) reviewed post-diagnosis pregnancies in a total of 175 women and compared them either with controls or pre-diagnosis pregnancies. There was a significantly increased risk of maternal and fetal complications in all those with a diagnosis of Takayasu arteritis. In general there were higher rates of maternal hypertension (new or worsening), intrauterine growth restriction, preeclampsia and prematurity [53–56]. The study from India suggests that early intervention prior to pregnancy to treat renal artery stenosis may reduce complications. Angioplasty rather than stenting is the treatment of choice for such stenosis as in stent restenosis is more common than restenosis after angioplasty [47]. Women with Takayasu arteritis need to be monitored very carefully through pregnancy – most have successful outcomes, but the rate of hypertension is up to 40 percent and when complications arise they can be very severe. These include the development of aortic aneurysms, stroke, heart failure and myocardial infarcts and aortic dissection – all rare but catastrophic when they occur [6].

GPA and MPA

There are only a handful of reports regarding pregnancies in women with small-vessel vasculitis. The consensus suggests that disease should be in stable remission prior to conception to ensure good outcomes. However, maternal and fetal complications appear to be common and flares are not infrequent [6]. A systematic review of 567 pregnancies among patients with primary systemic vasculitis highlighted a reciprocal influence between disease course and gestational outcome, although no definite effects could be shown [57]. A recent retrospective report followed 65 pregnancies in 50 women with systemic vasculitis in eight multi-specialist centers over a nearly 20-year period – again highlighting how uncommon it is to see pregnant women with vasculitis [58]. Importantly, they compared the outcomes for the women with vasculitis with those from a general obstetric population of 3,939 women. Only two of the women reported developed their vasculitis *de novo* during pregnancy and 59 of the remaining 63 had quiescent disease at conception. Despite this, complications were not infrequent. There were 59 live births, eight miscarriages and one fetal death. Preterm, particularly early preterm (< 34 weeks) deliveries and caesarean sections were significantly more frequent in the women with vasculitis than in the control group (11.3 percent versus 5.0 percent, p = 0.049 and 48.2 percent versus 31.0 percent, p = 0.009). Vasculitis-related complications occurred in 23 pregnancies (35.4 percent), with five severe events (7.7 percent), including three cases of transient ischemic attack. For the 56 pregnancies for which postpartum data were available, flares occurred in 12 (21.4 percent) women, with one severe event (1.8 percent). Overall, when the case reports and series are reviewed, pregnancy is perfectly feasible for women with small-vessel vasculitis but attention needs to be paid to systemic flares and women should be warned about the need to have quiescent disease at conception.

During Pregnancy

There are three key aspects to care during pregnancy for women with systemic vasculitis.

a) Monitoring of vasculitis

b) Diagnosing those with *de novo* vasculitis or flares of vasculitis

c) Treatment of *de novo* vasculitis or flares of vasculitis

Monitoring

Women should be cared for in centers where specialist multidisciplinary teams with relevant expertise are available. GPA and MPA should be in remission and women on pregnancy-safe medications – in reality most will be on steroids with or without azathioprine. Women should be advised to take low-dose aspirin to reduce the risk of preeclampsia. Women should be seen at least monthly and markers of disease activity monitored. These include CRP, full blood count, renal function, ANCA and urinalysis. It needs to be borne in mind that both acute vasculitis and pregnancy induce an acute phase response so serial monitoring to detect change is mandatory. Some extra-renal flares can be life threatening with minimal influence on blood tests – in particular the development of tracheal disease in women with GPA can lead to stridor and threatened ventilation. Although rare, if this is the first presentation of disease, diagnostic delay (leading to treatment delay) can be catastrophic.

Diagnosis

As in nonpregnant women, diagnosis is made on the combination of clinical findings and blood and urine tests. If renal disease presents for the first time during pregnancy in a woman not known to have vasculitis, the same criteria for undertaking a renal biopsy or not apply as discussed for lupus.

Treatment

Small-vessel vasculitis with organ-threatening involvement in some ways presents much more of a challenge in pregnancy than lupus as the consequences can be much more severe and rapid. For instance pulmonary hemorrhage is often life threatening and a renal flare can lead to renal failure within weeks. Prednisolone and azathioprine are inadequate to treat such flares. Plasma exchange can be considered. Beyond the stage of teratogenicity it is reasonable to consider standard treatment with cyclophosphamide. Rituximab could be considered in early pregnancy, but should be avoided in later pregnancy as it will persist in the fetus for at least six months [43].

Conclusions

There are simple messages to take on board – planning before pregnancy is vital for all women with known lupus or vasculitis in order to evaluate disease activity, optimize blood pressure control and medications and to discuss fully with the prospective parents the risks they face and the management and monitoring required. Disease should be quiescent well before conception and women should be monitored closely through pregnancy for complications due to their disease, their medications and flares. And above all, women should be managed in centers where collaborative multidisciplinary teams have the expertise to appropriately advise, monitor and treat women with these challenging diseases.

References

1. Andreoli L, Bertsias GK, Agmon-Levin N, Brown S, Cervera R, Costedoat-Chalumeau N, et al. EULAR recommendations for women's health and the management of family planning, assisted reproduction, pregnancy and menopause in patients with systemic lupus erythematosus and/or antiphospholipid syndrome. *Ann Rheum Dis.* 2017;**76**:476–485.

2. Østensen M, Andreoli L, Brucato A, Cetin I, Chambers C, Clowse MEB, et al. State of the art: Reproduction and pregnancy in rheumatic diseases. *Autoimmun Rev.* 2015 May;**14**:376–386.

3. Lazzaroni MG, Dall'Ara F, Fredi M, Nalli C, Reggia R, Lojacono A, Ramazzotto, F, Zatti, S, Andreoli L, Tincani A. A comprehensive review of the clinical approach to pregnancy and systemic lupus erythematosus. *J Autoimmun.* 2016;**74**:106–117.

4. Tincani A, Dall'Ara F, Lazzaroni MG, Reggia R, Andreoli L. Pregnancy in patients with autoimmune disease: A reality in 2016. *Autoimmun Rev.* 2016;**15**:975–977.

5. Knight CL, Nelson-Piercy C. Management of systemic lupus erythematosus during pregnancy: Challenges and solutions. *Open access Rheumatol Res Rev.* 2017;**9**:37–53.

6. Machen L, Clowse MEB. Vasculitis and pregnancy. *Rheum Dis Clin North Am.* 2017;**43**:239–247.

7. Petri M, Orbai A-M, Alarcón GS, Gordon C, Merrill JT, Fortin PR, et al. Derivation and validation of the Systemic Lupus International Collaborating Clinics Classification Criteria for Systemic Lupus Erythematosus. *Arthritis Rheum.* 2012;**64**(8):2677–2686.

8. Dooley MA, Jayne D, Ginzler EM, Isenberg D, Olsen NJ, Wofsy D, et al. Mycophenolate versus azathioprine as maintenance therapy for lupus nephritis. *N Engl J Med.* 2011;**365**:1886–1895.

9. Houssiau FA, D'Cruz D, Sangle S, Remy P, Vasconcelos C, Petrovic R, et al. Azathioprine versus mycophenolate mofetil for long-term immunosuppression in lupus nephritis: Results from the MAINTAIN Nephritis Trial. *Ann Rheum Dis.* 2010;**69**:2083–2089.

10. Buyon JP, Kim MY, Guerra MM, Laskin CA, Petri M, Lockshin MD, et al. Predictors of pregnancy outcomes in patients with lupus: A cohort study. *Ann Intern Med.* 2015;**163**:153–163.

11. Moroni G, Doria A, Giglio E, Imbasciati E, Tani C, Zen M, et al. Maternal outcome in pregnant women with lupus nephritis: A prospective multicenter study. *J Autoimmun.* 2016.

12. Moroni G, Doria A, Giglio E, Tani C, Zen M, Strigini F, et al. Fetal outcome and recommendations of pregnancies in lupus nephritis in the 21st century. A prospective multicenter study. *J Autoimmun.* 2016;**74**:6–12.

13. Manger K, Wildt L, Kalden JR, Manger B. Prevention of gonadal toxicity and preservation of gonadal function and fertility in young women with systemic lupus erythematosus treated by cyclophosphamide: The PREGO-Study. *Autoimmun Rev.* 2006;**5**:269–272.

14. Houssiau FA, Vasconcelos C, D'Cruz D, Sebastiani GD, Garrido E de R, Danieli MG, et al. The 10-year follow-up data of the Euro-Lupus Nephritis Trial comparing low-dose and high-dose intravenous cyclophosphamide. *Ann Rheum Dis.* 2010;**69**:61–64.

15. Tamirou F, Nieuwland Husson S, Gruson D, Debiève F, Lauwerys BR, Houssiau FA. The low-dose intravenous cyclophosphamide Euro-Lupus regimen does not impact the ovarian reserve, as measured by serum anti-Müllerian hormone levels. *Arthritis Rheumatol.* 2017. http://doi.wiley.com/10.1002/art.40079.

16. Nahata L, Sivaraman V, Quinn GP. Fertility counseling and preservation practices in youth with lupus and vasculitis undergoing gonadotoxic therapy. *Fertil Steril.* 2016;**106**:1470–1474.

17. Smyth A, Oliveira GHM, Lahr BD, Bailey KR, Norby SM, Garovic VD. A systematic review and meta-analysis of pregnancy outcomes in patients with systemic lupus erythematosus and lupus nephritis. *Clin J Am Soc Nephrol.* 2010; 5:2060–2068.

18. Götestam Skorpen C, Hoeltzenbein M, Tincani A, Fischer-Betz R, Elefant E, Chambers C, et al. The EULAR points to consider for use of antirheumatic drugs before pregnancy, and during pregnancy and lactation. *Ann Rheum Dis.* 2016;**75**:795–810.

19. Clowse MEB, Magder L, Witter F, Petri M. Hydroxychloroquine in lupus pregnancy. *Arthritis Rheum.* 2006;**54**:3640–3647.

20. Kaplan YC, Ozsarfati J, Nickel C, Koren G. Reproductive outcomes following hydroxychloroquine use for autoimmune diseases: A systematic review and meta-analysis. *Br J Clin Pharmacol*. 2016;81:835–848.

21. Levy R, Vilela V, Cataldo M, Ramos R, Duarte J, Tura B, et al. Hydroxychloroquine (HCQ) in lupus pregnancy: Double-blind and placebo-controlled study. *Lupus*. 2001;10:401–404.

22. Sperber K, Hom C, Chao CP, Shapiro D, Ash J, Aberientos C. Systematic review of hydroxychloroquine use in pregnant patients with autoimmune diseases. *Pediatr Rheumatol Online J*. 2009;7:9.

23. Fischer-Betz R, Specker C, Brinks R, Aringer M, Schneider M. Low risk of renal flares and negative outcomes in women with lupus nephritis conceiving after switching from mycophenolate mofetil to azathioprine. *Rheumatol*. 2013; 52:1070–1076.

24. Bateman BT, Patorno E, Desai RJ, Seely EW, Mogun H, Dejene SZ, et al. Angiotensin-converting enzyme inhibitors and the risk of congenital malformations. *Obstet Gynecol*. 2017;129:174–184.

25. Bundhun PK, Soogund MZS, Huang F. Impact of systemic lupus erythematosus on maternal and fetal outcomes following pregnancy: A meta-analysis of studies published between years 2001–2016. *J Autoimmun*. 2017. www.ncbi.nlm.nih.gov/pubmed/28256367.

26. Moroni G, Ponticelli C. Pregnancy in women with systemic lupus erythematosus (SLE). *Eur J Intern Med*. 2016;32:7–12.

27. Yelnik CM, Laskin CA, Porter TF, Branch DW, Buyon JP, Guerra MM, et al. Lupus anticoagulant is the main predictor of adverse pregnancy outcomes in aPL-positive patients: Validation of PROMISSE study results. *Lupus Sci Med*. 2016; 3.

28. Kim MY, Buyon JP, Guerra MM, Rana S, Zhang D, Laskin CA, et al. Angiogenic factor imbalance early in pregnancy predicts adverse outcomes in patients with lupus and antiphospholipid antibodies: Results of the PROMISSE study. *Am J Obstet Gynecol* 2016;214:108. e1-108.e14. http://dx.doi.org/10.1016/j.ajog.2015.09.066.

29. Imbasciati E, Surian M, Bottino S, Cosci P, Colussi G, Ambroso GC, et al. Lupus nephropathy and pregnancy: A study of 26 pregnancies in patients with systemic lupus erythematosus and nephritis. *Nephron*. 1984;36:46–51.

30. Day C, Hewins P, Hildebrand S, Sheikh L, Taylor G, Kilby M, et al. The role of renal biopsy in women with kidney disease identified in pregnancy. *Nephrol Dial Transplant*. 2008;23:201–206.

31. Webster P, Webster L, Cook H, Horsfield C, Seed P, Vaz R, et al. A multicentre cohort study of histological findings and long-term outcomes of kidney disease in women who have been pregnant. *Clin J Am Soc Nephrol*. 2017;12:408–416.

32. Bramham K, Seed PTPT, Lightstone L, Nelson-Piercy C, Gill C, Webster P, et al. Diagnostic and predictive biomarkers for pre-eclampsia in patients with established hypertension and chronic kidney disease. *Kidney Int*. 2016;89:874–885.

33. Bertsias GK, Tektonidou M, Amoura Z, Aringer M, Bajema I, Berden JH, Boletis J, Cervera R, Dorner T, Doria A, Ferrario F, Floege J, Houssiau FA, Ioannidis JP, Isenberg DA, Kallenberg CG, Lightstone L, Marks SD, Martini A, Moroni G, Neumann I, Praga M, Schneider M, Starra A, Tesar V, Vasconcelos C, van Vollenhoven RF, Zakharova H, Haubitz M, Gordon C, Jayne D, Boumpas DT. EULAR/ERA-EDTA recommendations for the management of adult and paediatric lupus nephritis. *Ann Rheum Dis*. 2012; 71: 1771–1782.

34. Edwards JCW, Snaith ML, Isenberg DA. A double blind controlled trial of methylprednisolone infusions in systemic lupus erythematosus using individualised outcome assessment. *Ann Rheum Dis*. 1987;46:773–776.

35. Badsha H, Kong KO, Lian TY, Chan SP, Edwards CJ, Chng HH. Low-dose pulse methylprednisolone for systemic lupus erythematosus flares is efficacious and has a decreased risk of infectious complications. *Lupus*. 2002;11:508–513.

36. Zeher M, Doria a., Lan J, Aroca G, Jayne D, Boletis I, et al. Efficacy and safety of enteric-coated mycophenolate sodium in combination with two glucocorticoid regimens for the treatment of active lupus nephritis. *Lupus*. 2011;20:1484–1493.

37. Webster P, Lightstone L, McKay D, Josephson MA. Pregnancy in chronic kidney disease and kidney transplantation. *Kidney Int*. 2017; 91:1047–1056.

38. Webster P, Wardle A, Bramham K, Webster L, Nelson-Piercy C, Lightstone L. Tacrolimus is an effective treatment for lupus nephritis in pregnancy. *Lupus*. 2015;23:1192–1196.

39. Perricone R, De Carolis C, Kroegler B, Greco E, Giacomelli R, Cipriani P, et al. Intravenous immunoglobulin therapy in pregnant patients affected with systemic lupus erythematosus and recurrent spontaneous abortion. *Rheumatology*. 2008;47:646–651.

40. Mulhearn B, Bruce IN. Indications for IVIG in rheumatic diseases. *Rheumatology (Oxford)*. 2015;54:383–391.

41. Webster P, Nelson-Piercy C, Lightstone L. A complicated multisystem flare of systemic lupus erythematosus during pregnancy. *BMJ Case Rep*. 2017.

42. Kronbichler A, Brezina B, Quintana LF, Jayne DRW. Efficacy of plasma exchange and immunoadsorption in systemic lupus erythematosus and antiphospholipid syndrome: A systematic review. *Autoimmun Rev.* 2016;**15**:38–49.

43. Nelson-Piercy C, Agarwal S, Lams B. Lesson of the month: Selective use of cyclophosphamide in pregnancy for severe autoimmune respiratory disease. *Thorax.* 2016;**71**:667–668.

44. Noviani M, Wasserman S, Clowse MEB. Breastfeeding in mothers with systemic lupus erythematosus. *Lupus.* 2016;**25**:973–979.

45. Bramham K, Chusney G, Lee J, Lightstone L, Nelson-Piercy C. Breastfeeding and tacrolimus: Serial monitoring in breast-fed and bottle-fed infants. *Clin J Am Soc Nephrol.* 2013;**8**:563–567.

46. Youngstein T, Mason JC. Interleukin 6 targeting in refractory Takayasu arteritis: Serial noninvasive imaging is mandatory to monitor efficacy. *J Rheumatol.* 2013;**40**:1941–1944.

47. Seyahi E. Takayasu arteritis: an update. *Curr Opin Rheumatol.* 2017;**29**:51–56.

48. Yates M, Watts RA, Bajema IM, Cid MC, Crestani B, Hauser T, et al. EULAR/ERA-EDTA recommendations for the management of ANCA-associated vasculitis. *Ann Rheum Dis.* 2016;**75**:1583–1594.

49. Pagnoux C, Guillevin L, French Vasculitis Study Group, MAINRITSAN Investigators. Rituximab or azathioprine maintenance in ANCA-associated vasculitis. *N Engl J Med.* 2015;**372**:386–387.

50. Soh MC, Nelson-Piercy C. High-risk pregnancy and the rheumatologist. *Rheumatology (Oxford).* 2015;**54**:572–587.

51. Flint J, Panchal S, Hurrell A, Van De Venne M, Gayed M, Schreiber K, et al. Guidelines BSR and BHPR guideline on prescribing drugs in pregnancy and breastfeeding – Part I: standard and biologic disease modifying anti-rheumatic drugs and corticosteroids. *Rheumatology (Oxford).* 2016;**55**:1693–1697.

52. Mahadevan U, Cucchiara S, Hyams JS, Steinwurz F, Nuti F, Travis SPL, et al. The London Position Statement of the World Congress of Gastroenterology on Biological Therapy for IBD with the European Crohn's and Colitis Organisation: Pregnancy and pediatrics. *Am J Gastroenterol.* 2011;**106**:214–223.

53. Comarmond C, Mirault T, Biard L, Nizard J, Lambert M, Wechsler B, et al. Takayasu arteritis and pregnancy. *Arthritis Rheumatol.* 2015;**67**:3262–3269.

54. Assad APL, da Silva TF, Bonfa E, Pereira RMR. Maternal and neonatal outcomes in 89 patients with Takayasu arteritis (TA): Comparison before and after the TA diagnosis. *J Rheumatol.* 2015;**42**:1861–1864.

55. Singh N, Tyagi S, Tripathi R, Mala YM. Maternal and fetal outcomes in pregnant women with Takayasu aortoarteritis: Does optimally timed intervention in women with renal artery involvement improve pregnancy outcome? *Taiwan J Obstet Gynecol.* 2015;**54**:597–602.

56. Alpay-Kanitez N, Omma A, Erer B, Artim-Esen B, Gül A, Inanç M, et al. Favourable pregnancy outcome in Takayasu arteritis: A single-centre experience. *Clin Exp Rheumatol.*;**33**(2 Suppl. 89):S-7–10.

57. Gatto M, Iaccarino L, Canova M, Zen M, Nalotto L, Ramonda R, et al. Pregnancy and vasculitis: A systematic review of the literature. *Autoimmunity Reviews.* 2012;**11**:A447–59.

58. Fredi M, Lazzaroni MG, Tani C, Ramoni V, Gerosa M, Inverardi F, et al. Systemic vasculitis and pregnancy: A multicenter study on maternal and neonatal outcome of 65 prospectively followed pregnancies. *Autoimmunity Reviews* 2015;**14**: 686–691.

Chapter 15

Diabetic Nephropathy in Pregnancy

Andrew McCarthy

Introduction

With the increasing prevalence of type II diabetes, and increased longevity, diabetes has become the most common cause of end-stage renal disease in the United Kingdom [1]. There is an increased rate of progression to end-stage renal disease in the United States, resulting in much higher numbers being on renal replacement therapy than in the United Kingdom. Approximately 20–30 percent of all patients with type I diabetes progress to nephropathy, and the incidence of nephropathy peaks 10–20 years after diagnosis. While a smaller proportion of type II diabetics will progress to renal failure than type I, they will contribute most cases as a reflection of the increasing prevalence of this condition. Genetic and racial factors influence progression to end-stage renal disease. Diabetic nephropathy is generally defined as albuminuria > 300 mg in 24 hours in a patient with diabetes in the absence of infection or other renal disease.

Diabetic nephropathy is manifest histologically as scattered sclerosis of glomeruli developing within years of the diagnosis. The progression of histological lesions from glomerular basement membrane thickening, increased mesangial matrix and mesangial expansion and progression to Kimmelstiel-Wilson nodules has been reviewed [2] alongside the development of arteriolar hyalinosis. Not all patients who develop glomerular structural changes develop nephropathy. Some patients progress to microalbuminuria (30–300 mg in 24 hours), marking a very substantial increase in risk of progression, and this may then be followed by overt nephropathy with further increasing proteinuria, and subsequent decline in renal function.

Microalbuminuria is the main predictor of nephropathy, and management strategies for microalbuminuria have developed with similar principles to diabetes care in general, and have been recently reviewed [3]. Treatment-induced and spontaneous remission of microalbuminuria can occur, and microalbuminuria marks the need for intensified treatment strategies to halt disease progression, including optimal glycemic control, control of blood pressure (the goal of therapy is a blood pressure of < 130/80 mmHg, American Diabetes Association (ADA [4]), blockade of the renin-angiotensin system and management of dyslipidemia [5]. Hypertension often manifests at the time of development of microalbuminuria in patients with type I diabetes.

Progression from micro- to macroalbuminuria has varied widely in the many studies performed, with estimates of 2.8 to 13 per 100 person-years. The EURODIAB study suggests that 14 percent (two per 100 person-years) of 352 patients with type I diabetes with microalbuminuria will progress to macroalbuminuria over seven years, and 51 percent regressed to normoalbuminuria [6]. HbA1 c, albumin excretion rate and body weight at baseline were associated with progression. End-stage renal disease develops in 50 percent of type I patients with overt nephropathy within 10 years and in > 75 percent within 20 years. The clinical and pathologic correlations are outlined in the review of Kitzmiller and Combs [7]. Long-term morbidity due to hypertension and cardiovascular risk, and end-stage renal disease impact life expectancy once nephropathy has developed. Microalbuminuria has some limitations in predicting long-term disease and Currie et al. review the development of other biomarkers to facilitate greater prevention of disease progression [8].

As type II diabetes may be unrecognized for years prior to diagnosis, microalbuminuria and nephropathy may be present from a very early stage after presentation, and will progress as outlined earlier. A smaller proportion of those with type II diabetes progress to end-stage renal disease, and death from cardiovascular disease is likely to precede progression in a substantial number of cases. It is thought that approximately 8 percent of renal failure in the diabetic population is due to causes other than diabetic nephropathy, and hence wider investigation may be required. Biopsy must be considered if disease progression is atypical, especially in the absence of retinopathy.

For a historical picture of the risk of complications associated with diabetic nephropathy in pregnancy, it is chastening to review the original publications of White that led to the clinical classification of women with diabetes in pregnancy [9, 10]. In a paper published in 1945, White refers to fetal mortality rates of 30 to 60 percent, the range depending on inclusion of early pregnancy loss. She describes a series of 181 consecutive women with diabetes managed personally between 1936 and 1944, resulting in one maternal death, and 29 fetal deaths. It is clear from the discussion that these loss rates are vastly better than her peers at the time. Subsequent publication in 1949 [10] reveals an 18 percent fetal mortality among 439 women with diabetes, excluding first-trimester loss.

Epidemiology

Nephropathy is defined in different ways in the published literature in pregnancy, some using 300 mg of protein excretion in 24 hours, others a 500 mg cut-off, assessed in the first half of pregnancy. Urinary albumin excretion before pregnancy and early in gestation has been studied by Ekbom et al. and shown to be comparable [11].

The Confidential Enquiry into Maternal and Child Health (CEMACH) [12] study in the United Kingdom gives a picture of how pregnancy is affected by diabetes: 73 percent of those with preexisting diabetes had type I diabetes, and 27 percent had type II. The latter group were more likely to be socially disadvantaged, older and multiparous and to belong to ethnic minority communities. In general, this population is at high risk of pregnancy-related complications with increased risks of preterm delivery (36 percent), caesarean section (67 percent), stillbirth (relative risk, RR, 5) and perinatal mortality (RR, 3), and it has a twofold increased risk of congenital abnormality compared with the general population.

Diabetes encapsulates all the arguments for preconceptual care and this is emphasized in a recent Cochrane review [13], which reported that preconceptual care was effective in reducing congenital abnormalities, preterm delivery and perinatal

mortality. Overall management of complications relating to diabetes in pregnancy has been reviewed elsewhere [14, 15], and this chapter focuses on the risks attributable to diabetic nephropathy specifically.

A recent UK population study suggests risk of congenital abnormality may be increased in patients with diabetic nephropathy [16] in addition to those associated with poor glycemic control, and this area needs further scrutiny. Klemetti et al. [17] describe an overall rate of congenital abnormality of 9.5 percent in a retrospective cohort of women with diabetic nephropathy. Overall improvements in blood glucose control were achieved within pregnancy, and it is interesting to speculate whether this rate could be reduced if the same intensity of care was provided prior to pregnancy.

Nephropathy is reported to complicate between 5 and 10 percent of pregnancies of women with preexisting diabetes. It has traditionally been associated with increased risks of preterm delivery, preeclampsia and general maternal morbidity. The risk of nephropathy may depend on which form of diabetes a woman suffers. In a separate subset of the CEMACH inquiry [12], 8 percent of women with type I diabetes had nephropathy, and 5 percent of women with type II. Damm et al. [18] more recently demonstrate a lower incidence of nephropathy in diabetic mothers, and comparable rates in type 1 and type II diabetes, 2.5 percent and 2.3 percent. A recent large retrospective review from Klemetti et al. [17] revealed an incidence of nephropathy in type I diabetic pregnancy of 14.7 percent up to 1999, and 6.5 percent in 2000–2011, suggestive of improvements in disease prevention.

It has always been a matter of great concern that pregnancy might exacerbate underlying nephropathy. There is general agreement that glomerular hyperfiltration contributes to progression of diabetic nephropathy, and if increased glomerular capillary pressure is present in pregnancy and not just increased renal blood flow, then there could be a subsequent loss of function. Glomerular filtration rate (GFR) increases by 50 percent in pregnancy and theoretically this could therefore increase the rate of progression of underlying nephropathy if accompanied by elevated intraglomerular pressure. The development of hypertension during pregnancy could also have a deleterious effect, as could increased protein intake, and any acute complication associated with a prerenal insult. The degree of glycemic control can also affect GFR and proteinuria.

Angiotensin-Converting Enzyme (ACE) Inhibitors

Medication exposure is covered in Chapter 7. However, there are specific issues relating to ACE inhibition in diabetic nephropathy. It has been demonstrated that ACE inhibition is associated with a 50 percent reduction in risk of death, dialysis and transplantation in patients with diabetic nephropathy [19], and it confers significant benefit in the absence of hypertension. These benefits are clearly very substantial and strategies of care around the time of conception must minimize the loss of such benefits.

Hod et al. [20] studied eight women with normotensive insulin-dependent diabetes with confirmed nephropathy (> 500 mg per day). The women took captopril, and vigorously pursued optimal blood sugar control, until a missed period followed by a positive pregnancy test. All patients had significantly lower urinary protein at conception following their captopril treatment (reduced from 1,633±666, to 273±146 mg daily), but then experienced increased protein excretion during the pregnancy, but not to pre-captopril levels. Postpartum, the level of protein excretion was still below the pretreatment levels. This study may be consistent with a sustained benefit of ACE inhibition prepregnancy, or markedly improved glycemic control. Glycemic control clearly has the potential to affect the development of nephropathy (Diabetes Control and Complications Trial Research Group) [21] and will have been an important influence in parallel with ACE inhibition.

Bar et al. [22] reported on a series of cases of 24 women with diabetic nephropathy treated with an ACE inhibitor until the first positive pregnancy test. In all patients in this study, the intensive prepregnancy regime resulted in a reduction in proteinuria to a range of 10 to 450 mg/day at conception, with sustained reduction in proteinuria during pregnancy.

Cooper et al. [23] in 2006 in the nondiabetic population reported a possible two- to threefold increase in the risk of congenital malformation in those exposed to ACE inhibitors in the first trimester. This was in contrast with a prior lack of substantive evidence of teratogenicity in the first trimester (for review, see How and Sibai) [24]. This prompted concern of a possibility of an even greater effect in the diabetic population, and hence considerable caution was then advised with prescribing of ACE inhibition in diabetic women of childbearing age. In the years following this paper, a number of important studies were published examining the effect of ACE inhibition and angiotensin receptor blockers (ARBs) in pregnancy. The study of Li et al. [25], and the review of Polifka [26], address many of the concerns of the Cooper study. The overall conclusion from these papers is that it is likely any increased congenital abnormality rate following exposure is explained by the effects of other maternal factors that typically coexist in this population, including the effects of hypertension itself.

The paper of Porta et al. [27] in 2011 provides evidence that strategies to continue such treatment (in this case candesartan) into early in the first trimester are relatively safe and not associated with adverse outcome specifically in a diabetic population. This is a prospective randomized study that provides powerful evidence that continuing treatment with these agents up to eight weeks' gestation is justified, and therefore policies of continuing such treatment until conception in diabetic nephropathic women who are planning pregnancy are reasonable.

Tenant et al. [28] have described overall loss rates due to stillbirth and infant death in the diabetic population, and in response to this paper Lewis and Maxwell [29] put forward the arguments for continuation of ACE inhibition and ARBs in this patient population in the hope that overall outcomes will be improved. The correspondence emphasizes the need for bigger trials prior to reaching comfort on this issue. The wider issue of fetal effects of ACE inhibition and ARBs is covered in the review of Bullo et al. [30].

It is not known if teratogenic risk due to this class of drug may be even greater in the diabetic group. However, the potential benefits are substantial and potentially lifesaving. Clearly strategies must be employed on an individual basis to maximize the potential benefits and to reduce risk. Such strategies may vary depending on background fertility, severity of nephropathy and comorbidities, and may entail cessation of ACE inhibition prior to attempts at conception, or a policy of regular pregnancy testing (in the presence of regular menses) with immediate cessation of treatment upon diagnosis of pregnancy. The recent data post Cooper suggest that such policies are reasonable, but one should be cautious to ensure that patients understand the wider issues and are capable of monitoring menstrual pattern with a view to ceasing treatment before eight weeks of gestation.

Table 15.1 Characteristics of patient populations with diabetic nephropathy

Author/ Pregnancies	Year/Country	% with nephropathy	% of nephropaths with hypertension	% with nephrotic range proteinuria	% with Creatinine > 125 umol/l
Klemetti [17] 108	1988–1999 (65) Finland	14.7	61		
	2000–2011(43)	6.5	65		
Khoury [31] 72	2002 United States	Unclear	60%		13%
Ekbom [11] 11	2001 Denmark	5%		55%	
Bar [32] 24	2000 Israel	All	46%	All	0
Reece [33] 315	1998 Review		42%		
Gordon [34] 49	1996 United States	12%	27%	13%	7%
Mackie [35] 24	1996 United Kingdom	9%	17%	13%	21%
Miodovnik [36] 46	1996 United States	25%	41%		
Purdy [37] 14	1996 United States	NA	82%	18%	All

Levels of Comorbidity

There are few data on levels of comorbidity in the pregnant diabetic nephropathic population. Retinopathy is often described, and the proportion of women with hypertension varies as shown in Table 15.1. Few of the studies make reference to comorbidities such as thromboembolic events or cardiac disease. The data on diabetic nephropathy are weighted toward milder degrees of renal impairment and there will be a clear aversion to pregnancy for those with serious comorbidities. Cardiovascular comorbidity is more frequently mentioned in studies of follow-up following pregnancy. Assessment of risk of coronary artery disease has been studied in this population in other contexts, and Manske et al. [38] found that there was a very low level of significant coronary disease where the patient was younger than 45, duration of diabetes less than 25 years, and no ST-T wave changes appeared on ECG.

Barak and Miodovnik [39] review the case reports of coronary events in pregnant diabetic women. They describe 20 cases between 1953 and 1998 who suffered a coronary event around the time of pregnancy. Of the 13 women who suffered an event during pregnancy or in the puerperium, 7 mothers and 7 infants died. These figures are largely historical, but nonetheless serve to define the natural history of such an event. Major changes in the treatment of coronary events have occurred since the majority of these case reports, but thrombolysis would still pose difficult issues in the perinatal period. The study of Klemetti [17] describes 2 of 65 patients in their pre-2000 cohort as having a history of myocardial infarction. The issue of ischemic heart disease in pregnancy more recently is addressed in the review of Hawthorne [14], and recommendations on management made with reference to stenting and mode and timing of delivery following an acute event.

It is clear from Table 15.1 that the literature is weakened by some lack of clarity of the patient population with varying reporting of hypertension, nephrotic range proteinuria and degree of renal failure. There is a clear paucity of data from prospective studies, particularly in those with more severe disease, which characterize the aforementioned features prepregnancy.

Screening for Comorbidity

An ECG should be performed in early pregnancy in this population. Assessment of cardiovascular and thromboembolic risk should be made. Relevant risk factors would include family or personal history of cardiac or thromboembolic disease, hypertension, raised body mass index (BMI), a history of smoking and degree of urinary protein leakage.

Klemetti [40] examined long-term trends in baseline blood pressure in pregnant women with type 1 diabetes without nephropathy and found an increase over recent decades in parallel with prepregnancy BMI. The same group in a more recent publication [17] describes the rate of smoking at 26–28 percent, and the prevalence of proliferative retinopathy at 50–65 percent with the higher rate reflecting more recent experience in women with type 1 diabetes with nephropathy. Yogev in 2010 [41] examined a cohort of 46 women with type I diabetes and nephropathy to determine which parameters may be associated with a greater risk of complications during pregnancy, and found BMI to be the only factor associated with greater risk of complicated pregnancy. This paper, as with other single-center studies confined to a nephropathic population, may be underpowered to definitively exclude other influences.

There are no specific data on thromboembolic risk in this group of pregnant women. Nonetheless a strategy to prevent thromboembolism needs to be employed. It would seem reasonable to suggest that all women with nephrotic range proteinuria receive low-molecular-weight heparin (LMWH) prophylaxis throughout pregnancy. Other women with more minor degrees of proteinuria should receive LMWH if other risk factors are present. The dose of LMWH employed will depend on degree of renal impairment.

Problems in Pregnancy

These data are summarized in Table 15.2. A number of recent helpful reviews have been published including Piccoli [48], Bramham [49] and Landon [50]. The following comments apply to complications from mid-trimester onward as most studies have excluded first-trimester complications. Reviews of diabetic nephropathy in pregnancy continue to emphasize the problems with this literature, almost invariably retrospective in nature, covering experience in single-site centers of excellence over decades, and still with relatively small numbers of patients. The situation is further complicated by the fact that level of glycemic control is a major determinant of outcome in such pregnancies. Furthermore the diabetic population is continuously changing, both in demography (increasing proportions of type II), and in exposure to treatments such as ACE inhibition. With reference to diabetic nephropathy, it is not possible to subdivide the data available according to prepregnancy treatment with ACE inhibition (approximately 60 percent in the study of Klemetti [17]), and a proportion of the published experience predates use of ACE inhibition. Summation of the data in such reviews give a picture of the relevant population, late twenties in age, with diabetes of 18 years' duration, and a mean age at onset of 12 years [33].

Caesarean rates are universally high, reflecting high degrees of intervention in such pregnancies, and possibly uncertainty regarding fetal status faced with the dual threats of renal impairment and diabetes, often in the presence of superimposed preeclampsia. The study of Klemetti [17] describes a move away from elective caesarean in more recent years, but resulting in a higher emergency caesarean rate, and no change in overall rate. Gestational age at delivery reflects the same concerns. Definitions of fetal growth restriction (FGR) are generally centile based, but caution is required with the confounding influences of diabetes and vascular disease [43]. There are strong arguments for regular ultrasound surveillance every two weeks, and more frequently in the presence of any acute concern. Perinatal loss rates vary from 0–10 percent, and the figures in the study of Klemetti [17] are likely to be representative at approximately 5 percent. Such figures are often viewed with optimism, but any perinatal loss in the context of such a high-risk pregnancy is clearly extremely disappointing. It is a double disaster for a woman with diabetic nephropathy to potentially compromise her long-term health and survival, and not achieve a healthy surviving infant.

Hypertension

There are good recent reviews of the issue of hypertension in diabetic pregnancy, which examine prevalence of hypertensive complications and also their ability to predict some long-term

Table 15.2 Complications of pregnancy affected by diabetic nephropathy

Authors Year	N	Caesarean section%	Mean gestational age (wks)	Prematurity N W = weeks	FGR	Perinatal death% (n)
Klemetti [17] Pre 2000		100	36	77 21 percent < 32 w		4.6 (3)
Klemetti [17] Post 2000		92	35	70 14 percent < 32 w		4.7 (2)
Damm [18] 2013 Type I	11	91	36	27 percent < 34 weeks	36 percent	(1)
Damm [18] 2013 Type II	5	60	36	40 percent < 34 weeks	40 percent	
Nielsen [42] 2009	7		36		29 percent	0
Howarth [43] 2007*	28	90	36		OR6	
Bagg [44] 2003	24	83	36			
Khoury [16] 2002	72	68	35	13 percent < 32 w		4 percent (3)
Rossing [45] 2002	31	39	37			10 percent (3)
Ekbom [11] 2001	11			45 percent before 34 w		0
Bar [32] 2000	24	62		17 percent < 37 w	21 percent	4 percent (1)
Biesenbach [46] 1999	14	50	34		64 percent	36 percent (5)
Dunne [47] 1999	21	90	34		14 percent	10 percent (2)
Reece [33] 1998**	315	74		22 percent < 34 w	15 percent	5 percent

N = number of pregnancies.
* Howarth et al. includes some women with hypertension but not nephropathy.
** Review article of papers from the 1980s and 1990s.

cardiovascular complications [51, 52, 53]. The paper of Jensen et al. [54] demonstrates that in women with type 1 diabetes with microalbuminuria (specifically excluding nephropathy) the incidence of preeclampsia is increased fourfold. Mathiesen [55] reviews the issue of hypertension with specific reference to diabetic nephropathy, and more recently with reference to temporal changes in blood pressure management and pregnancy outcome [56].

Carr et al. [57] address the issue of hypertensive control in pregnancy affected by diabetic nephropathy. This was a retrospective study that identified two groups, one achieving a target blood pressure of mean arterial pressure of less than 100 mm Hg, and another group failing to meet the target. Approximately 10 percent of the diabetic population in this study were deemed nephropathic. There was no difference in age or duration of diabetes between the two groups. The group with above-target control had greater urinary protein excretion and higher creatinine. Suboptimal control was associated with a significantly increased risk of delivering early i.e. less than 32 weeks' gestation, even after adjustment for blood glucose control and duration of diabetes.

The study of Carr et al. provides some specific data on hemodynamic measurement in pregnancy with diabetic nephropathy. Blood pressure and cardiac output were higher than expected, and total peripheral resistance elevated in the group with above-target blood pressure. The authors conclude that long-standing hypertension is likely to be more severe, characterized by vasoconstriction, and that treatment regimens should include vasodilators. The issue of target blood pressure is also addressed in the review of Kitzmiller and Combs, where they express a preference for blood pressure in the range of 120–130 / 80–85 mm Hg [7]. The wider issue of target blood pressure control in a hypertensive (long-term and gestational) population has been addressed in the Control of Hypertension in Pregnancy Study (CHIPS) [58] (see Chapter 8). This study examined outcome in two groups, one with a target diastolic blood pressure of 85 mmHg, while the less well-controlled group had a target diastolic of 100 mmHg. There were no deleterious effects of more rigid control, and there were less severe degrees of hypertension in the tightly controlled group. One cannot necessarily extrapolate the findings of this study to the diabetic nephropathic population, but it provides support for tighter control in these patients. The paper of Nielsen [42] would support the view that such management is associated with good outcomes, and may be an improvement on management with less effective blood pressure control. This topic is reviewed again by Mathiesen [56] and strong evidence presented to support a target of less than 130/80 mmHg.

Sibai et al. [59] report data on a large number of women with type I diabetes. The risk of preeclampsia increases with increasing white classification of diabetes, attaining a 36 percent risk in those with retinopathy or nephropathy, in comparison with an overall rate of 20 percent. Proteinuria at baseline, hypertension and nulliparity also predicted preeclampsia. The difficulty in diagnosing preeclampsia in a population with diabetic nephropathy is likely to be a significant factor explaining the varying rates of preeclampsia. The rate of diagnosis of preeclampsia is 40–60 percent in various studies, and more recently Klemetti describes a rate of 52 percent pre 2000, and 42 percent post 2000 [17]. The incidence of preeclampsia has been the subject of a separate review by Sibai [60]. In his review of seven publications there were 333 women with diabetic nephropathy, with an overall incidence of preeclampsia of 51 percent (range 35 percent–66 percent). The use of low-dose aspirin to prevent preeclampsia has not been adequately studied in this population, with the study of Caritis et al. [61] failing to show any benefit. Many clinicians would be reluctant to omit aspirin prophylaxis, however, given the vulnerability of this patient group to early-onset disease. Arguments for advising low-dose aspirin in such pregnancies include the potential to prevent mid-trimester preeclampsia, modest protection against thromboembolism in a high-risk group and prevention of coronary events.

Proteinuria

Once pregnant, women with nephropathy do not always adapt to pregnancy as do their controls with 50 percent increases in renal blood flow and glomerular filtration rate. Some will demonstrate the normal physiological rise in GFR, some will remain unchanged and in some a decrement will be noted [7]. As mentioned in that review, it is difficult to tease out the decline in function in pregnancy from the natural history of the condition with falls in GFR of 10–12mls per min per year.

Urinary protein is recognized to generally increase during the course of pregnancy in women with diabetic nephropathy. The study of Hod et al. [20] referred to earlier shows the progression of level of proteinuria in a subset of women with diabetes in the different trimesters and postnatally. Proteinuria can be substantial, but normally resolves following delivery. Much of the proteinuria must be caused by the hyperfiltration of pregnancy as it resolves reasonably consistently following delivery. Transient deterioration can of course arise as a result of superimposed preeclampsia. The greatest clinical concern arises from any subsequent fall in plasma oncotic pressure, with risk of pulmonary edema. Diuretic treatment may be required in such situations even though conceptually unattractive due to the potential to further reduce intravascular volume in compromised pregnancies. Patterns of weight gain in these pregnancies have not been described.

Urinary protein excretion was summarized in the review of Star and Carpenter in 1998 that evaluated nine studies [62]. Mean protein excretion was typically between one and three grams at baseline, but increased to between four and eight grams in the third trimester. This frequently fell postpartum, but not always to baseline values. It is unclear if those with persistently high levels postpartum were a reflection of a short follow-up period, or disease progression, or deterioration secondary to pregnancy. Klemetti et al. [17] also describe range of proteinuria with similar results to those quoted earlier, and median third-trimester protein excretion of 9.6 grams, emphasizing the vulnerability of this patient group to hypoalbuminemia and pulmonary edema.

Preterm Delivery

Rates of preterm delivery for this group must be compared with the diabetic population as a whole. These data are available from Sibai et al. [63] and from CEMACH [12]. Sibai breaks down rates of delivery as a result of spontaneous labor (16 percent at < 37 weeks, 9 percent at < 35 weeks), and from indicated delivery such as preeclampsia or FGR (22 percent at < 37 weeks, 7 percent at < 35 weeks). Steroids should generally be prescribed prior to 34 weeks albeit with caution i.e. with monitoring of the blood glucose response, urinary ketones and a temporary increase in insulin treatment as required. There is currently no consensus on use of steroids between 34 and 37 weeks, so any potential benefit has to be balanced against the disadvantage of loss of metabolic control. The greatest argument for steroids in this situation can be made when elective caesarean delivery is considered.

It is clear from many of the studies [34, 35] that those patients who enter pregnancy with the greatest impairment of renal function are most at risk of very preterm delivery, though mean gestational ages in all studies suggest most babies would be expected to do well, especially with current advances in management of neonatal lung disease. Many of the studies in this area are performed over a substantial time span, and many of the papers mentioned in this review include patients, and therefore preterm babies born in the early 1980s. Neonatal management has improved hugely over this time. While this may reassure us that the outcome should be substantially improved, it is also possible that thresholds for delivery have been moved forward to "protect renal function" or to improve overall perinatal survival. Influences likely to result in elective preterm delivery include concern about loss of renal function, presence of preeclampsia, or concern about risk of stillbirth. Amniocentesis may help provide reassurance about fetal lung maturity, while simultaneously assessing fetal status [64]. The latter method of assessment has yet to achieve widespread acceptance.

Factors Relating to Perinatal Outcome

Pregnancies complicated by diabetic nephropathy carry the added burdens of increased risk of congenital malformation, stillbirth and metabolic disturbance in comparison to other forms of renal disease in pregnancy. The literature in this area is more focused on those risks that arise as a result of the impaired renal function, as it is this that sets these women apart from the main diabetic population.

Khoury et al. [31] describe the problems inherent in calculating risks of complications in pregnancy with diabetic nephropathy, and they estimate that to assess an association between severity of diabetic nephropathy and perinatal death, a study of 850 pregnancies would be required. Ekbom et al. [11] have examined diabetic pregnancy with a range of urinary albumin excretion. Though the numbers of patients with nephropathy are low (n = 11), there is a clear association of increasing severity of urinary albumin excretion at baseline and preterm delivery due to preeclampsia (but not preterm delivery due to other causes). Lauenborg et al. [65] examined the characteristics of women with diabetes that increased risk of stillbirth across three tertiary centers in Denmark over a 10-year period. Twenty-seven percent of women with stillbirths suffered from diabetic nephropathy, as opposed to 5 percent overall in the reference group.

The CEMACH study [12] used a composite of poor clinical outcome (major anomaly at any gestation, intrauterine death from 20 weeks and any death up to 28 days after delivery). The odds ratio for such an outcome was 2.0 in the nephropathy group (95 percent CI 1.0, 4.2). Excluding congenital anomalies, the adjusted odds ratio for such a poor outcome was 2.6 (95 percent CI 1.1, 6.1). Haeri [66] examined the relationship of nephropathy to intrauterine growth restriction (IUGR) confirming this association, and this is further clarified in the study of Howarth et al. [43] demonstrating a bimodal distribution of custo-mized birth weight centiles.

Salvesen et al. [67] examined fetal well-being in a group of six fetuses where the mothers suffered diabetic nephropathy. Cordocentesis demonstrated that these fetuses were hypoxemic and acidemic in the absence of abnormal blood flow studies. This implies the lack of a placental cause, and may reflect wider metabolic disturbance. It emphasizes the diffi-culty in being confident regarding fetal outcome even in the presence of normal ultrasound assessment. This difficulty is compounded by the lack of data regarding background risks of placental abruption. It is likely that management of pregnancy in women with dia-betic nephropathy will always involve some conflict between stillbirth risk and neonatal morbidity as obstetricians struggle to decide on timing of delivery.

Long-Term Prognosis

• Mother

A major issue for women with diabetic nephropathy is the risk of a permanent deterioration in renal function attributable to pregnancy, bringing forward the need for renal replacement therapy. There are good reasons why pregnancy may increase the risk of progression of nephropathy, including increasing glomerular hyper-filtration and the risk of development of hypertension. Studies in this area have suffered from small numbers, changing outcome for progression of renal disease due to advances in management, and lack of appro-priate control groups. Most studies have found no effect of pregnancy on rate of decline in renal func-tion. The studies are summarized in Table 15.3. There is very wide variation in the follow-up periods reported in such studies, making the data on progres-sion to end-stage renal failure extremely difficult to interpret. These studies focus exclusively on renal outcome, and there is no formal assessment of the effect of pregnancy/preeclampsia on long-term risk of a cardiovascular event in this high-risk group. The study of Gordin et al. [69] adds weight to the general concern that women who suffer from pree-clampsia are at greater risk of long-term cardiovascu-lar morbidity. In this study women with type

I diabetes and a history of preeclampsia had a higher frequency of diabetic nephropathy at follow-up (41.9 percent versus 8.9 percent), were more likely to be on an antihypertensive treatment (50.0 percent versus 9.8 percent) and were more likely to have coronary artery disease (12.2 percent versus 2.2 percent).

The studies specifically in diabetic nephropathy tend to be retrospective cohort studies, though two major prospective cohort studies in diabetic pregnancy in general provide complementary information.

• Retrospective

The data on end-stage renal disease and maternal death in the review of Reece [33] reflect approximately three years of follow-up. The duration of follow-up in the different studies varies, and appears to be largely opportunistic. Biesenbach et al. [46] studied 14 preg-nancies in 12 women. All these women had preexist-ing hypertension. They subdivided pregnancies into those that had a physiological increase in creatinine clearance in early pregnancy, and those in whom it declined. This results in small numbers, in which the latter group is associated with longer duration of diabetes, greater proteinuria and worse renal function prior to conception. In six pregnancies there was an improvement in creatinine clearance of 36 percent up to 24 weeks. In another eight pregnancies it decreased by 16 percent over the same early period. In the latter group the deterioration in function persisted postpar-tum. In the group with a decline in renal function there was a greater increase in proteinuria during pregnancy, and more marked hypertension. In this study, seven out of eight women in the poor-prognosis group had a preconceptual creatinine clear-ance of < 70 ml/min, while all the women with a physiological increase in creatinine clearance had a clearance of > 70 ml/min. The groups in this study did not differ in metabolic control as demonstrated by HbA1c.

Gordon et al. in 1996 also found cause for concern related to severity and progression of renal impairment [34]. Women were categorized according to degree of renal impairment, and no difference in degree of change in the three groups was noted. It is noteworthy that the three women with the worst renal impairment progressed to transplantation after the pregnancy i.e. at intervals of 8, 15, and 41 months after delivery (no control data). Most of their population demonstrated

Table 15.3 Studies examining the effect of pregnancy on progression of renal disease

Authors	Year	N	Decline in function	Mortality	End-stage renal failure
Young [68] Brazil	2011	11	NS		NS
Bagg [44] New Zealand	2003	14	NS		36 percent
Rossing [45] Denmark	2002	26	NS	35 percent Mean follow up 16 years	19 percent
Bar [32] Israel	2000	24	None		
Biesenbach [46] Austria	1999	12	Yes	0	
Dunne [47] United Kingdom	1999	18	No	0	1
Reece [33] Review	1998	315	No	5 percent (mean 35 months)	17 percent (mean 33 months)
Gordon [34] United States	1996	45	Yes		3 (6 percent)
Mackie [35] United Kingdom	1996	24	No	0	4 (17 percent)
Miodovnik [36] United States	1996	56	No	1 Or 5*	26 percent at six years
Purdy [37] United States	1996	11	Yes		63 percent at two to three years

* dependent on duration of follow-up
N = number of pregnancies
NS = no significant difference

nephrotic-range proteinuria by the third trimester. At postnatal follow-up, mean creatinine clearance had decreased, but proteinuria was unchanged from early pregnancy measurement. The fall in creatinine clearance in ml/minute per year and the percent decline in creatinine clearance per year were assessed. Individuals entering pregnancy with proteinuria in excess of 1 g, and a creatinine clearance of less than 90 mls/minute fared worse by both criteria. The difference was not explained by mean HbA1c, mean arterial blood pressure or use of ACE inhibitor.

Purdy et al. [37] examined a group with poor renal function, all with a creatinine of 124 μmol/L or more.

They examined reciprocal of creatinine plots over time, but there is a clear paucity of data prior to the index pregnancies. Furthermore, there is a lack of clarity about inclusion criteria for the study. Nonetheless, the rate of progression of disease in this group with poor function is of concern.

Rossing et al. [45] evaluated the effect of pregnancy on renal function in women with diabetic nephropathy. They found no adverse effect compared with a control group of women with nephropathy but no pregnancies. No further details are given regarding the control group, raising the possibility that other comorbidities may have been present and sufficient to deter women from pregnancy. The study group did have a shorter duration of diabetes, but earlier onset of nephropathy. The pregnancy rate prior to the onset of nephropathy (similar in both groups) argues against any bias due to possible comorbidities.

Data in this study give a sense of the proportion of women who proceed to die prematurely, with 9 out of 26 dead at the end of the follow-up period. Half of these deaths were from cardiovascular disease and between 50 percent and 60 percent were smoking at the time of diagnosis of nephropathy. At the end of the follow-up period, 65 percent of the pregnant group and 53 percent of the nonpregnant group were still alive and without end-stage renal disease. In the review of Klemetti [17], 12 women out of 108 had died by the end of 2013 (25 years from first pregnancies recorded).

Bagg et al. [44] provide similar data from women managed from 1985 to 2000. Their study of 24 pregnancies in 14 women found at a median follow-up of six years postpartum, five (36 percent) had begun dialysis. Four had proliferative retinopathy (one blind), three had ischemic heart disease, three had stroke and two had peripheral vascular disease.

Bar et al. [32] found no deterioration in serum creatinine, or creatinine clearance, in their group of 24 women with diabetic nephropathy. Mackie et al. [35] plotted inverse creatinine over the long term in subjects with renal impairment and demonstrated a lack of any effect of pregnancy on long-term decline in renal function. More recently, the study of Young et al. would appear to confirm a good outcome where renal function does not fall in the moderately or severely impaired group [68].

- ### Studies on Parity

Miodovnik et al. [36] stratified the risk of developing nephropathy by parity using life-table analysis and showed no significant effects. They also examined the rate of decline in creatinine clearance and found no effect of pregnancy (decreasing at an annual rate of 8-10mls/min). No effect of parity on risk of end-stage renal disease was seen. Interestingly, the only factor that made progression to end-stage disease among the group with nephropathy more likely was black race. Retinopathy, development of hypertension in the pregnancy, development of nephrotic range proteinuria during the pregnancy or glycohemoglobin did not predict progression, though the study was not necessarily powered to address these issues specifically. While this study is reassuring, there was no nulliparous control group.

- ### Prospective Cohort Studies

The Diabetes Control and Complications Trial Group [70] allowed intensification of blood glucose control for pregnancy, and included 86 women (135 pregnancies) in the conventional treatment group and 94 (135 pregnancies) in the intensive treatment group. There was no difference in the rate of development of micro-albuminuria as a result of pregnancy, though some increases in albumin excretion rate were noted in relation to pregnancy.

The EURODIAB prospective complications study [71] examined risk factors for progression to nephropathy in a group of 425 childless diabetic women, and found that while HbA1c was a significant predictor of progression to microalbuminuria, pregnancy was not (102 gave birth in the study period). This applied to both the nulliparous and multiparous populations. In the same study, while duration of diabetes and HbA1c were predictive of retinopathy, pregnancy again was not. The study examined risk of neuropathy in addition to nephropathy and retinopathy and found that pregnancy was not a risk factor for the development or progression of any diabetic complication.

Some work has been published examining the relationship of pregnancy complications to subsequent morbidity in the diabetic population. Gordin [53] in follow-up of diabetic pregnancy in general, demonstrated that preeclampsia but not pregnancy-induced hypertension predicts subsequent development of diabetic nephropathy. Subsequently the same group showed [72] the predictive value of hypertensive complications in diabetic pregnancy for severe retinopathy. Sandvik in 2010 [73] similarly demonstrated the predictive value of preterm preeclampsia for end-stage renal disease in women with preexisting diabetes.

Neonate/Fetal

The data on neonatal outcome are limited. In the study of Bar et al. [22], there were two severely handicapped infants, both seemingly as a result of shoulder dystocia despite a caesarean rate of 62 percent. All other survivors to two years of age were free of disability. Reece et al. [33] in an earlier review provide data from three previous studies where the incidence of psychomotor impairment was 5.5 percent,

3.7 percent, and 9 percent, i.e. an overall incidence of 6 percent. The studies in question were published in 1981, 1988, and 1995, and one may therefore question their relevance today. However, it is the later study in 1995 that quotes the highest incidence. Mackie et al. [35] report that one baby delivered at 27 weeks went on to have cerebral palsy. As with the other studies, there was no formal neurodevelopmental follow-up of the infants involved. Khalil in 2010 [74] demonstrated decreased functional renal reserve in offspring of diabetic mothers, though not specifically those with nephropathy.

Omissions

There are clearly areas of clinical practice that are not addressed by the current literature. The world literature may be from very varied health care systems, with varying incidences of type II diabetes, access to health care and altered rate of progression of long-term complications, possibly with racial differences. There are few data on first-trimester complications, comorbidities and the potential impact of ACE inhibition prepregnancy, and the literature may not reflect the increasing proportion of women with type II diabetes.

Some guidance needs to be given about the reasons to advise against pregnancy. These would include evidence of untreated coronary artery disease, severity of cardiac disease, uncontrolled hypertension and proliferative retinopathy not in remission. Women with more severe renal impairment may be better served by assessment for transplantation, and consideration of pregnancy afterward, age allowing, or have discussion about intensive dialysis strategies (see Chapter 10).

Summary

The literature reviewed in this chapter spans a number of decades of experience. During this time there have been notable advances in diabetes and renal care. It is likely that the vast majority of women with diabetic nephropathy can consider a pregnancy without any threat to their long-term disease progression. There is a risk that those with the most severe disease may experience a significant deterioration in renal function, and ultimately, end-stage renal failure. The same patients will be most at risk of an adverse outcome to pregnancy, though most pregnancies will be successful. Caesarean delivery is likely and many deliveries are prior to full term as a result of preeclampsia. The demography of this population is changing continuously, and current cohorts of women may well have an improved outcome largely due to ACE inhibition and statins. The literature to date largely reflects experience with type I diabetes, and it is likely that type II diabetes will become more common in future.

In contemplating a pregnancy, women with diabetic nephropathy have to consider the dual risks of diabetes and their impaired renal function to a pregnancy. Furthermore, they need advice on the potential for such a pregnancy to further compromise their renal function. They will need to make a considered long-term judgment of the risks involved, which requires that they are well informed about their prognosis, even in the absence of pregnancy. It is most appropriate if this information is presented to them remote from pregnancy, emphasizing the importance of prepregnancy counseling. Given the pivotal role of control of blood glucose and hypertension, it may be that a series of visits reflecting an intensification of care is appropriate rather than a single preconceptual visit.

Management Box

Ensure informed decision about pregnancy (including maternal prognosis during and after pregnancy)
Advise on when to stop ACE/ARB

*** Intensification of care with emphasis on

Control of blood glucose

Control of blood pressure

Checking for retinopathy and treating accordingly

Check for other comorbidities such as cardiac disease or thromboembolic risk

Folic acid 5 mg commencing prior to conception

Aspirin 75–150 mg from end of first trimester

Review need for thromboprophylaxis regularly (early pregnancy, hospitalization, increasing proteinuria, preeclampsia)

Weigh the patient and document baseline renal function and albumin-creatinine ratio

Regular visits to a multidisciplinary team

Regular scans/monitoring for fetal growth and beware of confounding influences

Deliver for preeclampsia generally only if specific signs of preeclampsia

Caution with fluid overload peripartum

Restart ACE inhibition postnatally (+ statin if appropriate) (see Chapter 7)

References

1. Hill CJ, Fogarty DG. Changing trends in end-stage renal disease due to diabetes in the United Kingdom. *Journal of renal care* 2012;**38**(1):12–22.

2. Najafian B, Mauer M. Progression of diabetic nephropathy in type I diabetic patients. *Diabetes research and clinical practice* 2009;**83**: 1–8.

3. Parving H, Persson F, Rossing P. Microalbuminuria: A parameter that has changed diabetes care. *Diabetes research and clinical practice* 2015;**107**:1–8.

4. American Diabetes Association. Diabetic nephropathy. *Diabetes care* 2003;**26**(1):S94–S98.

5. Chan GC, Tang SCW. Diabetic nephropathy: Landmark clinical trials and tribulations. *Nephrol dial transplant* 2015;**0**:1–10.

6. Giorgino F, Laviola L, Cavallo Perin P, Solnica B, Fuller J, Chaturvedi N. Factors associated with progression to macroalbuminuria in microalbuminuric Type I diabetic patients: The EURODIAB Prospective Complications Study. *Diabetologia* 2004;**47**:1020–1028.

7. Kitzmiller JL, Combs A. Diabetic nephropathy and pregnancy. *Obstetric and gynecology clinics of North America* 1996;**23**:173–203.

8. Currie G, McKay G, Delles C. Biomarkers in diabetic nephropathy: Present and future. *World J diabetes* 2014;**5**(6):763–776.

9. White P. Pregnancy complicating diabetes. *JAMA* 1945;**128**(3):181–182.

10. White P. Pregnancy complicating diabetes. *American journal of medicine* 1949;November:609–616.

11. Ekbom P, Damm P, Feldt-Rasmussen B, Feldt-Rasmussen U, Molvig J, Mathiesen ER. Pregnancy outcome in Type I diabetic women with microalbuminuria. *Diabetes care* 2001;**24**:1739–1744.

12. Confidential enquiry into maternal and child health. *Diabetes in pregnancy: Are we providing the best care? Findings of a national enquiry: England, Wales and Northern Ireland*. London: CEMACH, 2007.

13. Wahabi HA et al. Preconception care for diabetic women for improving maternal and fetal outcomes: A systematic review and meta-analysis. *BMC pregnancy and childbirth* 2010;**10**:63.

14. Hawthorne G. Maternal complications in diabetic pregnancy. *Best practice and research clinical obstetrics and gynaecology* 2011:**25**:77–90.

15. Ali S and Dornhorst A. Diabetes in pregnancy: Health risks and management. *Postgrad med J* 2011;**87**: 417–427.

16. Bell R, Glinianaia SV, Tennant PWG, Bilous RW, Rankin J. Peri-conception hyperglycaemia and nephropathy are associated with risk of congenital anomaly in women with pre-existing diabetes: A population-based cohort study. *Diabetologia* 2012;**55**:936–947.

17. Klemetti MM et al. Obstetric and perinatal outcome in type I diabetes patients with diabetic nephropathy during 1988–2011. *Diabetologia* 2015;**58**:678–686.

18. Damm JA et al. Diabetic nephropathy and microalbuminuria in pregnant women with type I and type II diabetes. *Diabetes care* 2013;**36**: 3489–3494.

19. Lewis EJ, Hunsicker LG, Bain RP, et al. for the Collaborative Study Group. The effect of angiotensin-converting enzyme inhibition on diabetic nephropathy. *N Engl J med* 1993;**329**:1456–1462.

20. Hod M, van Dijk DJ, Karp M, Weintraub N, Rabinerson D, Bar J, et al. Diabetic nephropathy and pregnancy: The effect of ACE inhibitors prior to pregnancy on fetomaternal outcome. *Nephrol dial transplant* 1995;**10**:2328–2383.

21. The Diabetes Control and Complications Trial Research Group. The effect of intensive treatment of diabetes on the development and progression of long-term complications in insulin-dependent diabetes mellitus. *N Engl J med* 1993;**329**:977–986.

22. Bar J, Chen R, Schoenfeld A, Orvieto R, Yahav J, Ben-Rafael Z, et al. Pregnancy outcome in patients with insulin dependent diabetes mellitus and diabetic nephropathy treated with ACE inhibitors before pregnancy. *J pediatr endocrinol metab* 1999;**12**(5):659–665.

23. Cooper WO, Hernandez-Diaz S, Abrogast PG, Dudley JA, Dyer S, Gideon PS, et al. Major congenital malformations after first-trimester exposure to ACE inhibitors. *N Engl J med* 2006;**354**(23):2443–2451.

24. How HY, Sibai BM. Use of angiotensin-converting enzyme inhibitors in patients with diabetic nephropathy. *J matern fetal neonatal med* 2002;**12**(6):402–407.

25. Li D-K, Yang C, Andrade S, Tavares V, Ferber J. Maternal exposure to angiotensin converting enzyme inhibitors in the first trimester and risk of malformations in offspring: A retrospective cohort study. *BMJ* 2011;**343**:d5931.

26. Polifka JE (2012) Is there an embryopathy associated with first trimester exposure to angiotensin-converting enzyme inhibitors and angiotensin receptor antagonists? A critical review of the evidence. *Birth defects res A clin mol teratol* 94:576–598.

27. Porta M, Hainer JW, Jansson SO, et al. Exposure to candesartan during the first trimester of pregnancy in type 1 diabetes: Experience from the placebo-controlled Diabetic Retinopathy Candesartan Trials. *Diabetologia* 2011;**54**:1298–1303.

28. Tennant PWG, Newham JJ, Bell R, Rankin J (2011) Studies of congenital anomalies should capture all cases, not just live births. BMJ (electronic letter). Available from www.bmj.com/rapidresponse/2011/11/03/.

29. Lewis G, Maxwell AP. Should women with diabetic nephropathy considering pregnancy continue ACE inhibitor or angiotensin II receptor blocker therapy until pregnancy is confirmed? *Diabetologia* 2014.

30. Bullo M, et al. Pregnancy outcome following exposure to angiotensin converting enzyme inhibitors or angiotensin receptor antagonists: A systematic review. *Hypertension* 2012;**60**:444–450.

31. Khoury JC, Miodovnik M, LeMasters G, Sibai B. Pregnancy outcome and progression of diabetic nephropathy. *What's next? J matern fetal med* 2002;**11**:238–244.

32. Bar J, Ben-Rafael Z, Padoa A, Orvieto R, Boner G, Hod M. Prediction of pregnancy outcome in subgroups of women with renal disease. *Clin nephrol* 2000;**53**(6):437–444.

33. Reece EA, Leguizamon G, Homko C. Pregnancy performance and outcomes associated with diabetic nephropathy. *Am J Perinatol* 1998;**15**(7):413–421.

34. Gordon M, Landon MB, Samuels P, Hissrich S, Gabbe SG. Perinatal outcome and long-term follow-up associated with modern management of diabetic nephropathy. *Obstet Gynecol* 1996;**87**(3):401–409.

35. Mackie AD, Doddridge MC, Gamsu HR, Brudenell JM, Nicolaides KH, Drury PL. Outcome of pregnancy in patients with insulin-dependent diabetes mellitus and nephropathy with moderate renal impairment. *Diabetic medicine* 1996;**13**:90–96.

36. Miodovnik M, Roseen BM, Khoury JC, Grigsby JL, Siddiqi TA. Does pregnancy increase the risk of development and progression of diabetic nephropathy? *Am J obstet gynecol* 1996;**174**(4):1180–1189.

37. Purdy LP, Hantsch CE, Molitch ME, Metzger BE, Phelps RL, Dooley SL et al. Effect of pregnancy on renal function in patients with moderate-to-severe diabetic renal insufficiency. *Diabetes care* 1996;**19**(10):1067–1074.

38. Manske CL, Thomas W, Wang Y, et al. Screening diabetic transplant candidates for coronary artery disease: Identification of a low risk subgroup. *Kidney int* 1993;**44**:617–621.

39. Barak R, Miodovnic M. Medical complications of diabetes mellitus in pregnancy. *Clin obstet* 2000;**43**(1):17–31.

40. Klemetti MM et al. Blood pressure levels but not hypertensive complications have increased in Type I diabetes pregnancies during 1989–2010. *Diabet med* 2013;**30**:1087–1093.

41. Yogev Y, et al. Maternal overweight and pregnancy outcome in women with Type I diabetes mellitus and different degrees of nephropathy. *Journal of materno-fetal and neonatal medicine* 2010;**23**(9):999–1003.

42. Nielsen LR, Damm P, Mathiesen ER. Improved pregnancy outcome in Type I diabetic women with microalbuminuria or diabetic nephropathy. *Diabetes care* 2009;**32**:38–44.

43. Howarth C, Gazis A, James D. Associations of type I diabetes mellitus, maternal vascular disease and complications of pregnancy. *Diabetic medicine* 2007;**24**:1229–1234.

44. Bagg W, Neale L, Henley P, MacPherson P, Cundy T. Long-term maternal outcome after pregnancy in women with diabetic nephropathy. *N Z med J* 2003;**116**:1180.

45. Rossing K, Jacobsen P, Hommel E, Mathiesen E, Svenningsen A, Rossing P, et al. Pregnancy and progression of diabetic nephropathy. *Diabetologia* 2002;**45**:36–41.

46. Biesenbach G, Grafinger P, Stoger H, Zarzgornik J. How pregnancy influences renal function in nephropathic type I diabetic women depends on their pre-conceptual creatinine clearance. *J Nephrol* 1999;**12**(1):41–46.

47. Dunne FP, Chowdhury TA, Hartland A, Smith T, Brydon PA, McConkey C, et al. Pregnancy outcome in women with insulin-dependent diabetes mellitus complicated by nephropathy. *Q J Med* 1999;**92**:451–454.

48. Piccoli GB, et al. Type I diabetes, diabetic nephropathy, and pregnancy: A systematic review and meta-study. *Rev diabet stud* 2013;**10**:6–26.

49. Bramham K, Rajasingham D. Pregnancy in diabetes and kidney disease. *Journal of renal care* 2012;**38**(Suppl. 1):78–89.

50. Landon MB. Diabetic nephropathy and pregnancy. *Clinical obstetrics and gynaecology*. 2007;**50**:998–1006.

51. Colatrella A, et al. Hypertension in diabetic pregnancy: Impact and long term outlook. *Best practice and research clinical endocrinology and metabolism* 2010;**24**:635–651.

52. Sullivan SD, Umans JG, Ratner R. Hypertension complicating diabetic pregnancies: Pathophysiology, management and controversies. *J clin hypertens* 2011;**13**:275–284.

53. Gordin D, et al. Risk factors of hypertensive pregnancies in women with diabetes and the influence on their future life. *Annals of medicine* 2014;**46**:498–502.

54. Jensen DM, et al. Microalbuminuria, preeclampsia and preterm delivery in pregnant women with Type I diabetes. *Diabetes care* 2010;33:90–94.

55. Mathiesen ER et al. Obstetric nephrology: Pregnancy in women with diabetic nephropathy – The role of antihypertensive treatment. *Clin J Am Soc Nephrol* 2012;7:2081–2088.

56. Mathiesen ER. Diabetic nephropathy in pregnancy: New insights from a retrospective cohort study. *Diabetologia* 2015;58:649–650.

57. Carr DB, Koontz GL, Gardella C, Holing EV, Brateng DA, Brown ZA, et al. Diabetic nephropathy in pregnancy: Suboptimal hypertensive control associated with preterm delivery. *AJH* 2006;19:513–519.

58. Magee LA, et al. The control of hypertension in pregnancy study (CHIPS) randomised controlled trial. *Arch Dis Child Fetal Neonatal Ed* 2014;99(Suppl. 1): A1–A180.

59. Sibai BM, Caritis SN, Hauth JC, Lindheimer M, VanDorsten JP, MacPherson C, et al. for the National Institute of Child Health and Human Development Maternal-Fetal Medicine Units Network. Risks of preeclampsia and adverse neonatal outcomes among women with pregestational diabetes mellitus. *Am J obstet gynecol* 2000;182:364–369.

60. Sibai BM. Risk factors, pregnancy complications, and prevention of hypertensive disorders in women with pregravid diabetes mellitus. *J matern fetal med* 2000;9:62–65.

61. Caritis S, Sibai B, Hauth J, Lindheimer MD, Klebanoff M, Thom E, et al. Low-dose aspirin to prevent pre-eclampsia in women at high risk. *N Engl J med* 1998;338:701–705.

62. Star J, Carpenter MW. The effect of pregnancy on the natural history of diabetic retinopathy and nephropathy. *Clinics in perinatology* 1998;25(4):887–916.

63. Sibai BM, Caritis SN, Hauth JC, MacPherson C, VanDorsten JP, Klebanoff M, et al. Preterm delivery in women with pregestational diabetes mellitus or chronic hypertension relative to women with uncomplicated pregnancies. The National institute of Child health and Human Development Maternal- Fetal Medicine Units Network. *Am J obstet gynecol* 2000;183:1520–1524.

64. Teramo K, Kari MA, Eronen M, Markkanen H, Hiilesmaa V. High amniotic erythropoietin levels are associated with an increased frequency of fetal and neonatal morbidity in type I diabetic pregnancies. *Diabetologia* 2004;47:1695–1703.

65. Lauenborg J, Mathiesen E, Ovesen P, Westergard JG, Ekbom P, Molsted-Pedersen L, et al. Audit of stillbirths in women with pregestational type I diabetes. *Diabetes care* 2003;26:1385–1389.

66. Haeri S, et al. The association of intrauterine growth abnormalities in women with type I diabetes mellitus complicated by vasculopathy. *Am J obstet gynecol* 2008;199:278.1–278.e5.

67. Salvesen DR, Higueras MT, Brudenell JM, Drury PL, Nicolaides KH. Doppler velocimetry and fetal heart rate studies in nephropathic diabetics. *Am J obstet gynecol* 1992;167(5):1297–1303.

68. Young EC, et al. Effects of pregnancy on the onset and progression of diabetic nephropathy and of diabetic nephropathy on pregnancy outcomes. *Diabetes and metabolic syndrome: Clinical research and reviews* 2011;5:137–142.

69. Gordin D, Hiilesmaa V, Fagerudd J, Ronnback C, Kaaja R, Teramo K. Pre-eclampsia but not pregnancy-induced hypertension is a risk factor for diabetic nephropathy in type I diabetic women. *Diabetologia* 2007; 50:516–522.

70. The Diabetes Control and Complications Trial Research Group. Effect of pregnancy on microvascular complications in the diabetes control and complications trial. *Diabetes care* 2000;23:1084–1091.

71. Verier-Mine O, Chaturvedi N, Webb D, Fuller JH, the EURODIAB Prospective Complications Study Group. Is pregnancy a risk factor for microvascular complications? The EURODIAB Prospective Complications Study. *Diabetic medicine* 2005;22:1503–1509.

72. Gordin D, et al. Pre-eclampsia and pregnancy induced hypertension are associated with severe diabetic retinopathy in Type I diabetes in later life. *Acta diabetol* 2013;50: 781–787.

73. Sandvik MK, et al. Are adverse pregnancy outcomes risk factors for development of end-stage renal disease in women with diabetes? *Nephrol dial transplant* 2010;25: 3600–3607.

74. Khalil CA, et al. Fetal exposure to maternal Type I diabetes is associated with renal dysfunction at adult age. *Diabetes* 2010;59: 2631–2636.

Chapter 16

Urological Problems in Pregnancy

Jonathon Olsburgh and Susan Willis

Introduction

The most common urological symptoms in pregnancy are a consequence of pregnancy on a normal urinary tract, rather than specific urological diseases presenting in pregnancy. However, both the diagnosis and management of urological diseases in pregnancy can be complex. This review discusses etiology and management of loin pain, urinary frequency, urinary tract infection (UTI) and hematuria. Additionally, imaging of the renal tract, renal stone disease, urinary tract malignancy and the management of women with urinary tract diversion or reconstruction in pregnancy are specifically addressed. Postpartum complications affecting the urinary tract, such as fistulae and urinary incontinence, are not in the remit of this chapter.

Physiological Changes to the Urinary Tract in Pregnancy

Upper Tract

The increase in cardiac output, total vascular volume and renal blood flow in the first and second trimesters of pregnancy leads to a 40–65 percent increase in glomerular filtration rate (GFR) [1]. As a result, the kidneys increase by up to 1 cm in length and 30 percent in volume, with coincident hormonal and mechanical changes to the maternal renal pelvis and ureter [2]. A "physiological hydronephrosis" of pregnancy occurs in more than half of pregnancies in the middle trimester. Less commonly, ureteric dilation has been observed as early as seven weeks of pregnancy and may be due to a relaxant effect of progesterone. In a large prospective study of more than 1,000 women, dilatation of the right renal pelvis was evident by six weeks' gestation, with progressive expansion at a rate of 0.5 mm/week until weeks 24–26, then at a slower rate (0.3 mm/week) until term [3].

In early pregnancy, ureteric dilation does not equate with obstruction, whereas mechanical extrinsic compression can occur from the second trimester onward owing to both the gravid uterus and the engorged ovarian vein plexus crossing the ureter at the level of the pelvic brim. The ureter is usually dilated to the level of the true pelvis and of normal caliber at the level of the bladder. A fetus in the breech position in the third trimester may compress and obstruct the mid- or upper ureter. Dextrorotation of the gravid uterus may account for hydronephrosis being more common on the right side and the left ureter is protected by the sigmoid colon. Hydronephrosis resolves completely postpartum, but may take several weeks to be undetectable by renal ultrasound [4].

Lower Tract

As the gravid anteverted uterus enlarges, it increasingly indents the superior aspect or dome of the bladder. This changes the bladder shape and increases resistance to bladder stretching. In early pregnancy the functional bladder capacity remains fairly similar to the nonpregnant state, but, by the third trimester, crowding of the pelvis decreases the functional bladder capacity. These factors explain much of the increase in daytime urinary frequency and nocturia that are seen from early pregnancy onward.

Lower Urinary Tract Symptoms

Urinary frequency and nocturia can be considered normal physiological consequences of a healthy pregnancy. Urinary tract infection and glycosuria (from gestational diabetes) must be excluded on urine dipstick examination. Urinary urgency is common (in more than half of pregnant women) and, if severe, can lead to urinary urge incontinence, although this resolves postpartum in most women and, if incontinence persists, should be differentiated from stress urinary incontinence.

Stress urinary incontinence is also common, with between half and three-quarters of multiparous women having an episode during pregnancy [5]. Rates of stress urinary incontinence increase with increasing parity, previous vaginal delivery and obesity. Management should be supportive during pregnancy, with pelvic floor exercises and full evaluation for persistence of symptoms carried out in the postnatal period.

Urine retention in pregnancy is uncommon, occurring in less than 1 in 3,000 pregnancies. However, it presents as an emergency with pain and anuria. In early pregnancy, urinary retention may be due to failure of urethral relaxation and detrusor contractility secondary to progesterone. The retroverted uterus is more commonly associated with urinary retention occurring typically at 12–14 weeks' gestation, and is more common in women with fibroids or other uterine abnormalities. In the third trimester, urinary retention may occur if the uterus is incarcerated in the pelvis. Again, this can be associated with fibroids and other uterine abnormalities, as well as abnormal placentation such as placenta accreta. Management includes catheterization, intermittent self-catheterization and bimanual manipulation of a retroverted uterus to an anteverted position, which may require anesthesia.

Urinary Tract Infection

Bacterial UTI in pregnancy should be classified as asymptomatic bacteriuria (ABU), symptomatic lower tract UTI (cystitis) or symptomatic upper tract UTI (pyelonephritis). UTI is a urological emergency when coexistent with urinary tract obstruction.

Although the incidence of ABU in pregnancy is similar to that in age-matched non-pregnant women, the rates of cystitis and pyelonephritis in pregnancy are three- to four-fold higher than in the nonpregnant state [6, 7]. Furthermore, the consequences of pyelonephritis in pregnancy to both mother and fetus can be significant and include preterm birth and low birth weight. Hemorrhagic cystitis is also associated with preterm labor.

Meta-analysis of randomized controlled study data has shown that treating ABU with antibiotics leads to a 77 percent (95 percent CI 59–87 percent) relative risk reduction of pyelonephritis, with seven patients needing to be treated for one benefit [8]. Therefore it is widely accepted that screening for ABU in early pregnancy is beneficial, although the number needed to be screened to prevent one episode of pyelonephritis is 114. In the United Kingdom, screening occurs at the booking visit at approximately 12–16 weeks. Maternal risk factors for UTI include previous UTI, urinary tract abnormalities, including reflux and reconstruction, diabetes and immunosuppression.

Gram-negative bacteria, especially *Enterobacteriaceae*, including *Escherichia coli*, *Enterobacter* and *Klebsiella*, are the most common organisms causing UTI in pregnancy. Less commonly, other Gram-negative organisms such as *Pseudomonas*, *Proteus* and *Citrobacter* and Gram-positive organisms such as group B *streptococcus* are implicated. Other organisms that also need to be considered include *Chlamydia trachomatis*, *Gardnerella vaginalis*, *Ureaplasma urealyticum* and *lactobacilli*.

ABU is defined on midstream urine (MSU) culture as 10^5 colony-forming units of uropathogenic organisms (or greater) per milliliter of urine, in two consecutive specimens, without symptoms. However, it is likely that most physicians would treat on a single positive result during pregnancy: the UK National Institute of Health and Clinical Excellence guidelines do not specify one or two cultures [9]. A three-day antibiotic course for ABU is as effective as a seven-day course, with both regimens having a 70 percent eradication rate, and a single dose closely approximates this [7]. A repeat MSU should be done one week later and any persistence or recurrence should be treated with culture-specific antibiotics for 7–10 days. Following treatment of ABU, women with low risk and successful treatment with a three-day antibiotic course should have regular repeat MSU cultures to detect recurrent ABU. Women with low risk and recurrent ABU or with high risk of UTI should receive prophylaxis throughout pregnancy and an upper renal tract ultrasound scan. Women with high risk of UTI in pregnancy but a clear first MSU should have regular repeat MSUs to ensure that ABU does not go untreated.

Cystitis should be treated with empirical antibiotic therapy pending the results of an MSU collected prior to commencing treatment. In women in low-risk groups, an initial three-day course and a repeat MSU a week later is appropriate, followed by regular screening for ABU. In high-risk patients, a baseline upper renal tract ultrasound scan should be arranged and consideration given to prophylaxis throughout pregnancy.

Occasionally, severe visible hematuria can occur in pregnancy with cystitis (hemorrhagic cystitis), perhaps owing to the engorgement of the bladder mucosa in pregnancy. It may require parenteral antibiotics, bladder irrigation and cystoscopy to evacuate blood clot in the bladder.

Pyelonephritis should be managed initially with hospital admission for blood and urine cultures and 48–72 hours of parenteral antibiotics. If there has been clinical improvement, antibiotic therapy can be switched to a further 11–12-day oral antibiotic course. This should be followed by a repeat MSU a week later to ensure eradication of infection and then consideration given to low-dose antibiotic therapy for the remainder of pregnancy.

A renal tract ultrasound scan should be performed to exclude perinephric abscess. This should be managed with a percutaneous drain. As most pyelonephritis occurs in the third trimester, hydronephrosis is likely to be present. If systemic features are prominent (tachycardia, hypotension), then pyonephrosis should be suspected and percutaneous aspiration for culture and nephrostomy placement advised. Management should focus on the causes and relief of urinary tract obstruction (see later in this chapter).

Loin Pain, Hydronephrosis and Imaging

Loin pain in pregnancy has a variety of etiologies. Ureteric obstruction may be due to the fetus, urolithiasis or a number of less common causes such as intrinsic pelviureteric junction obstruction (PUJO). Loin pain may occur with urolithiasis, a bleed into a renal angiomyolipoma (AML), renal vein compressive hypertension, rupture of a renal artery aneurysm and non-urinary tract conditions.

Loin pain in pregnancy may be associated with hydronephrosis and, conversely, asymptomatic maternal hydronephrosis may be observed on routine ultrasound imaging. Non-radiation-based imaging of the urinary tract is clearly the preferred choice in pregnancy, with ultrasound scanning being the first-line investigation [10, 11]. A comparison of fetal exposure doses from urinary tract imaging is provided in Table 16.1.

A transabdominal ultrasound scan can detect dilation of the maternal renal pelvis and collecting system

and an antero-posterior (AP) diameter of 1 cm or more together with calyceal dilation is defined as hydronephrosis. However, dilation does not equate with obstruction. In physiological hydronephrosis of pregnancy, dilation of the upper ureter should also be seen. If dilation is confined to the renal pelvis, it may be due to a renal pelvis calculus or PUJO that may be preexistent. The common scenario on transabdominal ultrasound is dilation to the mid- or lower ureter. The differential diagnosis is an obstruction either from an intraluminal cause, most commonly a calculus, or an extrinsic cause such as the gravid uterus, fibroids, ovarian hyperstimulation after IVF and, rarely, uterine artery aneurysm, or non-obstructive hydronephrosis (physiological hydronephrosis of pregnancy).

The specificity of (B mode) ultrasound in pregnancy to diagnose a ureteric stone is poor (around 50 percent) and may be increased by a number of techniques. First, color flow Doppler can be used to determine the level of the iliac vessels in relation to the dilated ureter. Second, scanning can be initially performed in a supine position and then repeated after 30 minutes in an "all fours" position (in physiological hydronephrosis the AP renal diameter should be less than 1 cm after this maneuver) [15]. Third, use transvaginal scanning to help to determine the level of the dilated ureter and detection of distal ureteric calculi. A 5 MHz vaginal transducer with a 90° sector angle and 30° off-axis beam is used. The renal resistive index (RI) has been investigated for its sensitivity to predict urinary tract obstruction in pregnancy. The RI is best at separating obstructed from non-obstructed systems, but may also help to differentiate acute from chronic obstruction. In an obstructing process that develops over weeks, such as the enlarging fetus, adaptive processes in the renal vasculature maintain a near normal RI, whereas in an acute process, such as a complete obstruction from a ureteric stone, the RI is likely to be raised above 0.7.

Currently, after a non-diagnostic ultrasound scan in the second or third trimester, magnetic resonance urography (MRU) should be considered the second-line investigation of choice. Historically, MR imaging has been hampered by slow image acquisition times; recent reports have described the use of half-Fournier single shot turbo spin-echo (HASTE) MRU – MR scans that previously took 45 minutes now take just 15 [16]. Ultrafast T2-weighted sequences to image the abdomen and pelvis in the axial, sagittal and coronal

Table 16.1 Fetal exposure doses from urinary tract imaging

Examination	Fetal radiation dose	mSv equivalent	Reference
Ultrasound	nil	nil	
MRI	nil	nil	
CXR	0.02 rad	0.2	[10][7]
KUB X-ray	0.05 rad	0.5	[10][7],[12][8]
	1.4 – 4.2 mGy	1.4–4.2	[13][18]
Limited IVU (3-4 films)	0.2–0.25 rad	2.0–2.5	[10][7],[14]
	1–2 cGy	10–20	[14]
Standard IVU	0.4–0.5 rad	4–5	[10][7],[14][8]
	1.7–10 mGy	1.7–10	[13][18]
Fluoroscopy	1.5–2 rad/minute	15–20/minute	[10][7]
CT standard	2–2.5 rad	20–25	[10][7]
CT abdomen	8–49 mGy	8–49	[12][8],[13][18]
CT pelvis	25–79 mGy	25–79	[12][8],[13][18]
Conventional CT KUB	3.5 cGy	35	[14][12]
Multidetector CT KUB	0.8–1.2 cGy	8–12	[14][12]
Low-dose/ultra-low-dose CT KUB	0.72 cGy	7	[14][12]
Tc-99m DTPA	1.5–4 mGy	1.5–4	[12][8],[13][18]
Tc-99m MAG-3	0.7 mGy	0.7	[12][8],[13][18]
Lethal fetal dose (conception to first trimester)	100–500 mGy	100–500	[12][8],[13][18]

CT = computed tomography; CXR = chest X-ray; DTPA = diethylenetriamine pentaacetic acid; IVU = intravenous urogram; KUB = kidneys, ureters and bladder; MAG-3 = mercaptoacetyltriglycine; MSU = midstream urine; NRPB = National Radiological Protection Board

The National Radiological Protection Board (now Health Protection Agency, HPA) gives fetal doses in mGy (milliGray), whereas the standard international unit for X-ray exposure is now the mSv (milliSievert). The conversion factor to equivalent dose is 1, i.e. 1 mGy = 1 mSv for X-rays. Older and overseas literature report dose exposure in other units for which the conversion is 1 rad = 1 cGy = 10 mGy = 10 mSv.

planes are utilized. MRU does not require Gadolinium contrast. MRU provides high-quality images that permits identification of and differentiation between extrinsic and luminal causes of ureteric obstruction. MRU may also demonstrate other non-urinary tract causes of pain such as ovarian torsion or appendicitis. The exact cause of an intraluminal obstructing lesion is not specific with MRU as it appears as a "filling defect" and could be a stone, clot or sloughed papilla (in a patient with diabetes or sickle cell disease). A further limitation of MRU is that most MR scanners are closed-ring systems, with an internal radius of approximately 60 cm. Therefore, some women in the third trimester may not fit inside a closed-ring system; there are a small number of open-ring MRI scanners in the United Kingdom. Present data have not conclusively demonstrated any deleterious effects of MR imaging exposure on the developing fetus at any stage of pregnancy [17]. Access to MRU may not be available in all UK centers and, as the next investigations involve limited fetal exposure to radiation, discussion between urologist, radiologist, obstetrician and patient is advised regarding the treatment plan.

Dynamic radionuclide renography, such as technetium-labelled MAG-3, exposes the fetus to very low radiation doses and is a widely available test, though infrequently used in pregnancy. It is best at diagnosing obstruction in the upper rather than lower ureter and requires an overall GFR of greater than 15ml/minute [18].

The intravenous urogram (IVU) may expose the fetus to an unacceptably high radiation dose, particularly if a comprehensive series of follow-up plain films are required to delineate a level of ureteric obstruction. The IVU is rapidly becoming obsolete in contemporary urological practice, having been replaced by CT scanning, and as such is unlikely to be requested in pregnancy.

Cystoscopy with retrograde ureteropyelography is generally performed under general anesthesia, although in women it can be performed under local anesthetic. It is important to limit fluoroscopy to the minimum required using coned beam and to shield the fetus. General anesthesia in pregnancy is associated with increased risks of gastric aspiration, decreased respiratory reserve and increased risk of thromboembolic events. To improve venous return the patient should be placed in a modified Trendelenburg position with left uterine displacement.

The advantages of retrograde ureteropyelography are that it allows both diagnosis of obstruction, definition of the level of obstruction and the opportunity to insert a double-J ureteric stent without the trauma to the kidney associated with percutaneous nephrostomy (PCN). This is a particularly important consideration in a patient with a solitary kidney. Retrograde ureteropyelography will diagnose or refute suspected obstruction if there is minimal or no pelvicalyceal dilation on ultrasound.

The gold-standard imaging test for the detection of ureteric calculi in the general population is non-contrast computed tomography (NCCT), with a sensitivity of 94–100 percent and a specificity of 92–100 percent [19]. The American College of Radiologists states that the deterministic effects of 50mGy or less of ionizing radiation is safe at all gestational ages; however stochastic effects are suspected, if not conclusively demonstrated [20]. Over the past decade, the radiation dose required for NCCT has dropped significantly due to rapid technological developments in CT: in 2008 the average effective dose of an abdominal X-ray and NCCT was 0.7mSv and 8mSv respectively; in 2013 this might have been as low as 0.4mSv for a NCCT [21]. At low dose, the higher image noise is clearly visible but does not impair the recognition of the pathology under evaluation. Clearly, CT will remain a third-line investigation after US and MRU for the detection of ureteric calculi, but its use in pregnancy may become increasingly acceptable to both patients and clinicians.

Urolithiasis

Symptomatic urolithiasis in pregnancy is reported to affect between 1 in 250 to 1 in 3,000 women [22]. However, recent reports show that although the incidence of nephrolithiasis has been increasing in the general population, in pregnancy there has been no increase in incidence over the past two decades [23]. This suggests a fundamental difference in the pathophysiology of stone formation in pregnancy.

In the general population, stones are often diagnosed incidentally on imaging for another condition. Incidental presentation in pregnancy is less frequent and most renal stones present when symptomatic. An exact comparison of incidence and prevalence rates is thus difficult. Stones tend to present in the second or third trimester [24]. There are significant metabolic changes in pregnancy that relate to stone disease:

- circulating 1,25-dihydroxyvitamin D concentration increases (produced by the placenta), which results in a higher gastrointestinal absorption of calcium
- renal calcium excretion therefore increases up to twice the normal concentration; there is reduced renal tubular reabsorption of calcium
- a combination of these two events leads to a physiological hypercalciuria with normocalcemia
- filtered sodium and uric acid increase
- net sodium excretion is unchanged as there is increased tubular reabsorption
- the filtered load of urinary citrate and magnesium stone inhibitors increases
- increased urinary excretion of glycosaminoglycans and acidic glycoproteins inhibits oxalate stone formation
- respiratory alkalosis, which leads to relatively alkaline urine, inhibits uric acid stone formation but may enhance calcium phosphate stone formation

The overall situation is an increase in both stone-promoting and stone-inhibiting factors so that there is probably no increase in stone formation. However, there appears to be an increase in the rate of encrustation of urinary tract stents and nephrostomy tubes compared with the nonpregnant state, with encrustation seen as early as two weeks of tube placement [25].

The severe pain of renal/ureteric colic has been associated with preterm labor in the second and third trimesters. Treatment can range from conservative measures to temporizing measures until after delivery, to definitive treatment during pregnancy. Renal/ureteric colic should not be treated with nonsteroidal anti-inflammatory drugs (NSAIDs) in pregnancy if at all possible and especially not in the third trimester. Options include paracetamol, opiate analgesia and epidural anesthesia. Painful hydronephrosis that does not settle with these measures may require urinary tract decompression with a PCN. Sepsis associated with renal tract obstruction is a surgical emergency and a PCN should be placed promptly under ultrasound guidance by an experienced interventional radiologist.

The majority of stones are smaller than 5 mm and will pass spontaneously with analgesia, bed rest and hydration. Medical expulsive therapy with the use of alpha-blockers and calcium channel antagonists is not recommended in pregnancy; indeed this form of stone management is not currently advocated in the general population following publication of a large, multicenter RCT showing no difference in the rate of stone passage with medical expulsive therapy compared to placebo [26]. Epidural anesthesia placed for pain relief may give additional benefit by allowing smooth muscle relaxation of the lower ureter facilitating stone passage [27].

The management of symptomatic stones that do not respond to conservative measures is based on a number of factors: size, number and location of stone(s) and the stage of pregnancy [11, 14]. Extracorporeal shockwave lithotripsy is contraindicated in pregnancy due to its potentially damaging effects to the fetus.

The most direct temporizing method is external urinary drainage with a PCN. PCN is safe, placed under local anesthetic and ultrasound guidance (+/- fluoroscopic screening), relieves the pain of obstruction and allows immediate drainage and culture of infected urine. It avoids manipulation of the obstructed ureter with associated risks of perforation and further sepsis. PCN tubes can become blocked, requiring flushing, or dislodged or encrusted, requiring replacement. Limitations of PCN are that placement is operator dependent and requires an experienced interventional radiologist, and there is potential for bleeding both at the time of PCN insertion and at exchange. Consideration should be given to PCN as a route for subsequent antegrade internal double-J stent placement, and an appropriately placed PCN track can be dilated to permit access for percutaneous nephrolithotomy (PCNL) or antegrade ureteroscopic stone removal. PCNL requires prolonged general anesthesia and fluoroscopic screening, and is generally not recommended in pregnancy. Individual patient experience of a PCN tube or a double-J stent varies, with some tolerating a PCN better and others preferring a stent. PCN tubes can be uncomfortable and cumbersome, with an external urine drainage bag requiring regular emptying. A double-J stent can be extremely uncomfortable both in the kidney and bladder regions, with urinary frequency and urgency being potentially intensely bothersome.

Cystoscopy, retrograde imaging and double-J stent placement have been discussed earlier. An impacted stone may not be able to be stented from below, requiring PCN placement. It is well recognized that stent and PCN encrustation can be rapid in pregnancy, and tubes should therefore be exchanged at approximately four to six weekly intervals [25, 28]. This can be a significant inconvenience and undertaking.

Advances in instrument design and fiber-optic technology have permitted the development of small-caliber semi-rigid and flexible ureteroscopes that have revolutionized endourological stone management. New semi-rigid scopes are 6.5F caliber and flexible scopes 6.8F caliber. Ureteroscopy permits definitive stone removal (with baskets) and fragmentation using holmium laser technology, which appears to be safe in pregnancy [19]. Ureteroscopic stone extraction is becoming more common in pregnancy; a recent systematic review concluded that ureteroscopy has been shown to be safe and effective during pregnancy, and can be performed under local or regional anesthesia without the use of fluoroscopy [29].

Although ureteroscopy is becoming the standard of care for ureteric stones in pregnancy, ureteroscopy in pregnancy is difficult and should only be undertaken by expert operators. Stones in the lower third of the ureter are most amenable to treatment and the ureteric orifice may not require dilation owing to the dilating effects of progesterone. Following successful ureteroscopic stone fragmentation it was conventional to place a double-J stent. However, if there has been minimal ureteric wall trauma, it may be possible either not to place a double-J stent or to place a "stent on a string" that can be removed 24 hours later on the ward.

Ureteroscopy in pregnancy is contraindicated with multiple stones, stones greater than 1 cm and in the presence of sepsis, when placement of a double-J stent or PCN with treatment of infection is the first priority. Women with a known history of renal stone disease, for example, those with cystinuria who are contemplating pregnancy should be seen by their urologist prior to conception. An up-to-date CT KUB (kidneys, ureters and bladder), MSU and metabolic stone profile should be arranged to determine stone burden, urine infection and a baseline metabolic risk profile prior to pregnancy. There is benefit in treating asymptomatic stones prior to pregnancy that otherwise might be observed. Women with previous struvite "infection" stones should have antibiotic prophylaxis throughout pregnancy.

Hematuria and Urinary Tract Tumors

Nonvisible Hematuria (NVH)

In a study by Brown and colleagues [30], asymptomatic nonvisible hematuria (NVH) detected on dipstick was found to be common, occurring on at least two occasions in 3–20 percent of pregnant women, and resolving postpartum in the majority. Ultrasound evaluation of the renal tract was normal in all cases and NVH did not confer any additional risk of gestational hypertension. Retesting at three months postpartum is recommended to detect the small minority who may have mild glomerular disease or who may require further urological investigation. Clearly the presence of NVH with proteinuria, in the absence of infection, requires a complete nephrological assessment. Renal stone disease is associated with NVH in approximately 90 percent of cases.

Visible Hematuria

Visible hematuria in pregnancy should be differentiated from vaginal bleeding, and renal tract ultrasound scan is the investigation of choice together with MSU. Consideration should be given to both the upper and lower urinary tracts as the source of the bleeding.

Upper Tract

Significant renal trauma can cause hematuria; the method of diagnosis and treatment will depend upon the severity of maternal injuries, the scope of which is outside of this chapter.

The uncommon, benign renal tumor angiomyolipoma (AML) may grow rapidly in pregnancy with increased risk of rupture, although the mechanisms of this are speculative. This can present as visible hematuria with or without loin pain and can be life threatening. Ruptured AML in pregnancy requires either selective renal embolization [31] or nephrectomy, depending on the individual case. The average size of tumor in cases of rupture has been reported to be around 11cm [32]. A woman contemplating pregnancy with ≥ 4 cm AML should be advised to have selective renal embolization prior to conception. Where the AML is less than 4 cm, it may be prudent to observe the tumor with ultrasound scanning at regular intervals during pregnancy, although there are no suggested guidelines.

Malignant renal tumors are not more common in pregnancy than in the nonpregnant population [33]. However, there are at least 50 reported cases of renal cell carcinoma (RCC) in pregnancy. Depending on the size of the lesion and the stage of pregnancy when the tumor is detected, management may be either observation with postnatal treatment (for a 4 cm or smaller lesion found in the third trimester) or nephrectomy. Laparoscopic nephrectomy for RCC has been described in both first and second trimesters with favorable maternal and fetal outcomes.

Occasionally, renal vein compression occurs secondary to the gravid uterus, leading to profuse hematuria and loin pain. On the left side this is an aggravation of the classic "nutcracker syndrome" in which the left renal vein lies between the aorta and superior mesenteric artery. Treatment of this rare condition depends on severity and symptoms, but can be managed with vascular stent placement, low molecular weight heparin and serial renal vein flow Doppler studies [34].

Lower Tract

Pregnant women are typically younger than the age range in which bladder cancer occurs. However, as women are delaying pregnancy until older ages and more women are smoking, the likelihood of bladder cancer developing during pregnancy is increased. Occupational exposure to aromatic amines in permanent hair dyes may occur in women's hairdressing and an occupational history should be taken. Bladder tumors usually present with hematuria that may be confused by the patient as "vaginal bleeding" [35]. Another confounding factor is that carcinoma in situ of the bladder presents with urine frequency and urgency, symptoms typically present in pregnancy. Carcinoma of the bladder may be transitional cell, squamous cell or adenocarcinoma. Tumors greater than 0.5 cm can be visualized on transabdominal ultrasound scan with a full bladder. Flexible cystoscopy is safe at all stages of pregnancy. The majority of bladder tumors are superficial, i.e. papillary noninvasive or papillary superficially invasive. However, poorly differentiated superficial and muscle-invasive transitional cell carcinomas have a rapid tumor doubling time and a poor prognosis.

An initial transurethral resection of bladder tumor (TURBT) under general anesthesia appears to be safe in pregnancy and allows accurate staging and grading of the disease so that an appropriate diagnostic and management plan can be formulated, depending on histology results and what stage of pregnancy has been reached. These decisions need to be individualized, but maternal health and safety are paramount and delaying definitive treatment for aggressive transitional cell carcinoma beyond 8–12 weeks from TURBT may have poor long-term prognostic implications. Follow-up cystoscopy for noninvasive transitional cell carcinoma may be delayed until after delivery.

Pregnancy in Women with Urinary Tract Reconstruction

Vesicoureteric reflux is considered in Chapter 12. However, distal obstruction at the site of previous ureteric re-implantation has been reported as presenting in pregnancy. The timing of this presentation may relate to the physiological changes in pregnancy revealing a previously subclinical narrowing. Therefore, it has been suggested that women with a history of ureteric re-implantation who are considering pregnancy should be evaluated with either a dynamic radionucleotide renogram or cystoscopy and retrograde ureteropyelogram to exclude obstruction prior to conception.

The indications for urinary tract diversion or reconstruction in women of childbearing age are due to benign rather than malignant disease [36]. These include congenital disease such as spina bifida (including myelomeningocele) and bladder extrophy, or acquired neurological or fibrotic (including tuberculosis and schistosomiasis) diseases. The congenital diseases may be associated with other urogenital abnormalities, including solitary kidney and uterine abnormalities. Furthermore, many of the conditions may be associated with some degree of renal impairment and all are associated with bacterial UTI. Nevertheless, the majority of these women are fertile. It is important to note that urine-based pregnancy tests in women with a bowel segment incorporated into the urinary tract are likely to give a false positive result and it is recommended that serum human chorionic gonadotrophin is used instead. Pregnancy should be managed in a joint obstetric–urology clinic with intensive monitoring and easy access to specialist help.

There is a diverse range of urinary tract reconstructions that a pregnant woman may have, including incontinent urinary diversion (ileal or colonic conduit), continent urinary diversion that may be either to the colon (ureterosigmoidostomy or Mainz II pouch) or continent catheterizable bowel pouch (Koch and Indiana pouch), enterocystoplasty (native bladder augmented with bowel that drains either via the urethra or via a continent catheterizable stoma – *Mitrofanoff*) or orthotopic neobladder.

ABU is present in all patients with a bowel segment incorporated into the urinary tract. Some of the aforementioned configurations are also freely refluxing to the upper tract. Women who are prone to recurrent, symptomatic UTI are recommended to take antibiotic prophylaxis for the duration of pregnancy [37]. In a review of spinal cord–injured women, a quarter needed to change their bladder management during pregnancy (usually increasing the frequency of CISC), and one third were affected by pyelonephritis [38].

Vaginal delivery may be possible in women with urinary tract reconstruction and should be judged on the merits of both obstetric and urological factors. Breech presentation is very common in women with history of bladder extrophy. Neurological conditions that affect the bladder may also affect coordinated muscle activity required in the final stage of vaginal delivery. However, vaginal delivery is contraindicated in women with an artificial urinary sphincter and cautioned against in patients with orthotopic neobladder and ureterosigmoidostomy.

Ureterosigmoidostomy or Mainz II pouch depend on an intact anal sphincter for continence and, if a vaginal delivery is attempted, care must be taken to make lateral episiotomies. For all women with complex urinary tract reconstruction, if caesarean section is likely, it should be anticipated and performed electively with an experienced urologist present. Some patients with spina bifida and myelomeningocele may have a ventricular-peritoneal shunt to treat hydrocephalus – the shunt can be compressed by the gravid uterus and is at risk of bacterial infection if the peritoneum is opened during caesarean section.

An important mechanical factor that needs to be considered during pregnancy is the points of fixation of the ureters, the mesentery (that supplies the urinary tract reconstruction) and the efferent drainage. The mesentery stretches and is lateralized as the gravid uterus enlarges and can usually be safely moved laterally during upper-segment caesarean section.

An ileal conduit in a woman of childbearing age when formed should be fixed to the retroperitoneum. The enlarging uterus may compress the conduit, leading to dilation of the upper tracts, but this is rarely seen. Retroperitonealizing the conduit prevents the conduit from being stretched, which may need return to prepregnancy size postpartum and require self-catheterization or revision. The conduit skin appliances may require adjustment to maintain a water-tight seal as the position of the stoma changes with uterine enlargement. A pouch or Mitrofanoff catheterizable stoma can be stretched during pregnancy, leading to difficulties with self-catheterization, which usually resolves postpartum.

The leading British experience in this field report that there are no long-term adverse effects of pregnancy on renal function or the reconstructed urinary tract in 29 live births in 20 women [39]. Pregnancy-related complications were encountered, particularly UTI in at least half, and upper tract obstruction and preeclampsia in 10 percent. The majority of babies were delivered by caesarean section.

Patients with refractory overactive bladder syndrome or intractable urinary retention are occasionally managed with sacral nerve stimulators (SNS); there may be some effect on uterine activity [40] and manufacturers advise that they should be turned off for the duration of pregnancy. However, women may see a return of their symptoms with deactivation of their SNS, and case reports of women choosing to keep their SNS activated during pregnancy seem to have done so safely [41].

Although their use is not widespread in women desiring further pregnancies, mid-urethral slings and other surgical interventions for stress urinary incontinence may occasionally be encountered in the pregnant patient. The published data are limited, but a recent systematic review found the incidence of urinary retention in these patients to be low [42].

Conclusion

The most common urological symptoms in pregnancy are urine frequency and urgency, but the most common reason for a urological consultation is loin pain associated with hydronephrosis. There is often difficulty in diagnosing the specific cause of hydronephrosis in pregnancy. Ultrasound scanning remains the first investigation and a number of specific measures to increase the sensitivity to differentiate between non-obstructive physiological hydronephrosis of pregnancy, obstruction by the gravid uterus and ureteric calculus are described. New ureteroscope instrument design and fiber-optic technology have permitted ureteroscopy to be used in expert hands during pregnancy to provide definitive stone treatment and reduce the problems associated with a number of temporizing measures.

Visible and persisting nonvisible hematuria should be investigated initially with ultrasound scan and, when indicated, flexible cystoscopy, which is safe throughout pregnancy.

The rate of pyelonephritis in pregnancy can be reduced by screening and treating ABU, and this is recommended. Certain at-risk groups benefit from low-dose antibiotic prophylaxis during pregnancy to reduce the risk of UTI.

Careful planning of pregnancy with joint urology and obstetric care is recommended for women with previous urinary tract reconstruction. Experience suggests that the majority can have healthy, successful pregnancies without compromise to the urinary tract reconstruction or renal function.

References

1. Jeyabalan A, Lain KY. Anatomic and functional changes of the upper urinary tract during pregnancy. *Urol Clin North Am* 2007;34: 1–6.

2. Rasmussen PE, Nielsen FR. Hydronephrosis during pregnancy: A literature survey. *Eur J Obstet Gynecol Reprod Biol* 1988:249–259.

3. Faundes A, Bricola-Filho M, Pinto e Silva JL. Dilatation of the urinary tract during pregnancy: Proposal of a curve of maximal caliceal diameter by gestational age. *Am J Obstet Gynecol* 1998:1082–1086.

4. Au KK, Woo JS, Tang LC, et al. Aetiological factors in the genesis of pregnancy hydronephrosis. *Aust N Z J Obstet Gynaecol* 1985:248–251.

5. Chaliha C, Stanton SL. Urological problems in pregnancy. *BJU Int* 2002;**89**:469–476.

6. Macejko AM, Schaeffer AJ. Asymptomatic bacteriuria and symptomatic urinary tract infections during pregnancy. *Urol Clin North Am* 2007;**34**:35–42.

7. Nicolle LE. Screening for asymptomatic bacteriuria in pregnancy. In *Canadian Guide to Clinical Preventive Health Care*. Ottawa: Health Canada; 1994. pp. 100–106.

8. Smaill F, Vazquez JC. Antibiotics for asymptomatic bacteriuria in pregnancy. *Cochrane Database Syst Rev* 2007;**2**:CD000490.

9. NICE clinical guideline 62: Antenatal care for uncomplicated deliveries. www.nice.org.uk/guidance/cg62/chapter/1-guidance.

10. Loughlin KR. Urologic radiology during pregnancy. *Urol Clin North Am* 2007;**34**:23–26.

11. Biyani CS, Joyce AD. Urolithiasis in pregnancy. I: Pathophysiology, fetal considerations and diagnosis. *BJU Int* 2002;**89**;811–818.

12. Biyani CS, Joyce AD. Urolithiasis in pregnancy. II: Management. *BJU Int* 2002;**89**:819–923.

13. Sharp C, Shrimpton JA, Bury RF. Advice on exposure to ionizing radiation during pregnancy. National Radiological Protection Board. 2008. www.hullrad.org.uk/DocumentMirror/health&safety/HPA/1998_NRPB_diagnostic%20&%20pregnancy.pdf. Accessed January 2018.

14. Pais VM, Payton AL, LaGrange CA. Urolithiasis in pregnancy. *Urol Clin North Am* 2007;**34**:43–52.

15. Isfahani M, Haghighat M. Measurable changes in hydronephrosis during pregnancy induced by positional changes: Ultrasonic assessment and its diagnostic implication. *Urology Journal* 2005:2;97–101.

16. Mullins JK, Semins MJ, Hyams ES, Bohlman ME, Matlaga BR. Half Fourier single-shot turbo spin-echo magnetic resonance urography for the evaluation of suspected renal colic in pregnancy. *J Urol* 2012;**79**:1252–1255.

17. American College of Obstetricians and Gynecologists' Committee on Obstetric Practice. Committee Opinion No. 656: Guidelines for diagnostic imaging during pregnancy and lactation. *Obstet Gynecol.* 2016 Feb;**127**(2):e75–80.

18. *Grainger and Allison's diagnostic radiology.* 6th edn., 2015. London: Elsevier.

19. Turk C, Knoll T, Petrik A, Sarica K, Skolaricos A, Straub M, Seitz C. Guidelines on urolithiasis. European Association of Urology 2016. http://uroweb.org/guideline/urolithiasis/.

20. ACR-SPR practice parameter for the performance of computed tomography (CT) of the abdomen and computed tomography (CT) of the pelvis. Amended 2014 (Resolution 39). www.acr.org/~/media/ACR/Documents/PGTS/guidelines/CT_Abdomen_Pelvis.pdf.

21. McLaughlin PD, Ouellette HA, Louis L, Mallinson PI, O'Connell T, Mayo J, Muck PL, Nicoaou S. The emergence of ultra-low-dose computed Tomography and the impending obsolescence of the plain radiograph? *Can Assoc Radiol J* 2013;**64**:314–318.

22. *Campbell-Walsh Urology.* 11th edn., 2016. Philadelphia, PA: Elsevier.

23. Riley JM, Dudley AG, Semins MJ. Nephrolithiasis and pregnancy: Has the incidence been rising? *J Endourol* 2014;**28**:383–386.

24. Horowitz E, Schmidt JD. Renal calculi in pregnancy. *Clin Obstet Gynaecol*, 1985.

25. Kavoussi LR, Albala DM, Basler JW, Apte S, Clayman RV. Percutaneous management of urolithiasis during pregnancy. *J Urol* 1992;**148**:1069–1071.

26. Pickard R, Starr, K, MacLennan G, Lam T, Thomas R, et al. Medical expulsive therapy in adults with ureteric colic: A multicentre, randomized, placebo-controlled trial. *Lancet* 2015;**386**(9991):341–349.

27. Maikranz P, Coe FL, Parks J, Lindheimer MD. Nephrolithiasis in pregnancy. *Am J Kidney Dis* 1987; **9**: 354–358.

28. Rodriguez PN, Klein AS. Management of urolithiasis during pregnancy. *Surg Gynecol Obstet* 1998; **166**:103–106.

29. Laing KA, Lam TBL, McClinton S, Cohen NP, Traxer O, Somani BK. Outcomes of ureteroscopy for stone disease in pregnancy: Results from a systematic review of the literature. *Urol Int* 2012;**89**:380–386.

30. Brown MA, Holt JL, Mangos GJ, Murray N, Curtis J, Homer C. Microscopic hematuria in pregnancy: Relevance to pregnancy outcome. *Am J Kidney Dis* 2005;**45**: 667–673.

31. Morales JP, Georganas M, Khan MS, Dasgupta P, Reidy JF. Embolization of a bleeding renal angiomyolipoma in pregnancy: Case report and review. *Cardiovasc Intervent Radiol* 2005;**28**: 265–268.

32. Zapardiel I, Delafuente-Valero J, Bajo-Arenas JM. Renal angiomyolipoma during pregnancy: Review of the literature. *Gynec Obstet Inv* 2011;**72**:217–219.

33. Martin FM, Rowland RG. Urologic malignancies in pregnancy. *Urol Clin North Am* 2007;**34**:53–59.

34. Zapardiel I, Sanfrutos S, Perez-Medina T, Godoy-Tundidor V, Delafuente-Valero J, et al. Clinical

management of Nutcracker's syndrome during pregnancy. *J Matern Fetal Neonatal Med* 2010;**23**(7):589–592.

35. Spahn M, Bader P, Westermann D, Echtle D, Frohneberg D. Bladder carcinoma during pregnancy. *Urol Int* 2005;**74**:153–159.

36. Hautmann RE, Volkmer BG. Pregnancy and urinary diversion. *Urol Clin North Am* 2007;**34**:71–88.

37. Huck N, Schweizerhof S, Honeck P, Neisius A, Thuroff J et al. Pregnancy after urinary diversion at young ages – risks and outcome. *Urology* 2017;**104**:220–224.

38. Le Liepvre, Dinh A, Idiard-Chamois B, Chartier-Kastler E, Phe V, et al. Pregnancy in spinal-cord injured women, a cohort study of 37 pregnancies in 25 women. *Spinal Cord* 2017;**55**: 167–171.

39. Greenwell TJ, Venn SN, Creighton S, Leaver RB, Woodhouse CR. Pregnancy after lower urinary tract reconstruction for congenital abnormalities. *BJU Int* 2003;**92**:773–7. Erratum in: BJU Int 2004;93: 655.

40. Govaert B, Melenhorst J, Link G, Hoogland H, van Gemert W, Baeten C. The effect of sacral nerve stimulation on uterine activity: A pilot study. *Colorectal Dis* 2010;**12**(5):448–451.

41. Mahran A, Soriano A, Safwat A, Hijaz A, Mahajan S, et al. The effect of sacral neuromodulation on pregnancy: a systematic review. *Int Urogynecol J*; Epub 03 February 2017.

42. Pollard ME, Morrisroe S, Anger JT. Outcomes of pregnancy following surgery for stress urinary incontinence: A systematic review. *J Urol* 2012;**187**:1966–1970.

17

Acute Kidney Injury in Pregnancy
Causes not Due to Preeclampsia

Anita Banerjee

Introduction

Acute kidney injury (AKI) in pregnancy is a medical emergency. AKI is associated with an increase in maternal and fetal mortality and morbidity regardless of the underlying etiology [1]. AKI in pregnancy is characterized by a rise in creatinine or decreased urine output or both. The recent international classifications of AKI in non-obstetric patients are not validated in pregnancy [2, 3]. Diagnosis of AKI in pregnancy remains a challenge due to a lack of evidence-based guidance, since no consensus or uniform definition of AKI in pregnancy has been reached.

Renal Physiology in Normal Pregnancy

The anatomical and physiological adaptations during pregnancy lead to an increase in glomerular filtration rate (GFR). Renal blood flow increases by 80 percent and GFR increases by 40–60 percent. A rise in plasma volume and GFR leads to a fall in creatinine in normal pregnancy. The kidney size increases by 1.0–1.5 cm due to an increase in blood flow. The dilatation of the calyces, renal pelvis and ureters are driven by the hormonal changes during pregnancy. A mild respiratory alkalosis, secondary to an increase in minute ventilation, results in a compensatory increase in kidney bicarbonate excretion and a fall in serum bicarbonate to 18–22 mmol/L (see Chapter 1). The diagnostic criteria for AKI differ in pregnancy due to these alterations. The rise in creatinine clearance may mask AKI in pregnancy and because of the renal adaptations the recognition of AKI in pregnancy may be more subtle.

A creatinine rise greater than 26 μmol/L is defined as AKI in the non-obstetric population. The mean creatinine during the second half of pregnancy is approximately 56 μmol/L. There is a suggestion that a creatinine greater than 90 μmol/L would capture the majority of cases with AKI during pregnancy [4–7]. Others have suggested a creatinine value greater than

97 μmol/L or doubling of the creatinine as a definition of AKI in pregnancy [8]. Some have suggested an even lower value of creatinine of 88 μmol/L be used as the definition of AKI in pregnancy [9].

Epidemiology

Epidemiology of AKI in pregnancy has changed over the past four decades. The most common causes of AKI in pregnancy in the developed world four decades ago were septic abortion and puerperal sepsis. Now due to improved antenatal care and abortion laws, the causes of AKI in pregnancy have altered and the incidence has fallen. Accurate data are difficult to obtain in view of the variable definitions of AKI in pregnancy used in the literature. In general in developed countries, a fall in the incidence has been described from 1 in 3,000 to 1 in 15,000 [10–11]. A recent Canadian study, however, has described an increased rate of obstetric AKI limited to women with hypertensive disorders of pregnancy [15]. However in developing countries, the incidence of AKI remains higher and the causes are different [12–13].

The incidence of AKI was 1 in 68 cases in our tertiary obstetric unit, which is 1.4 percent of 6,500 deliveries [7]. A creatinine greater than 90 μmol/L was used in this study to define AKI in pregnancy. The commonest causes of AKI in the obstetric unit were preeclampsia and postpartum hemorrhage. The majority of AKI was observed in the third trimester and postpartum. However, not all the AKI had improved prior to discharge. Fewer than one in six cases had no follow-up arranged to ensure renal function had returned to normal. AKI had been recognized in less than 50 percent of the cases. There were 100 percent live births in these women. The reasons behind the lack of recognition and follow-up of AKI in pregnancy include unfamiliarity and paucity of consensus of guidelines for AKI in pregnancy.

Table 17.1 Causes of AKI in Pregnancy (permission from Clin Med 2015) [16]

Renal Insult	Diagnosis	Clinical Features
Pre-renal	Hyperemesis gravidarum	First-trimester nausea, vomiting, ptyalism
	Placental abruption	Vaginal bleeding, abdominal pain, uterine tenderness
	Postpartum hemorrhage	Bleeding postpartum leading to hemodynamic instability
	Septic abortion/miscarriage	Uterus is the source of infection. Can present with septic shock.
Renal	Preeclampsia	New-onset hypertension and proteinuria after 20 weeks' gestation.
	HELLP	Hemolysis, elevated liver enzymes and low platelets. A variant of severe preeclampsia.
	Microangiopathic hemolytic anemia (TTP/HUS)	Platelet consumption leading to hemolysis and end-organ damage. Presents in second and third trimesters and postpartum.
	Acute fatty liver of pregnancy	Fatty infiltration of hepatocytes leading to liver failure
	Lupus nephritis	Autoimmune renal damage with proteinuria ± hematuria
Post-renal	Obstructive nephropathy	Increased risk if single kidney (including transplant), autonomic neuropathy (MS, Type 1 DM), polyhydramnios, multiple pregnancy. Need to distinguish from physiological dilatation of renal tract.

Abbreviations: TTP = thrombotic thrombocytopenic purpura, HUS = hemolytic uremic syndrome, MS = multiple sclerosis, Type 1 DM = Type 1 diabetes mellitus

Etiology of AKI in Pregnancy

The causes of AKI in pregnancy are divided into pre-renal, renal and post-renal causes. The incidence of AKI is higher postpartum and in the third trimester. Some causes are pregnancy specific or are more common during pregnancy, and many will be expanded in other chapters. Pre-existing hypertension is a significant risk factor for AKI in pregnancy [14–15]. More than one cause may coexist in the same case, for example, postpartum hemorrhage and preeclampsia. During pregnancy preeclampsia remains the most common cause of AKI (see Chapter 18). Outside of pregnancy, sepsis and hypotension remain the most common causes for AKI, both of which may occur during pregnancy. *De novo* presentation of primary glomerular diseases in pregnancy is less common, but deterioration of preexisting renal disease may lead to superimposed AKI. Sepsis and pyelonephritis can cause AKI in pregnancy and can be a challenge to treat. Obstructive nephropathy is uncommon, but may be difficult to diagnose due to possible dilation of the upper urinary tract due to physiological reasons as stated earlier. Table 17.1 summarizes the common causes of AKI in pregnancy.

Thrombotic Microangopathies

Thrombotic microangiopathies are rare in pregnancy, estimated to occur in 1 in 25,000 pregnancies [17]. The hallmark is thrombi in the microvasculature causing mechanical hemolysis and consumptive thrombocytopenia. Thrombotic thrombocytopenic purpura (TTP) and hemolytic uremic syndrome (HUS) are the most common microangiopathies that may both masquerade as and coexist with preeclampsia. Other conditions such as catastrophic antiphospholipid syndrome have similar clinical manifestations [18]. Table 17.2 provides a comparison of the clinical features and management of these conditions.

Thrombotic Thrombocytopenic Purpura

TTP is classically described as a pentad of microangiopathic hemolysis with red cell fragments, thrombocytopenia, neurological signs, AKI and pyrexia. Depending upon the severity of the clinical phenotype, it commonly presents either early in life or after the third decade of life, when pregnancy may be

Table 17.2 Clinical Features of Thrombotic Thrombocytopenic Purpura, Hemolytic Uremic Syndrome, Acute Fatty Liver of Pregnancy, Catastrophic Anti-phospholipid Syndrome and HELLP

Conditions	TTP	aHUS	AFLP	CAPS	HELLP
Incidence	1 in 25,000 cases	1 in 25,000 cases	1 in 20,000 cases	Rare	10–20 percent of PET
Time of presentation	Second trimester	Three-fourths occur postpartum	Third trimester and postpartum	Postpartum	Third trimester and postpartum
AKI	30–80%	70% dialysis dependent	60%	70%	3–15%
Neurological sequelae	Common	Uncommon	Encephalopathy Common	Common	Eclampsia
ADAMTS-13	Deficient	Present	Reduced marginally	Reduced marginally	Reduced marginally
Platelets	$<10 \times 10^9$/L	$10–30 \times 10^9$/L	$<100 \times 10^9$/L	$<150 \times 10^9$/L	$>30 \times 10^9$/L
Coagulopathy	No	No	Yes	Yes	Yes 20 percent
Elevated Transaminases	No	No	Yes	Yes	Yes
Treatment	Plasmapheresis	Disease specific	Supportive	Full Anticoagulation	Supportive
Delivery	Unaffected	Unaffected	Affected	Unaffected	Affected

TTP: thrombotic thrombocytopenic purpura; aHUS: atypical HUS; AFLP: acute fatty liver of pregnancy; CAPS: catastrophic antiphospholipid syndrome; HELLP: hemolysis, elevated liver enzymes and low platelets

a trigger. The underlying mechanism is a functional deficiency of the von Willebrand factor (vWF) cleaving protease ADAMTS-13 (A Disintegrin and Metalloproteinase with Thrombospondin type 1 motif, member-13). Due to the ADAMTS-13 deficiency, the large multimers of vWF that are released from the endothelium are not cleaved appropriately, leading to the formation of spontaneous platelet aggregates in multiple organs, including cardiac, renal and cerebral microvasculature. The mechanical fragmentation of erythrocytes through the partially occluded microvasculature causes a microangiopathic hemolytic anemia (MAHA). Congenital TTP is an inherited constitutional deficiency of ADAMTS-13, whereas acquired immune TTP is due to the reduction of ADAMTS-13 by auto-antibodies against it which may be triggered in pregnancy. The median time of presentation of TTP in pregnancy is around 24 weeks of gestation [19].

The initial diagnosis is based upon the clinical history and examination with routine laboratory investigations, including a blood film. The AKI is usually not as severe as that seen in HUS; it is more common than in the nonpregnant TTP population

and found in 30–80 percent of pregnancy-related TTP [20]. There are schistocytes on the blood film due to red blood cell fragmentation. The hemolysis leads to a fall in hemoglobin to 80–100 g/L with raised reticulocytes and low haptoglobin levels. The combination of the hemolysis and tissue ischemia leads to a raised LDH. The median platelet count is in the order of $10–30 \times 10^9$/L [21]. An important discriminatory feature is that of normal clotting parameters found in TTP.

Pregnancy is a trigger for congenital TTP associated with significant maternal and fetal morbidity and mortality due to thrombi occurring in the placenta, leading to fetal growth restriction, intrauterine death and severe early-onset preeclampsia [22].

Plasma exchange remains the mainstay of treatment for TTP during pregnancy. It is effective in restoring ADAMTS-13 enzymatic activity by removing the antibodies. Early treatment with plasma exchange should be initiated within four to eight hours of the assumed diagnosis [23]. Second-line treatment for TTP is rituximab, an anti-CD20 monoclonal antibody. This is a B-cell-depleting antibody, raising concerns for the immunity of the neonate if given in pregnancy. Live vaccines such as BCG should be avoided in the first six months of life [24] (see Chapter 7). Fetal loss remains high in TTP in pregnancy as the placenta is usually involved with infarcts, leading to a growth-restricted fetus with placental insufficiency and signs of preeclampsia.

Prepregnancy counseling and a multidisciplinary approach are required for future pregnancies. The risk of relapse in a future pregnancy of congenital TTP is 100 percent and for acquired TTP around 45 percent [25]. Regular plasma exchange commenced early in pregnancy will reduce acute TTP flares in future pregnancies.

Hemolytic Uremic Syndrome

HUS is caused by excessive complement activation. HUS most commonly presents in childhood and is precipitated by a shigatoxin-producing enterpathogenic E. coli or Shigella. HUS is now subclassified into toxin-related HUS and non-toxin-related atypical HUS. Toxin-related HUS is associated with contaminated food and bloody diarrhea, whereas atypical HUS (aHUS) is associated with the activation of the alternate complement pathway. Atypical HUS is either an acquired or inherited imbalance between factors involved in the regulation of the complement pathway.

The hallmarks of aHUS include evidence of hemolysis with severe anemia, schistocytes on the blood film and markedly raised LDH. Hemoglobin is usually less than 100 g/L and as low as 30–40 g/L. As with TTP, there is an absence of a coagulopathy. Distinguishing factors from TTP include a more severe AKI and more than three-quarters of women with aHUS will progress to end-stage renal disease [26]. Unlike TTP, there is detectable ADAMTS-13 activity. The platelet count is low, but not usually as low as with TTP and usually between $30–60 \times 10^9$/L. Of note more than 75 percent of aHUS occurs in the postpartum period when complementary proteins are decreased.

Supportive treatment is the mainstay of management with some requiring renal dialysis/hemofiltration. Secondary aHUS is when a causative factor is identified, such as pregnancy. Management of aHUS is with the use of Eculizumab, a monoclonal antibody that inhibits complement activation [27]. Eculizumab is considered safe in pregnancy and is already licensed in pregnancy for paroxysmal nocturnal hemoglobinuria; however, placental transfer is recognized.

Catastrophic Anti-phospholipid Syndrome

Anti-phospholipid syndrome (APS) is defined as a syndrome with arterial, venous or capillary vascular thrombosis, and/or recurrent early or single late fetal loss and the presence of the following antibodies on two or more occasions 12 weeks apart; lupus anticoagulant (LA), anticardiolipin antibodies (aCL) and/or anti-ß2 glycoprotein-I antibodies. Catastrophic APS (CAPS) is life-threatening and is characterized by a thrombotic storm with widespread multi-organ microvascular occlusions occurring over a short period of time within days of each other. In a large APS multicenter prospective study, 0.9 percent of cases manifested CAPS and more than half of them died [28]. A high index of suspicion should remain for CAPS when a mother with APS develops HELLP syndrome in pregnancy, improves and postpartum deteriorates again, as she manifests with CAPS [29].

Full anticoagulation remains the mainstay of treatment. The management of CAPS includes an aggressive approach requiring urgent multidisciplinary input with treatment that includes anticoagulation, high-dose steroids, plasma exchange and/or intravenous immunoglobulin. More recently Eculizumab has been used successfully for the management of CAPS [30].

Acute Fatty Liver of Pregnancy

Acute fatty liver of pregnancy (AFLP) is uncommon. In the United Kingdom, the largest prospective, population-based study found the incidence of AFLP to be 5 cases per 100,000 maternities, or approximately 1 case per 20,000 births [31]. The case fatality was 1.8 percent in this study.

The pathogenesis of the disease is thought to involve impaired ß-oxidation of fatty acids in hepatic mitochondria, and in some cases the fetal autosomal recessive defect of the long-chain 3-hydroxyl coenzyme A dehydrogenase (LCHAD) has been reported [32]. Without mitochondrial ß-oxidation of the fatty acids ketogenesis is impaired, leading to severe hypoglycemia. The histology findings of the liver include microvesicular steatosis.

AKI was associated with 58 percent of cases of AFLP and the median creatinine was 169 µmol/L in the aforementioned study, with 3.5 percent (2/57 cases) requiring renal replacement therapy. The clinical features of AFLP are nonspecific, including anorexia, nausea, vomiting, fatigue, polyuria, polydipsia and lactic acidosis with hypoglycemia. Hepatic enzymes are markedly raised; with hyperbilirubinemia, leukocytosis and thrombocytopenia. There is a prolonged prothrombin time, causing a coagulopathy. Six or more characteristics of the Swansea criteria of AFLP support the diagnosis [33]. The onset of symptoms is usually in the third trimester after 35 weeks' gestation.

A multidisciplinary team approach and prompt delivery is advocated. The management thereafter is supportive with blood products, hydration and surveillance in an intensive care or high-dependence unit. Mainstay of treatment includes administration of 10–20 percent dextrose infusion to treat the hypoglycemia and fresh frozen plasma and vitamin K to treat the coagulopathy. N-acetylcysteine infusion is commenced to protect from further hepatoxicity. Reasons to transfer to a specialist liver unit for further management include features of fulminant hepatic failure and encephalopathy.

Sepsis

Sepsis remains a common cause of morbidity and mortality in pregnancy. A prospective case-control study of 365 confirmed cases of severe maternal sepsis in obstetrician-led maternity units was undertaken [34]. The incidence of severe sepsis was 4.7 (95 percent CI 4.2–5.2) per 10,000 maternities; 71 (19.5 percent) women developed septic shock, and five (1.4 percent) women died. *Escherichia coli* was the most common causative organism in severe maternal sepsis, whereas group A streptococcus was most strongly associated with progression to septic shock. It is the hypo-perfusion because of sepsis that leads to acute tubular necrosis and AKI in pregnancy.

- **Urinary tract infections**
The common microorganisms in urinary tract infections in pregnancy are similar pathogens found in the non-obstetric population. Most infections are caused by *Enterobacteriaceae*, commonly found in the gastrointestinal tract, with *Escherichia coli* responsible for 63–85 percent of cases. The others include: *Klebsiella pneumoniae* (8 percent), coagulase-negative *Staphylococcus* (up to 15 percent), *S. aureus* (up to 8 percent) and group B streptococci (GBS) (2–7 percent) [35]. Asymptomatic bacteremia, if not treated in early pregnancy, has been found in later pregnancy to be associated with pyelonephritis and preterm delivery. Symptomatic bacteremia should be treated as per local guidelines (see Chapter 7).

- **Acute pyelonephritis**
The clinical signs and symptoms of pyelonephritis include pyrexia, rigors, flank pain, nausea and vomiting and lower urinary tract symptoms such as cystitis [36]. The complications of pyelonephritis include increased risks for AKI, transfusion, need for mechanical ventilation, acute heart failure, pneumonia, pulmonary edema, acute respiratory distress syndrome, sepsis, preterm labor and chorioamnionitis [37]. All mothers should be admitted for at least 24 hours to treat the pyelonephritis with intravenous antibiotics. Risks to the pregnancy include preterm labor and a pathological cardiotocography (CTG) secondary to severe sepsis. Early intervention and administration of intravenous antibiotics is required. Supportive measures including fluid resuscitation are warranted.

- **Bilateral renal cortical necrosis**
Bilateral renal cortical necrosis in the majority of cases leads to irreversible kidney injury [38]. Abruption, septic abortion, postpartum hemorrhage or any hypotensive crisis can cause bilateral renal cortical necrosis. One single center in India found the incidence of renal cortical necrosis in obstetrics has reduced over 20 years [12]. There were more 32/57 (56.2 percent) cases of renal cortical necrosis in their obstetric population than non-obstetric population. The overall incidence is decreasing due to better access to health care and improved guidelines.

Drugs

Drug-induced AKI does occur in pregnancy. Common culprits include nonsteroidal anti-inflammatory drugs (NSAIDs) and the aminoglycosides e.g. gentamicin. Caution is required when NSAIDs are used postpartum for analgesia. NSAIDs should be avoided in mothers with chronic renal disease or those who may have recently suffered a renal insult leading to AKI e.g. postpartum hemorrhage and/or preeclampsia. The use of magnesium sulphate infusion, a standard treatment in the management of preeclampsia, can cause hyperkalemia or toxic magnesium levels in the presence of AKI [39]. The guidelines for hyperkalemia for non-obstetric adults should be followed in this situation, including dextrose/insulin, and to consider calcium gluconate infusion, if there are ECG changes consistent with hyperkalemia.

Antibiotics and NSAIDs may cause an interstitial nephritis, which will usually recover on stopping the medication. In kidney transplant recipients regular monitoring of immunosuppressant levels such as tacrolimus and ciclosporine is required to prevent rejection and avoid drug toxicity that may cause AKI during pregnancy (see Chapters 7 and 8).

De novo Renal Diseases during Pregnancy

The importance of considering *de novo* glomerular disease causing AKI is very important as timely investigations and disease-specific treatment may prevent a poor outcome. Dipstick urinalysis with microscopic hematuria and protein are key to the diagnosis of *de novo* glomerular disease. Differentials include systemic lupus erythematosus and other causes of glomerulonephritis.

• Systemic lupus erythematosus

Systemic lupus erythematosus (SLE) (see Chapter 14) is a multisystem autoimmune condition. Severe lupus flares occur in 25–30 percent of pregnancies and lupus nephritis may present for the first time during the pregnancy or in the postpartum period. One needs to distinguish this from preeclampsia as many clinical features are similar. Deteriorating renal function, hypertension and worsening proteinuria and thrombocytopenia in the presence of an active urinary sediment, positive/rising anti dsDNA titers and hypocomplementemia suggests a diagnosis of lupus nephritis. Other features that may strengthen the diagnosis of SLE include a skin rash (malar rash), arthritis or a serositis. A kidney biopsy may be necessary to confirm the diagnosis and subtype of lupus nephritis (see Chapter 19 for risks versus benefits of biopsy in pregnancy).

• Glomerulonephritidies

Limited data are available regarding *de novo* glomerulonephritis in pregnancy. Causes of rapidly progressive AKI include glomerulonephritis such as *de novo* Goodpasture's disease, ANCA vasculitis (see Chapter 14) membranoproliferative and poststreptococcal glomerulonephritis. Further investigations will be required and early liaison with nephrologists and a multidisciplinary approach is necessary.

Preexisting Chronic Kidney Diseases

Preexisting chronic kidney diseases such as lupus nephritis and diabetic nephropathy can worsen in pregnancy, causing superimposed AKI. However, it may be difficult to distinguish deterioration of chronic kidney disease (CKD) from superimposed preeclampsia. It is important to have a prepregnancy renal profile measurement and then continued surveillance of renal function and protein leak during pregnancy with pre-existing CKD. Disease activity and disease duration prior to pregnancy influences the risk of relapse postpartum of SLE [40]. Preexisting comorbidities such as diabetes mellitus are risk factors for AKI in pregnancy. Fetal outcomes are influenced by the underlying etiology. The data regarding preexisting CKD and fetal outcomes may not reflect AKI-related pregnancies and fetal outcomes.

Urinary Tract Obstruction

• Acute renal obstruction

Bilateral acute renal obstruction is a very rare event in pregnancy. Risk factors for acute obstruction include polyhydramnios, multiple pregnancies and a single kidney or transplanted kidney [41]. In the context of loin pain or reduced amount of urine with an AKI, acute obstruction should be considered. The urine sediment is bland in this context. An urgent ultrasound is *key* to confirming the diagnosis. Reasons for intervention include a worsening AKI and the presence of infection. Nephrostomy tubes and occasional ureteric stents have been used to treat the hydronephrosis and prolong the pregnancy (see Chapter 16) [42].

• Bladder injury

Iatrogenic injuries to the bladder and ureter are uncommon, 0.006–0.94 percent, and rare causes of AKI in pregnancy [43]. The risk is higher in an emergency caesarean section. The early recognition and repair of damage to the urinary tract will provide the best outcomes.

• Acute tubular necrosis

AKI due to acute tubular necrosis (ATN) occurs in the context of severe hypoperfusion to the kidneys. Therefore it may develop in the context of postpartum hemorrhage, sepsis, placental abruption and any fluid deplete state. At presentation there is hypotension, tachycardia and oliguria. The skin turgor is poor and the mucous membranes dry. If diagnosed early when the condition is still pre-renal, the AKI is reversible. Once ATN is established, there is a delay in renal function recovery. In such cases the management is supportive.

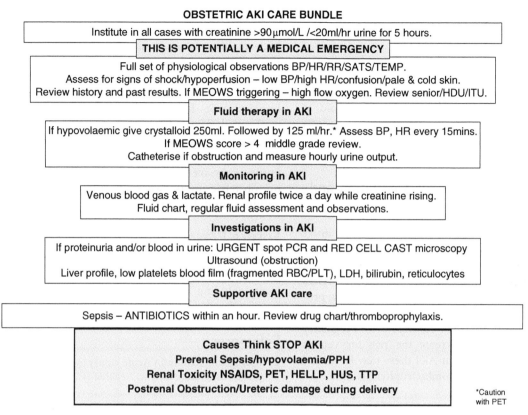

OBSTETRIC AKI CARE BUNDLE

Institute in all cases with creatinine >90 µmol/L /<20ml/hr urine for 5 hours.

THIS IS POTENTIALLY A MEDICAL EMERGENCY

Full set of physiological observations BP/HR/RR/SATS/TEMP.
Assess for signs of shock/hypoperfusion – low BP/high HR/confusion/pale & cold skin.
Review history and past results. If MEOWS triggering – high flow oxygen. Review senior/HDU/ITU.

Fluid therapy in AKI

If hypovolaemic give crystalloid 250ml. Followed by 125 ml/hr.* Assess BP, HR every 15mins.
If MEOWS score > 4 middle grade review.
Catheterise if obstruction and measure hourly urine output.

Monitoring in AKI

Venous blood gas & lactate. Renal profile twice a day while creatinine rising.
Fluid chart, regular fluid assessment and observations.

Investigations in AKI

If proteinuria and/or blood in urine: URGENT spot PCR and RED CELL CAST microscopy
Ultrasound (obstruction)
Liver profile, low platelets blood film (fragmented RBC/PLT), LDH, bilirubin, reticulocytes

Supportive AKI care

Sepsis – ANTIBIOTICS within an hour. Review drug chart/thromboprophylaxis.

Causes Think STOP AKI
Prerenal Sepsis/hypovolaemia/PPH
Renal Toxicity NSAIDS, PET, HELLP, HUS, TTP
Postrenal Obstruction/Ureteric damage during delivery

*Caution with PET

Figure 17.1 Proposed obstetric AKI bundle [44]

The Approach to AKI in Pregnancy

The objective is to have a structured approach to a diagnosis of AKI and provide goal-directed treatment. Supportive management includes the maintenance of fluid balance, frequent reassessment and review of medication chart.

The development of an AKI obstetric bundle (refer to Figure 17.1) involves the following factors:

i)   Initial recognition of AKI
ii) Assessment of fluid balance status in the mother
iii) Appropriate fluid replacement to the mother
iv) Avoidance of nephrotoxic medication and review of the medication chart
v)   Timely and appropriate uniform diagnostic work-up to be provided
vi) Timely management and reassessment of the AKI

Initial Recognition of AKI

A creatinine >90µmmol/L or serial creatinine rise of 26µmmol/L or 20 ml/hr urine for 12 hours (if PET excluded) is diagnostic of AKI in pregnancy. However, most pregnant women do not have a prepregnancy or early pregnancy renal profile as a baseline; hence this may confound the diagnosis as some may have preexisting CKD. It is important to be aware of the oliguric phase of preeclampsia and rapid fluid administration would be contraindicated in this setting. Women with preeclampsia will likely have a care plan already in place (see Chapter 18).

Assessment of Fluid Balance Status in the Mother

An accurate assessment will enable appropriate fluid resuscitation. An "ABCDE" approach allows for this assessment. The fluid balance chart at the best of times may be challenging and accurate recording is essential. The measurement of a lying and standing blood pressure is important as this will unmask a hypovolemic state, if the systolic difference in blood pressure is greater than 20 mmHg.

Appropriate Fluid Replacement to the Mother

Fluid volume repletion needs to be timely. If hypovolemic, and preeclampsia is excluded, immediately administer 250 ml of crystalloid intravenously. This should be followed by further crystalloid at 125 ml/h, and continuing reassessment. Preeclampsia is a contraindication for rapid fluid administration as there is a high risk of pulmonary edema in the mother.

Avoidance of Nephrotoxic Medication and Review of the Medication Chart

On reviewing the drug chart, nephrotoxic drugs should be stopped. Common drugs on the obstetric units to avoid in AKI in pregnancy and postpartum include aminoglycosides such as gentamicin, NSAIDS that are regularly found in postpartum analgesia protocols and, when considering imaging modality, to avoid the use of iodinated contrast dyes. Pregnancy and the puerperium increase the risk for venous thromboembolism, and in AKI there may be a need to reduce the LMWH thromboprophylaxis dose.

A Timely and Appropriate Uniform Diagnostic Work-Up

If dipstick urinalysis confirms proteinuria and/or blood in urine, then an urgent spot protein creatinine ratio and microscopy to look for red cell casts should be requested. An early renal ultrasound should be requested and performed within four to six hours if obstruction is being considered. The biochemical investigations should be requested in a timely fashion and for specific causes. This would include a liver profile, full blood count, blood film to look for fragmented red blood cells and platelets, lactate dehydrogenase, bilirubin and reticulocytes.

Timely Management and Reassessment of AKI

Adherence to the sepsis bundle and early administration of antibiotics within an hour of recognition of sepsis is important. Reassessment and early multidisciplinary input is required.

The indications for renal replacement therapy are similar to those outside pregnancy when hyperkalemia, fluid overload, metabolic acidosis and uremia are refractory to medical treatment (see Chapter 10).

An obstetric AKI care bundle may help to provide a means of standardizing care and provide high-quality care from all health professionals in the obstetric units. Care bundles have been reported to improve outcomes and provide a recognized approach and definitive AKI care bundles have been previously defined and are established for non-obstetric AKI [44–45]. We have proposed an obstetric AKI bundle to parallel these non-obstetric AKI guidelines to ensure cohesive and well-structured management on obstetric units, where women are managed within a multidisciplinary team.

Future Perspectives

The public health burden of AKI in pregnancy long term remains unknown. More studies and future tools including biomarkers to detect AKI may be beneficial.

References

1. Murugan R, Kellum JA Acute kidney injury: What's the prognosis? *Nature reviews. Nephrology* 2011; 7:4: 209–217.

2. Bellomo R, Ronco C, Kellum JA, et al. Acute renal failure – definition, outcome measures, animal models, fluid therapy and information technology needs: The Second International Consensus Conference of the Acute Dialysis Quality Initiative (ADQI) Group. *Critical care (London, England)* 2004; 8:4: R204–R212.

3. Levin A, Warnock DG, Mehta RL, et al. Improving outcomes from acute kidney injury: Report of an initiative. *American journal of kidney diseases: The official journal of the National Kidney Foundation* 2007; 50:1: 1–4.

4. Girling JC Re-evaluation of plasma creatinine concentration in normal pregnancy. *Journal of obstetrics and gynaecology: The journal of the Institute of Obstetrics and Gynaecology* 2000; 20:2: 128–131.

5. Bayliss D, Davison JM *Pregnancy and renal disease.* In *Comprehensive clinical nephrology.*, ed. Jurgen F, Johnson RJ, Feehally J 2014. 5th edn., Elsevier, New York. 498–505.

6. Brown MA, Mangos GJ, Peek M, Plaat F Renal disease In *De Swiet's medical disorders in obstetric practice.* ed. Powrie R, Greene MF, Camann W 2010. 5th edn., Chichester: Blackwell, 182–209.

7. Millache A, Ateka O, Palma Reis I, et al. Acute kidney injury in pregnancy: Experience from a large tertiary care referral centre. *American Society of Nephrology, San Diego, CA, USA.* Oct 30–Nov 4, 2012.

8. American College of Obstetricians and Gynecologists & Task Force on Hypertension in Pregnancy. Hypertension in pregnancy. Report of the American College of Obstetricians and Gynecologists' Task Force on Hypertension in Pregnancy *Obstetrics and gynecology* 2013; **122**:5: 1122–1131.

9. Acharya A, Santos J, Linde B, et al. Acute kidney injury in pregnancy-current status. *Advances in chronic kidney disease* 2013; **20**:3: 215–222.

10. Beaman M, Turney JH, Rodger, RS, et al. Changing pattern of acute renal failure. *The quarterly journal of medicine* 1987; **62**:237: 15–23.

11. Stratta P, Besso L, Canavese C, et al. Is pregnancy-related acute renal failure a disappearing clinical entity? *Renal failure* 1996; **18**:4: 575–584.

12. Prakash J, Niwas SS, Parekh A, et al. Acute kidney injury in late pregnancy in developing countries. *Renal failure* 2010; **32**:3: 309–313.

13. Sivakumar V, Sivaramakrishna G, Sainaresh VV, et al. Pregnancy-related acute renal failure: A ten-year experience. *Saudi journal of kidney diseases and transplantation: An official publication of the Saudi Center for Organ Transplantation, Saudi Arabia* 2011; **22**:2: 352–353.

14. Gurrieri C, Garovic VD, Gullo A, et al. Kidney injury during pregnancy: Associated comorbid conditions and outcomes. *Archives of gynecology and obstetrics* 2012; **286**:3: 567–573.

15. Mehrabadi A, Liu S, Bartholomew S, Hutcheon JA, et al. Hypertensive disorders of pregnancy and the recent increase in obstetric acute renal failure in Canada: Population based retrospective cohort study. *BMJ (Clinical research ed.)* 2014; **349**: 4731.

16. Palma-Reis I, Vais A, Nelson-Piercy C, et al. Renal disease and hypertension in pregnancy. *Clin Med (Lond)*. 2013; Feb;13(1):57–62.

17. Dashe JS, Ramin SM, Cunningham FG The long-term consequences of thrombotic microangiopathy (thrombotic thrombocytopenic purpura and hemolytic uremic syndrome) in pregnancy. *Obstetrics and gynecology* 1998; **91**:5:P1: 662–668.

18. Sibai BM. Imitators of severe preeclampsia. *Obstetrics and gynecology* 2007; **109**:4: 956–966.

19. Martin JN, Jr, Bailey AP, Rehberg JF et al. Thrombotic thrombocytopenic purpura in 166 pregnancies: 1955–2006. *American journal of obstetrics and gynecology* 2008; **199**:2: 98–104.

20. Ganesan C, Maynard SE Acute kidney injury in pregnancy: The thrombotic microangiopathies. *Journal of nephrology* 2011; **24**:5: 554–563.

21. Scully M, Yarranton H, Liesner R, et al. Regional UK TTP registry: Correlation with laboratory ADAMTS 13 analysis and clinical features. *British journal of haematology* 2008; **142** 5: 819–826.

22. Fujimura Y, Matsumoto M, Kokame K, et al. Pregnancy-induced thrombocytopenia and TTP, and the risk of fetal death, in Upshaw-Schulman syndrome: A series of 15 pregnancies in 9 genotyped patients. *British journal of haematology* 2009; **144**:5: 742–754.

23. Scully M, Hunt BJ, Benjamin S, Liesner R, et al. Guidelines on the diagnosis and management of thrombotic thrombocytopenic purpura and other thrombotic microangiopathies. *British journal of haematology* 2012; **58**:3: 323–335.

24. Hyrich KL, Verstappen SM Biologic therapies and pregnancy: The story so far. *Rheumatology (Oxford, England)* 2014; **53**:8: 1377–1385.

25. Vesely SK, Li X, McMinn JR, et al. Pregnancy outcomes after recovery from thrombotic thrombocytopenic purpura-hemolytic uremic syndrome. *Transfusion* 2004; **44**: 1149–1158.

26. Fakhouri F, Roumenina L, Provot F, et al. Pregnancy-associated hemolytic uremic syndrome revisited in the era of complement gene mutations. *Journal of the American Society of Nephrology: JASN* 2010; **21**:5: 859–867.

27. De Sousa Amorim, E, Blasco, M, Quintana, L, Sole, M, de Cordoba, SR, Campistol, JM Eculizumab in pregnancy-associated atypical hemolytic uremic syndrome: insights for optimizing management. *Journal of nephrology* 2015; Feb 25: [Epub ahead of print].

28. Cervera R, Serrano R, Pons-Estel GJ, et al. Morbidity and mortality in the antiphospholipid syndrome during a 10-year period: A multicentre prospective study of 1000 patients. *Annals of the rheumatic diseases* 2015; **74**:6: 1011–1018.

29. Hanouna G, Morel N, Le Thi Huong D, et al. Catastrophic antiphospholipid syndrome and pregnancy: An experience of 13 cases. *Rheumatology (Oxford, England)* 2013; **52**:9: 1635–1641.

30. Kronbichler, A, Frank, R, Kirschfink, M, Szilagyi, A, Csuka, D, Prohaszka, Z, Schratzberger, P, Lhotta, K, Mayer, G Efficacy of eculizumab in a patient with immunoadsorption-dependent catastrophic antiphospholipid syndrome: A case report. *Medicine* 2014; **93**:26: pp. e143.

31. Knight M, Nelson-Piercy C, Kurinczuk JJ, et al. A prospective national study of acute fatty liver of pregnancy in the UK. *Gut* 2008; **57**:7: 951–956.

32. Wilcken B, Leung LC, Hammond J, et al. Pregnancy and fetal long-chain 3-hydroxyacyl coenzyme A dehydrogenase deficiency. *Lancet* 1993; **341**:8842: 407–408.

33. Ch'ng CL, Morgan M, Hainsworth I, et al. Prospective study of liver dysfunction in pregnancy in Southwest Wales. *Gut* 2002; **51**:6: 876–880.

34. Acosta CD, Kurinczuk JJ, Lucas DN, et al. Severe maternal sepsis in the UK, 2011–2012: A national case-control study. *PLoS medicine* 2014; **11**:7: e1001672.

35. Matuszkiewicz-Rowinska J, Malyszko J, Wieliczko M Urinary tract infections in pregnancy: Old and new unresolved diagnostic and therapeutic problems. *Archives of medical science: AMS* 2015; **11**:1: 67–77.

36. Jolley JA, Wing DA Pyelonephritis in pregnancy: An update on treatment options for optimal outcomes. *Drugs* 2010; **70**:13: 1643–1655.

37. Dotters-Katz, SK, Heine RP, Grotegut CA Medical and infectious complications associated with pyelonephritis among pregnant women at delivery. *Infectious diseases in obstetrics and gynecology* 2013; **124102**:6.

38. Chugh KS, Singhal PC, Sharma BK, et al. Acute renal failure of obstetric origin. *Obstetrics and gynecology* 1976; **48**:6: 642–646.

39. Iglesias MH, Giesbrecht EM, von Dadelszen P, et al. Postpartum hyperkalemia associated with magnesium sulfate. *Hypertension in pregnancy* 2011; **30**:4: 481–484.

40. Andrade R., McGwin G, Jr, Alarcon GS, et al. Predictors of post-partum damage accrual in systemic lupus erythematosus: Data from LUMINA, a multiethnic US cohort (XXXVIII). *Rheumatology (Oxford, England)* 2006; **45**:11: 1380–1384.

41. Jena M, Mitch WE Rapidly reversible acute renal failure from ureteral obstruction in pregnancy. *American journal of kidney diseases: The official journal of the National Kidney Foundation* 1996; **28**:3: 457–460.

42. Brandes JC, Fritsche C Obstructive acute renal failure by a gravid uterus: A case report and review. *American journal of kidney diseases: The official journal of the National Kidney Foundation* 1991; **18**:3: 398–401.

43. Yossepowitch O, Baniel J, Livne PM Urological injuries during cesarean section: Intraoperative diagnosis and management. *The journal of urology* 2004; **172**:1: 196–199.

44. London Acute Kidney Injury Network. 2016. *Obstetric AKI*. Available at: http://londonaki.net/downloads/LondonAKInetwork-obstetric.pdf. (Accessed 8 February 2018).

45. Tsui A, Rajani C, Doshi R, et al. Improving recognition and management of acute kidney injury. *Acute medicine* 2013; **13**:3: 108–112.

Chapter 18

Preeclampsia-Related Renal Impairment

Louise C. Kenny

Introduction

Preeclampsia is a pregnancy-specific, multisystem disorder that affects 3–5 percent of pregnant women. Globally, the disorder is a leading cause of maternal and neonatal morbidity and mortality. There is a major interplay between renal disease and preeclampsia. The disease is defined by the presence of new-onset hypertension and proteinuria, which typically arises in the third trimester. Preeclampsia is the most common form of renal impairment arising *de novo* in late pregnancy, and, furthermore, it is well recognized that underlying renal disease is an independent risk factor for the development of preeclampsia. In recent years, a deeper understanding of the renal pathophysiology of preeclampsia has led to improved clinical management of severe cases, particularly with respect to fluid balance and consequently morbidity secondary to fluid overload has fallen significantly. In this chapter, the renal pathophysiology of preeclampsia and the differential diagnosis of renal impairment, particularly in late pregnancy, are discussed. The investigation and management of preeclampsia-related renal impairment, particularly with respect to intrapartum and postpartum care, are described.

Renal Pathophysiology in Preeclampsia

Normal pregnancy is characterized by marked glomerular hyperfiltration. The glomerular filtration rate (GFR) begins to increase in the first trimester and peaks in the second trimester at approximately 40–60 percent above nonpregnant levels [1, 2] (see Chapter 1). The hyperfiltration of normal pregnancy results from increased renal blood flow, which increases by approximately 80 percent in the first trimester of pregnancy and from a fall in oncotic pressure in the plasma entering the glomerular capillaries that occurs secondary to plasma volume expansion and hemodilution. This hyperfiltration results in a fall in serum markers of renal clearance, urea, creatinine and uric acid [3].

In preeclampsia, both GFR and renal plasma flow are decreased by 30–40 percent compared with normal pregnancy of the same duration [4, 5], and this results in a corresponding relative increase in serum urea and creatinine. However, it is important to note serum levels of creatinine considered normal in a nonpregnant woman can represent renal impairment in a pregnant woman with preeclampsia [6].

In normal pregnancy, urinary protein excretion doubles [7]. Preeclampsia is characterized and indeed is defined by the presence of more significant proteinuria. The International Society for the Study of Hypertension in Pregnancy (ISSHP) defines significant proteinuria as 300mg/day or more of protein in a 24-hour urine collection or a spot urine protein/creatinine ratio (PCR) of 30mg/mmol or more [8]. The American Congress of Obstetricians and Gynecologists (ACOG) classification of severe preeclampsia includes proteinuria in excess of 5 g/day as one of the qualifying criteria [9]. However, these cutoff levels are somewhat arbitrary and without a sound rationale. Moreover, although increased protein loss suggests the presence of more significant renal injury, the actual amount and the rate of increase of proteinuria have not been found to be consistent predictors of either adverse maternal or fetal/neonatal outcomes [10, 11, 12].

The mechanism for proteinuria in preeclampsia is not well understood. Recent data suggest that a loss of both size and charges selectivity of the glomerular barrier contribute to the development of albuminuria [5]. Morphometric studies of the kidney in preeclampsia have focused on the renal glomerulus and a characteristic non-inflammatory lesion commonly referred to as the glomerular endotheliosis [13, 14, 15]. It primarily involves swelling and the hypertrophy of the glomerular endothelial and mesangial cells,

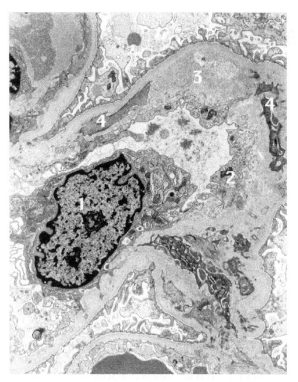

Figure 18.1 Transmission electron microscopy of a representative glomerular capillary enumerating pathological changes associated with pre-eclampsia; these include: (1) hypertrophied endothelial cells, (2) swollen segments of endothelial cytoplasmic rim in which fenestrae are not discernible, (3) sub-endothelial fibrinoid and granular deposits, and (4) interposition of mesangial cells; reproduced by permission from Macmillan Publishers Ltd: *Kidney International*, Lafayette et al.[4] © 1998

which encroach on and occlude the glomerular capillary lumen, giving rise to the typical bloodless appearance. Mesangial interposition may occur in severe cases or in the healing stages. Glomerular sub-endothelial and occasional mesangial electron-dense deposits can be seen. These likely relate to fibrin or related breakdown products. Immunofluorescence may reveal deposition of fibrin or fibrinogen derivatives, particularly in biopsies done within two weeks postpartum [16]. Electron microscopy demonstrates the loss of endothelial fenestrae (Figure 18.1).

Despite heavy proteinuria, the podocyte foot processes have traditionally been thought to be relatively preserved [17]. Recent data, however, suggest preeclampsia is associated with subtle damage to the foot process as evidenced by the appearance of podocyturia – the excretion of glomerular visceral epithelial cells or podocytes into the urine of women with preeclampsia [18]. It has been speculated that subtle

damage to the foot processes may actually be a significant pathological event in preeclampsia [19] as the epithelial podocytes secretes vascular endothelial growth factor (VEGF) and at least certain VEGF receptors, such as neuropilins, are expressed on podocytes [20]. Increasing soluble fms-like tyrosine kinase-1 (sFlt1) (a soluble VEGF antagonist) levels in rodents produces a renal lesion similar in appearance to glomerular endotheliosis characteristic of preeclampsia, which suggests that impairment of VEGF signaling in the kidney may be responsible for this lesion [21]. Indeed, genetic deficiency of VEGF production in the podocytes also leads to glomerular endotheliosis [22]. Finally, dramatic decreases in nephrin (a podocyte markers) have been noted in the glomerular podocytes of animals that are exposed to sFlt1 or VEGF antibody and in the glomeruli that are obtained from human preeclamptic renal biopsy specimens [23].

It has been claimed [13] and refuted [24] that glomerular endotheliosis is pathognomonic. The former view would suggest that preeclampsia is primarily a renal disease. It is now accepted that renal involvement in preeclampsia can vary markedly and always occurs secondary to the primary uteroplacental pathology. In support of this, normal renal histology has been found in some cases of eclampsia [25] and previous biopsy studies have found biopsy-proven glomerular capillary endotheliosis in only 84 percent of nulliparae with a clinical diagnosis of preeclampsia and in only 38 percent of multiparae [15]. Interestingly, a recent study reported that glomerular endotheliosis is present in the kidneys of approximately 40 percent of normotensive pregnant women [24]. This study was unique for several reasons, but particularly because of the major ethical debate triggered by its publication [26]. It involved renal biopsy, a procedure with a well-documented risk profile, of healthy pregnant women. The role of renal biopsy in pregnancy is discussed in detail in Chapter 19. Suffice it to say that renal biopsy is rarely helpful in the differential diagnosis of preeclampsia, least of all in the nulliparous woman in the third trimester.

Glomerular enlargement and endothelial swelling usually disappear within eight weeks of delivery, coinciding with resolution of the hypertension and proteinuria. Further investigation, including renal biopsy, may be indicated in women with persisting signs in the puerperium (see Chapter 5).

Differential Diagnosis of Preeclampsia-Related Renal Impairment

Preexisting Renal Disease and Preeclampsia

In a primigravid woman with no antecedent history, the onset of hypertension and proteinuria during the third trimester is almost synonymous with preeclampsia. However, preeclampsia can mimic a variety of conditions that can manifest with the same symptoms and signs. Thus, on occasion the presentation of proteinuria and hypertension in pregnancy may pose a diagnostic dilemma. This is particularly true in the case of an unbooked woman without a clearly documented normal blood pressure urinalysis in whom hypertension and proteinuria may represent an exacerbation or onset of an underlying renal condition. The issue is further complicated by the fact that preeclampsia can be superimposed on preexisting renal disorders and it can be difficult to distinguish between the two. It is imperative, wherever possible, to make a rapid diagnosis of preeclampsia as the condition remains a leading cause of maternal mortality in the developed world and delayed diagnosis and inappropriate clinical management contribute to the mortality rates.

In women of childbearing age, the most common causes of renal impairment are:

- reflux nephropathy
- diabetic nephropathy
- systemic lupus erythematous (SLE)
- other forms of glomerulonephritis
- polycystic kidney disease

All of these predispose to the development of superimposed preeclampsia. In women presenting with renal impairment in pregnancy, the aggressive nature and attendant morbidity of preeclampsia may render it dangerous and inadvisable to conduct an exhaustive search for an underlying renal disorder. If there is doubt about the diagnosis, preeclampsia should be overdiagnosed [27] and a search for a definitive diagnosis delayed until the postpartum period.

The one possible exception to this rule is lupus nephritis (see Chapter 14). This is a common cause of renal insufficiency in women of childbearing age. Exacerbations increase the risk of renal failure.

Approximately half of women experience an exacerbation of lupus during pregnancy (although it is much less common in women who have been in remission for more than six months). Fetal loss rates are high. Wherever possible a full history and investigation should seek to exclude (or implicate) this from the list of differential diagnoses of renal impairment in pregnancy because the treatment, particularly remote from term, is different from that of other forms of renal impairment. Treatment for lupus flares, aimed at inducing remission, includes prednisolone and azathioprine. It is important to have a high degree of confidence that worsening renal function in a woman with lupus reflects an exacerbation of the underlying disease and is not the development of superimposed preeclampsia because prednisolone, although usually well tolerated, may worsen hypertension and lead to further complications. Furthermore, continuing the pregnancy in the presence of established preeclampsia may be fatal for mother and infant. There is increasing data on newer biologic agents in pregnancy, in particular B-cell depletion therapy (see Chapter 7). Rituximab (a chimeric anti-CD20 monoclonal B cell-depleting antibody) was initially developed for hematologic malignancies and active rheumatoid arthritis, but has been used with some success in patients with lupus. Despite counseling to avoid pregnancy, women have inadvertently become pregnant during or after rituximab treatment. The Rituximab Global Drug Safety Database details 153 pregnancies with known outcomes. Ninety resulted in live births. Twenty-two infants were born prematurely, with one neonatal death at six weeks. Eleven neonates had hematologic abnormalities; none had corresponding infections. Two congenital malformations were identified: clubfoot in one twin, and cardiac malformation in a singleton birth [28]. These are good outcomes considering the indications for which rituximab was used (predominantly for hematological malignancies and often combined with other chemotherapeutic agents). Belimumab is the first targeted biologic agent developed specifically for SLE. Use in pregnancy is limited and a pregnancy registry has been set up by the manufacturer [29].

The presence of lupus anticoagulant and/or anticardiolipin antibodies increases the risk and the likelihood of renal lupus flares. Therefore all women with lupus should be screened for these antibodies.

Table 18.1 Laboratory differential diagnosis in pregnancy-associated thrombotic microangiopathies

Abnormality	HUS/TTP	AFLP	Preeclampsia/HELLP syndrome
Abnormal PT/PTT	No	Yes	No
Hemolysis	Yes	Yes	Yes
Thrombocytopenia	Yes	Yes	Yes
Abnormal liver function tests	No	Yes	Yes
Abnormal renal function tests	Yes	No/Yes	No/Yes

AFLP = acute fatty liver of pregnancy; HELLP syndrome = hemolytic anemia, elevated liver enzymes and low platelet count; HUS = hemolytic uremic syndrome; PT = prothrombin time; PTT = partial thromboplastin time; TTP = thrombotic thrombocytopenic purpura

Recent advances in the understanding of the role circulating angiogenic factors (sFlt1 and placental growth factor [PlGF]) play in the pathogenesis of preeclampsia offer the potential of more accurate diagnostic tools. Levels of these factors correlate with the diagnosis and adverse outcomes, particularly when the disease presents prematurely (< 34 weeks). Consequently, there has been much interest in whether measurement of these angiogenic biomarkers further helps differentiate preeclampsia and its complications from other disorders that present with similar clinical profiles. Emerging data suggests that the sFlt1/PlGF ratio can distinguish women with developing superimposed preeclampsia in women with preexisting renal disease [30], particularly in those with lupus nephritis [31], although further large studies are need to confirm this.

Acute Renal Failure and Preeclampsia

Acute renal failure in the presence of preeclampsia is rare and when it occurs it is usually precipitated by hemolysis, elevated liver enzymes and low platelets (HELLP) syndrome or significant obstetric hemorrhage. Acute renal failure caused by hypovolemic states is often reversible if renal perfusion is restored. Acute tubular necrosis follows more prolonged ischemia. It is also reversible and damage is limited to the metabolically active tubular cells. More prolonged or severe renal ischemia gives rise to acute cortical necrosis characterized by disintegration of both glomeruli and tubules in the renal cortex. Although the process is irreversible, it is the incomplete or patchy variety that occurs more often in pregnancy.

There are several rare but important and difficult differential diagnoses of oliguric acute renal failure in late pregnancy and the puerperium. These include acute fatty liver of pregnancy (AFLP), thrombotic thrombocytopenic purpura (TTP) and atypical hemolytic uremic syndrome (aHUS) (Table 18.1) (see Chapter 17). Differentiating among these conditions is critical because they respond to different therapeutic modalities. However, the clinical and histological features are so similar that establishing the correct diagnosis is often difficult. Most important is the history (e.g. preceding proteinuria and hypertension favor preeclampsia) and time of onset. Preeclampsia typically develops in the third trimester, but may rarely present before 20 weeks with only a few percent of cases developing postpartum usually in the first two days. TTP almost always occurs antepartum; many cases begin before 24 weeks, but the disease also occurs in the third trimester. Atypical HUS is generally a postpartum disease. Symptoms can begin before delivery, but the onset in most cases is delayed for 48 hours or more after delivery (mean about four days). AFLP is characterized by acute hepatic failure with a significant elevation of liver function tests and renal function abnormalities tend to be mild unless disseminated intravascular coagulation (DIC) and hemorrhage intervene. These conditions often share clinical and laboratory features and, at times, progress from one to another.

Antenatal and Intrapartum Management of Renal Impairment in Preeclampsia

Management of Hypertension

Antenatal Control of Blood Pressure

The pharmacological treatment of high blood pressure in pregnancy in women with preexisting renal disease and/or chronic hypertension is an important and contentious issue (see Chapter 8). Blood pressure targets for women with hypertension in pregnancy have been much debated and there is little consensus. International guidelines vary, with some recommending treatment goals consistent with either "less-tight control" (blood pressure that is higher than normal but not severely elevated) or "tight control" (the use of antihypertensive therapy to normalize blood pressure).

Many clinicians believe that women with evidence of end-organ disease should be treated as aggressively as nonpregnant women to achieve blood pressures averaging below 140/80 mmHg. Previous randomized controlled trials (RCTs) have been small and of moderate or poor quality. Tight control has been associated with maternal benefits (e.g. a decrease in the frequency of severe hypertension and possibly in the rate of antenatal hospitalization). However, a meta-regression showed that every 10 mmHg fall in mean arterial pressure in women taking antihypertensives was associated with a 145 g decrease in birth weight [32].

The Control of Hypertension in Pregnancy Study (CHIPS) trial, a large RCT designed to compare less-tight control with tight control of non-proteinuric, non-severe hypertension in pregnancy recently reported. The investigators found no significant differences in the risk of pregnancy loss, high-level neonatal care or overall maternal complications between the tight and less-tight group, although less-tight control was associated with a significantly higher frequency of severe maternal hypertension [33].

This evidence would suggest that women with renal disease and/or chronic hypertension in pregnancy can be managed with antihypertensive therapies to obtain tight control without an increased risk of adverse outcome for the fetus. Lowering blood pressure does not cure or prevent the onset of superimposed preeclampsia, but it may permit prolongation of pregnancy because uncontrolled blood pressure is frequently an indication for delivery.

A variety of antihypertensive agents are available for use in pregnant women and a summary of commonly used agents is provided in Table 8.1. A discussion of these agents focusing on their pharmacokinetics and dynamics can be found in Chapter 8 [34]. The use of angiotensin-converting enzyme (ACE) inhibitors in pregnancy has been associated with increased rates of congenital malformations,

intrauterine growth restriction, hypoglycemia, kidney disease and preterm birth [35]. Similarly, studies have linked the use of angiotensin II receptor blockers (ARBs) in pregnancy with an increased risk of congenital malformations [36]. The diuretic chlorothiazide may also increase the risk of congenital abnormality, neonatal thrombocytopenia, hypoglycemia and hypovolemia [37]. Despite the relatively poor quality of these studies, there is sufficient concern to avoid the use of ACE inhibitors, ARBs and chlorothiazide both in women with preexisting renal disease and/or chronic hypertension planning pregnancy and for the treatment of hypertension in pregnancy.

For antihypertensive drugs currently in use, other than the aforementioned agents, there is no evidence for teratogenicity, although the quality of the data is generally poor.

There are limited good-quality trials to evaluate the effectiveness of alpha- and beta-blockers, methyldopa and calcium channel antagonists for the treatment of chronic hypertension during pregnancy and very few head-to-head comparisons. Consequently, international guidelines vary.

Control of Blood Pressure in Severe Preeclampsia

In women with severe preeclampsia, there is an urgent need to lower blood pressure. Uncontrolled systolic blood pressure in severe preeclampsia is associated with cerebrovascular and cardiovascular complications. Lowering blood pressure leads to a decrease in maternal death.

The aim of stabilization of blood pressure is to reduce the blood pressure to below 160/105 mmHg in the first instance (mean arterial pressure below 125 mmHg) and maintain the blood pressure at or below that level. There are two agents of choice: labetalol and hydralazine.

If the woman can tolerate oral therapy, an initial 200 mg dose of labetalol can be given. This can be done immediately before venous access is obtained and so can achieve as quick a result as an initial intravenous dose. This should lead to a reduction in blood pressure in about half an hour. A second of those can be given if needed.

If there is no initial response to oral therapy, or if it cannot be tolerated, control should be achieved with repeated boluses of intravenous labetalol followed by a labetalol infusion. A bolus infusion of 50 mg should be given over at least five minutes. This should have an effect by 10 minutes and should be repeated if diastolic blood pressure has not been reduced to below 160/105 mmHg. This can be repeated in doses of 50 mg to a maximum dose of 200 mg at 10-minute intervals. Following this, or as an initial treatment in moderate hypertension, a labetalol infusion should be commenced at an initial rate of 20mg/hour, doubled thereafter every half hour to a maximum of 160 mg/hour until the blood pressure has dropped and stabilized at an acceptable level. Labetalol is contraindicated in women with asthma and should be used with caution in women with preexisting cardiac disease.

If labetalol is contraindicated or fails to control the blood pressure, hydralazine is an alternative agent. A second agent should be considered where mean arterial pressure is persistently over 120 mmHg. In such cases, it is normally appropriate to continue the first drug i.e. labetalol while administering the second.

Hydralazine is given as a bolus infusion of 5 mg over five minutes measuring the blood pressure every five minutes. This can be repeated every 20 minutes to a maximum dose of 20 mg. This may be followed by an infusion of 40 mg of hydralazine at any rate of 1–5mg/hour. However, the labetalol infusion is continued; the hydralazine may not be required as the blood pressure will probably settle with the bolus dose.

Fluid Balance

Inappropriate management of renal impairment in preeclampsia can be fatal. Left ventricle dysfunction and capillary leak complicate fluid management in severe preeclampsia. A review of the last five triennial reports of the Confidential Enquiries into Maternal in Child Health illustrates the declining mortality rates from acute respiratory distress syndrome and pulmonary edema as awareness of the importance of appropriate fluid management has grown.

Clinical guidelines, both national and local, regarding the management of preeclampsia emphasize the need for careful fluid balance aimed at avoiding fluid overload. While there is some variation, there is a consensus that in severe preeclampsia total input should be limited to 80ml an hour of a crystalloid solution. If oxytocin is used, then it should be at a high concentration and the volume of fluid included in a total input. Such a "dry" regime provokes oliguria, particularly if the woman is still undelivered or laboring. This should not precipitate any specific intervention except to encourage early delivery. Even with this "dry" approach, acute renal shutdown is extremely unlikely unless there is a concomitant hypotension, coagulopathy or the use of nonsteroidal anti-inflammatory agents such as diclofenac.

As women with preeclampsia tend to maintain their blood pressure despite regional blockade, fluid load prior to regional anesthesia is unnecessary and may complicate fluid balance. For this reason fluid loading in preeclampsia should always be controlled and should never be done prophylactically or routinely. Hypotension when it occurs can be easily controlled with small doses of ephedrine.

Following delivery series restriction should continue until a natural diuresis occurs, usually around 36 to 48 hours post delivery. The total amount of fluid (the total of intravenous and oral fluids) should be given at 80 mL an hour. It is important to remember that this must include the volume of fluid in drug infusions such as magnesium and labetalol.

Urine output should be recorded hourly and each four-hour block should be summated and recorded. Each four-hour block should total in excess of 80 ml. If two consecutive blocks fail to achieve 80 ml, then further action is appropriate. This would either be:

- If total input is more than 750 ml in excess of output in the previous 24 hours (or since starting the regime), 20 mg of intravenous furosemide should be given. Colloid should then be given as follows if a diuresis of more than 200 ml in the next hour occurs.

Or

- If total input is less than 750 ml in excess of output in the previous 24 hours (or since starting the regime), then an infusion of 250 mL of colloid over 20 minutes should be given. The urine output should then be watched until the end of the next four-hour block. If the urine output is still low, then individual unit policies for fluid management in preeclampsia should be followed and liaison with and referral to a renal physician would be advisable.

Central Venous Pressure Monitoring

Central venous pressure (CVP) monitoring may mislead in preeclampsia as it does not correlate well with the pulmonary capillary wedge pressure in these women [38]. Owing to the fact that pulmonary wedge pressure may be high in the absence of an elevated CVP, assessment of whether the myocardium is handling the therapeutic volume expansion can be assessed only after placement of a pulmonary artery catheter. The risks of pulmonary artery catheterization are well described and evidence supporting benefit is subjective at best [39]. It will only be necessary in very selected cases. CVP monitoring may occasionally be useful to exclude volume depletion as a cause of severe or prolonged postpartum oliguria that requires total interpretation.

Dialysis

Most of the problems linked to acute renal failure will respond to conservative management, but if this approach is unsuccessful, dialysis will be necessary. Both hemodialysis and peritoneal dialysis can be used in pregnant or recently delivered women (see Chapter 10). The main indications for the dialysis are:

- Volume overload with congestive heart failure
- Severe hyperkalemia (K more than 7.0mmol/l)
- Severe acidosis
- Uremic symptoms not manageable by conventional methods

Seizure Prophylaxis

The drug of choice for the treatment and prevention of eclampsia is magnesium sulphate, but 97 percent of magnesium is excreted in the urine and therefore the presence of oliguria can lead to toxic levels. In the presence of oliguria or chronic kidney disease, following the normal loading dose of magnesium, further administration should be reduced or withheld. If magnesium is not being excreted, then levels should not fall and no other anticonvulsant is needed. Magnesium should be reintroduced if urine output improves.

Postnatal Follow-Up

Hypertension frequently persists after delivery in women with antenatal hypertension or preeclampsia and blood pressure may be labile in the initial postpartum days. Some of this lability may reflect the redistribution of fluids from the extracellular to the intravascular space. However, postpartum hypertension that persists beyond 12 weeks postpartum may represent previously undiagnosed chronic hypertension, which should be investigated, followed and treated appropriately.

Postpartum evaluation should be considered for women with preeclampsia who developed the condition early (before 34 weeks of gestation), had severe or recurrent preeclampsia or who have persistent proteinuria. In these cases, underlying renal disease, secondary hypertension and thrombophilias (e.g. factor V Leiden, prothrombin 20201, anticardiolipin antibodies and lupus anticoagulant) may be considered. Studies report varying rates of underlying and previously undiagnosed renal disease in women with severe preeclampsia ranging from 12.1 percent to 71.7 percent [40].

Counseling for future pregnancies requires consideration of different recurrence rates for preeclampsia, depending on the pathogenesis and population characteristics. The earlier in gestation, the higher the risk of recurrence: before 30 weeks, recurrence rates may be as high as 40 percent [41]. If preeclampsia has developed in a nulliparous woman close to term (i.e. after 36 weeks), the risk or recurrence is thought to be about 10 percent. Women who have had HELLP syndrome have a high risk of subsequent obstetric complications with preeclampsia occurring in 55 percent, although the rate of recurrent HELLP syndrome appears to be low at only 6 percent [42].

Hypertensive diseases of pregnancy have been associated with an elevated risk of hypertension and stroke in later life. In one study gestational hypertension was associated with the relative risk (RR) of 3.72 subsequent hypertension and preeclampsia, with an RR of 3.98 for subsequent hypertension and 3.59 for stroke [43]. Preeclampsia associated with preterm birth is also a risk factor for ischemic heart disease when studied retrospectively [44]. These associations may serve to increase awareness of the need to monitor for future hypertensive and cardiovascular disorders [45].

References

1. Sims, E. A. and K. E. Krantz, Serial studies of renal function during pregnancy and the puerperium in normal women. *J Clin Invest*, 1958. 37(12): pp. 1764–1774.

2. Davison, J. M. and M. C. Noble, Serial changes in 24 hour creatinine clearance during normal menstrual cycles and the first trimester of pregnancy. *Br J Obstet Gynaecol*, 1981. 88(1): pp. 10–17.

3. Karumanchi, S. A., et al., Preeclampsia: A renal perspective. *Kidney Int*, 2005. 67(6): pp. 2101–2113.

4. Lafayette, R. A., et al., Nature of glomerular dysfunction in pre-eclampsia. *Kidney Int*, 1998. 54(4): pp. 1240–1249.

5. Moran, P., et al., Glomerular ultrafiltration in normal and preeclamptic pregnancy. *J Am Soc Nephrol*, 2003. 14(3): pp. 648–652.

6. Fischer, M. J., Chronic kidney disease and pregnancy: Maternal and fetal outcomes. *Adv Chronic Kidney Dis*, 2007. 14(2): pp. 132–145.

7. Roberts, M., M. D. Lindheimer and J. M. Davison, Altered glomerular permselectivity to neutral dextrans and heteroporous membrane modeling in human pregnancy. *Am J Physiol*, 1996. 270(2 Pt 2): pp. F338–F343.

8. Tranquilli, A. L., et al., The definition of severe and early-onset preeclampsia. Statements from the International Society for the Study of Hypertension in Pregnancy (ISSHP). *Pregnancy Hypertens*, 2013. 3(1): pp. 44–47.

9. Bulletins–Obstetrics, A. C. O. P., ACOG practice bulletin. Diagnosis and management of preeclampsia and eclampsia. Number 33, January 2002. *Obstet Gynecol*, 2002. 99(1): pp. 159–167.

10. Schiff, E., et al., The importance of urinary protein excretion during conservative management of severe preeclampsia. *Am J Obstet Gynecol*, 1996. 175(5): pp. 1313–1316.

11. Payne, B., et al., PIERS proteinuria: Relationship with adverse maternal and perinatal outcome. *J Obstet Gynaecol Can*, 2011. 33(6): pp. 588–597.

12. von Dadelszen, P., et al., Prediction of adverse maternal outcomes in pre-eclampsia: Development and validation of the full PIERS model. *Lancet*, 2011. 377(9761): pp. 219–227.

13. Spargo, B., C. P. McCartney, and R. Winemiller, Glomerular capillary endotheliosis in toxemia of pregnancy. *Arch Pathol*, 1959. 68: pp. 593–599.

14. Pollak, V. E. and J. B. Nettles, The kidney in toxemia of pregnancy: A clinical and pathologic study based on renal biopsies. *Medicine (Baltimore)*, 1960. 39: pp. 469–526.

15. Fisher, K. A., et al., Hypertension in pregnancy: Clinical-pathological correlations and remote prognosis. *Medicine (Baltimore)*, 1981. 60(4): pp. 267–276.

16. Morris, R. H., et al., Immunofluorescent Studies of Renal Biopsies in the Diagnosis of Toxemia of Pregnancy. *Obstet Gynecol*, 1964. 24: pp. 32–46.

17. Mautner, W., et al., Preeclamptic nephropathy: An electron microscopic study. *Lab Invest*, 1962. 11: pp. 518–530.

18. Garovic, V. D., et al., Urinary podocyte excretion as a marker for preeclampsia. *Am J Obstet Gynecol*, 2007. 196(4): pp. 320 e1-7.

19. Karumanchi, S. A. and M. D. Lindheimer, Preeclampsia and the kidney: Footprints in the urine. *Am J Obstet Gynecol*, 2007. 196(4): pp. 287–288.

20. Harper, S. J., et al., Expression of neuropilin-1 by human glomerular epithelial cells in vitro and in vivo. *Clin Sci (Lond)*, 2001. 101(4): pp. 439–446.

21. Maynard, S. E., et al., Excess placental soluble fms-like tyrosine kinase 1 (sFlt1) may contribute to endothelial dysfunction, hypertension, and proteinuria in preeclampsia. *J Clin Invest*, 2003. 111(5): pp. 649–658.

22. Eremina, V., et al., Glomerular-specific alterations of VEGF-A expression lead to distinct congenital and acquired renal diseases. *J Clin Invest*, 2003. 111(5): pp. 707–716.

23. Sugimoto, H., et al., Neutralization of circulating vascular endothelial growth factor (VEGF) by anti-VEGF antibodies and soluble VEGF receptor 1 (sFlt-1) induces proteinuria. *J Biol Chem*, 2003. 278(15): pp. 12605–12608.

24. Strevens, H., et al., Glomerular endotheliosis in normal pregnancy and pre-eclampsia. *BJOG*, 2003. 110(9): pp. 831–836.

25. Dennis, E. J., 3rd, et al., Percutaneous renal biopsy in eclampsia. *Am J Obstet Gynecol*, 1963. 87: pp. 364–371.

26. Lupton, M. G. and D. J. Williams, The ethics of research on pregnant women: is maternal consent sufficient? *BJOG*, 2004. 111(12): pp. 1307–1312.

27. Report of the National High Blood Pressure Education Program Working Group on High Blood Pressure in Pregnancy. *American Journal of Obstetrics & Gynecology*. 183(1): pp. s1–s22.

28. Chakravarty, E. F., et al., Pregnancy outcomes after maternal exposure to rituximab. *Blood*, 2011. 117(5): pp. 1499–1506.

29. http://pregnancyregistry.gsk.com/belimumab.html.

30. Rolfo, A., et al., Chronic kidney disease may be differentially diagnosed from preeclampsia by serum biomarkers. *Kidney Int*, 2013. 83(1): pp. 177–181.

31. Qazi, U., et al., Soluble Fms-like tyrosine kinase associated with preeclampsia in pregnancy in systemic lupus erythematosus. *J Rheumatol*, 2008. 35(4): pp. 631–634.

32. von Dadelszen, P., et al., Fall in mean arterial pressure and fetal growth restriction in pregnancy hypertension: a meta-analysis. *Lancet*, 2000. 355(9198): pp. 87–92.

33. Magee, L. A., et al., Less-tight versus tight control of hypertension in pregnancy. *N Engl J Med*, 2015. 372(5): pp. 407–417.

34. Umans, J. G., Medications during pregnancy: antihypertensives and immunosuppressives. *Adv Chronic Kidney Dis*, 2007. 14(2): pp. 191–198.

35. Lip, G. Y., et al., Angiotensin-converting-enzyme inhibitors in early pregnancy. *Lancet*, 1997. 350(9089): p. 1446–7.

36. Velazquez-Armenta, E. Y., et al., Angiotensin II receptor blockers in pregnancy: a case report and systematic review of the literature. *Hypertens Pregnancy*, 2007. 26(1): pp. 51–66.

37. Maren, T. H. and A. C. Ellison, The teratological effect of certain thiadiazoles related to acetazolamide, with a note on sulfanilamide and thiazide diuretics. *Johns Hopkins Med J*, 1972. 130(2): pp. 95–104.

38. Bolte, A. C., et al., Lack of agreement between central venous pressure and pulmonary capillary wedge pressure in preeclampsia. *Hypertens Pregnancy*, 2000. 19(3): pp. 261–271.

39. Gilbert, W. M., et al., The safety and utility of pulmonary artery catheterization in severe preeclampsia and eclampsia. *Am J Obstet Gynecol*, 2000. 182(6): pp. 1397–1403.

40. Beller, F. K., W. R. Dame, and C. Witting, Renal disease diagnosed by renal biopsy: Prognostic evaluation. *Contrib Nephrol*, 1981. 25: pp. 61–70.

41. Sibai, B. M., B. Mercer and C. Sarinoglu, Severe preeclampsia in the second trimester: recurrence risk and long-term prognosis. *Am J Obstet Gynecol*, 1991. 165(5 Pt 1): pp. 1408–1412.

42. Sibai, B. M., et al., Aggressive versus expectant management of severe preeclampsia at 28 to 32 weeks' gestation: a randomized controlled trial. *Am J Obstet Gynecol*, 1994. 171(3): pp. 818–822.

43. Wilson, B. J., et al., Hypertensive diseases of pregnancy and risk of hypertension and stroke in later life: results from cohort study. *BMJ*, 2003. 326(7394): p. 845.

44. Haukkamaa, L., et al., Risk for subsequent coronary artery disease after preeclampsia. *Am J Cardiol*, 2004. 93(6): pp. 805–808.

45. Bellamy, L., et al., Pre-eclampsia and risk of cardiovascular disease and cancer in later life: Systematic review and meta-analysis. *BMJ*, 2007. 335 (7627): p. 974.

Chapter 19

Renal Biopsy in Pregnancy

Nigel Brunskill

Renal Biopsy in General Nephrological Practice

Since its first description in the early 1950s [1], percutaneous renal biopsy has evolved to become an indispensable tool in the management of patients with kidney disease. In general nephrological practice, the commonest indications for performing native kidney biopsy are in some patients with nephrotic syndrome, unexplained urinary dipstick abnormalities, acute kidney injury, renal dysfunction in the setting of systemic immunological diseases such as lupus or vasculitis, unexplained chronic kidney disease (CKD) and familial renal disease. Ideally, the biopsy should provide specific diagnostic and prognostic information, and facilitate informed management decisions. Recent prospective studies show that the pathological diagnosis provided by kidney biopsy results in altered patient management in 50–80 percent of cases [2].

In some situations, renal biopsy may be unsafe or technically impossible. An uncorrectable bleeding diathesis is an absolute contraindication to percutaneous renal biopsy, whereas hyper- (blood pressure > 160/95) or hypotension, urinary infection, low platelet count, single kidney, renal cysts or tumor, severe anemia, uremia, obesity and an uncooperative patient are relative contraindications [2].

In general, renal biopsy is performed with the patient in the prone position using local anesthesia. Ultrasonography is used to locate the lower pole of the kidney and a biopsy needle advanced to the kidney under direct ultrasound guidance. This may be more challenging in large or obese patients. The disposable biopsy needle is attached to a spring loaded biopsy "gun" with a trigger mechanism that, when released with the patient's breath held, instantly advances the needle tip into the kidney. The biopsy needle is then withdrawn and the sample of renal tissue removed from the sample notch of the needle. This procedure

may need to be repeated to obtain sufficient tissue for analysis.

Renal biopsy is not an uncomplicated procedure [3, 4, 5, 6]. Pain around the biopsy site is common, but severe pain should raise the possibility of significant peri-renal hemorrhage. Bleeding may also occur into the urine with macroscopic hematuria (3 percent) and painful clot colic. Some degree of peri-renal bleeding is inevitable after every biopsy and a mean fall in hemoglobin of 1 g/dL has been reported [2]. More severe bleeding complications requiring transfusion, renal embolization or surgery occur in approximately 0.1 percent of procedures. Other organs (liver, spleen, pancreas, gallbladder, large and small bowel) may be inadvertently biopsied or injured. Hematoma may rupture into the peritoneal cavity or track along the psoas muscle into the groin. Trauma to renal, mesenteric and lumbar arteries are all described, as are pneumo- and hemothorax and calyceal-peritoneal fistula [3]. Renal arteriovenous fistulae are also described [7]. Death following severe hemorrhage is rare, but reported.

Evidence suggests that serious biopsy complications are more likely to occur in patients with severe illness, particularly severe acute kidney injury and poorly controlled blood pressure, or in those who have other relative contraindications. In some series, renal amyloidosis is associated with a greater bleeding tendency after renal biopsy [6]. Careful patient selection is suggested to minimize risks [4]. Therefore, although renal biopsy is regarded as a safe procedure, it should be performed only under the supervision of experienced operators after careful patient evaluation.

Experience of Renal Biopsy in Pregnancy

Pregnancy in women with CKD is associated with adverse maternal and fetal outcomes [8, 9], and there is an understandable desire of carers to fully understand underlying nephrological conditions in these patients. Despite the rarity of significant renal biopsy complications in nonpregnant individuals, most experienced clinicians will have encountered these problems, and decisions around renal biopsy are often difficult and the source of considerable anxiety. These feelings of anxiety are exacerbated when the performance of a potentially morbid, invasive diagnostic intervention is considered in pregnancy when the "stakes" may be higher. Therefore, it is important when considering renal biopsy in the special situation of pregnancy to ask: i) is renal biopsy safe with a complication rate no worse than that in the non-pregnant situation? and ii) does the information obtained by renal biopsy affect the management of the mother or the pregnancy?

A few studies have specifically evaluated indications for renal biopsy in pregnancy with its subsequent outcomes, and it is useful to consider the evidence from this work in chronological sequence. Initial reports were encouraging. Macroscopic hematuria occurred in just 3.5 percent of several hundred renal biopsies performed in pregnancy or shortly thereafter in an effort to establish the importance of chronic renal disease as a cause of hypertension in pregnancy [10], although the renal biopsy itself was not the focus of the author's interest. The first series concentrating on complications of renal biopsies in pregnancy was provided by Schewitz [11] and is widely referenced. The complication rate in their series was unacceptably high – a greater than 16 percent rate of macroscopic hematuria, nearly 5 percent perirenal hematomas and one maternal death. It must be borne in mind, however, that the patients reported by these authors were biopsied during the formative years of the biopsy procedure, and that biopsy techniques were very different from those in use today. Also, indications and contraindications were less well developed, and therefore patient selection was less stringent than may be the case currently. Indeed, other workers demonstrated that complications may be considerably less than indicated by the study of Schewitz [11] and suggested guidelines for the use of renal biopsy in pregnancy [12].

Packham and Fairley [13] reported the outcomes of 111 renal biopsies performed in the first or second trimester of pregnancy over a 21-year period up to 1985. Of these women, 22 had a preexisting diagnosis of glomerulonephritis and were biopsied in pregnancy to assess progress of this condition. The most common indications for biopsy in the remainder were hematuria and proteinuria (36 percent of all biopsies), nephrotic syndrome (12 percent), hematuria, proteinuria and hypertension (10.5 percent) and impaired renal function (8 percent). Four patients underwent renal biopsy because of severe early preeclampsia and fetal death in an earlier pregnancy but in the absence of hypertension or renal abnormalities in the index pregnancy, and none of these yielded a positive diagnosis of glomerulonephritis. In 80 percent of those biopsied in pregnancy for the first time, a positive diagnosis of glomerulonephritis was revealed. In the nine nephrotic patients, seven had membranous nephropathy, one had focal segmental glomerulosclerosis and one had IgA nephropathy. How often this information altered clinical management was not discussed. The complication rate, including failure to obtain tissue, was very low at 7.2 percent. There were no serious complications. The authors concluded that renal biopsy was safe in pregnancy, advocated a relaxed approach to renal biopsy in pregnancy and proposed increasing its use. However this suggestion was challenged in an accompanying editorial where a more moderate interventional approach was advanced [14].

Kuller, D'Andrea and McMahon [15] reported results collected from 18 women biopsied at ≤30 weeks or immediately postpartum (three biopsies). The complication rate was relatively high with seven identifiable hematomas (38 percent) and two patients (11 percent) requiring blood transfusion as a consequence. Again, precisely how often biopsy diagnosis altered management is not clear, although the absence of glomerular endotheliosis in some women may have resulted in prolongation of their pregnancy. In a series of 15 renal biopsies prior to 30 weeks' gestation performed because of renal impairment of obscure cause or nephrotic syndrome, the only complication was macroscopic hematuria in one patient. As a result of these interventions, 11 patients were treated with glucocorticoids [16]. Experience of 20 renal biopsies in pregnancy from the Queen Elizabeth Hospital, Birmingham, UK, indicates that in carefully selected patients, the procedure yields a positive diagnosis of glomerular disease in 95 percent, a change in management in 40 percent and no serious complications [17].

Strevens and colleagues [18] biopsied 36 women with hypertension in pregnancy to compare glomerular endothelial changes with those observed in contemporaneous biopsies from 12 women with normal control pregnancies. The mean blood pressure of the proteinuric hypertensives in this study was 150/101 mmHg. One woman with early-onset severe preeclampsia developed a hemodynamically significant hematoma and required blood transfusion. Glomerular endotheliosis was found in most healthy controls in addition to all the hypertensive women, and the authors concluded that this lesion is not specific for preeclampsia. This series was also reported by Wide-Swensson, Strevens and Willner [19], who provided more details of biopsy-related complications. Three women complained of pain after their biopsy and one had a small peri-renal hematoma. One woman with severe pregnancy-induced hypertension, proteinuria, oliguria and pulmonary edema at 25 weeks of a twin pregnancy suffered a large retroperitoneal bleed requiring renal embolization following renal biopsy. This represents a 1.8 percent rate of serious complications, and it is unsurprising that a patient with severe hypertension should be affected.

Several questions exist about the ethics of the studies reported by these authors [18, 19]. Few medical practitioners consider renal biopsy an appropriate diagnostic investigation in preeclampsia because management is insufficiently altered to justify the risks involved, regardless of any perceived uncertainties about underlying pathology. Women with poorly controlled blood pressure in the setting of preeclampsia, such as those deliberately enrolled in this study, fall into a group at high risk of complications. In fact, generally accepted clinical criteria (see earlier in this chapter) contraindicate the renal biopsy procedure in individuals with this degree of hypertension. Generally speaking, given the unavoidable risks of renal biopsy, this author believes that subjecting normal controls to the procedure in any study is ethically unacceptable. Despite these concerns, the study was reported twice by the same group in 2003 and 2007. The data in the two papers are very similar, although the latter publication [19] fails to reference the former [18].

Han and colleagues [20] reported a series of renal biopsies performed to assess preeclampsia/eclampsia in the antepartum or immediate postpartum periods. In three antepartum biopsies (28–30 weeks' gestation) and five postpartum biopsies, typical findings of enotheliosis were observed and no serious complications were encountered. Whether patient management was significantly altered by this information is unclear [20].

A recent systematic review [21], focusing on risks and timing of kidney biopsy in pregnancy, has examined data available in 39 published references reporting 243 biopsies in pregnancy and 1,236 after delivery. Evidence was heterogeneous but suggested that, compared to postpartum biopsy, biopsy in pregnancy is likely more risky with a peak risk around 25 weeks.

When Should Renal Biopsy Be Performed in Pregnancy?

Overall the available published evidence from studies of contemporary practice suggests that the complication rate of renal biopsy in pregnancy is broadly similar to that encountered with this intervention in general nephrological practice. It is possible that the pro-thrombotic environment engendered by pregnancy may mitigate bleeding. Nonetheless, because the reported experience of renal biopsy in pregnancy in the modern era amounts to only a few hundred cases, compared to thousands in the nonpregnant setting, it is not possible to conclude with complete confidence that rates of unusual but serious complications are equivalent. Clearly, if enough biopsies of pregnant women are performed, a serious complication will eventually follow. Therefore, in pregnancy, consideration should be given to the same absolute and relative contraindications to the biopsy procedure that apply to the nonpregnant situation (see earlier in this chapter). Potential operators should not be tempted to perform a renal biopsy in an unfamiliar manner, for example, with the patient seated rather than prone. This may be of particular relevance in pregnancies over 24 weeks' of gestation when it may be difficult or uncomfortable for women to lie prone. Also, as in the nonpregnant setting, renal biopsy should not be performed in the presence of hypertension (> 160/95) [2].

Given these caveats, what indications necessitate renal biopsy in pregnancy? It can be difficult to distinguish between preeclampsia and primary renal disease in pregnancy, and often the two may coexist. However, it is usually possible to distinguish between the two conditions by observing other clinical parameters. In preeclampsia, proteinuria generally develops rapidly after 20 weeks' gestation, and other features such as falling platelet count and abnormal liver enzymes and placental and fetal Dopplers may point to this diagnosis. Considering this, and in the knowledge that those bleeding complications that have been observed with renal biopsy in pregnancy particularly afflict hypertensive preeclamptics, renal biopsy cannot be recommended routinely as an investigation for preeclampsia.

In non-preeclamptic women with nephrotic syndrome after 32 weeks' gestation, delivery should be expedited and renal investigations postponed to the postpartum period. Before 28 weeks of gestation, renal biopsy should be performed to make a histological diagnosis and to guide therapy since some lesions may be amenable to steroid therapy. Between 28 and 32 weeks of gestation, the decision is less straightforward. The major question is whether the mother has a condition, predominantly minimal change disease, that may respond promptly to steroids. In adults of childbearing age, minimal change disease comprises only ~25 percent of all nephrotic syndrome and may respond more slowly to therapy than the same condition diagnosed in children. It may be difficult to justify antepartum biopsy simply in order to prolong pregnancy for a couple of weeks to improve fetal outcome, when any maternal intervention is unlikely to have had a therapeutic effect. A trial of steroids is a possibility, but many clinicians are uncomfortable with blind glucocorticoid treatment given the potential maternal complications such as hypertension, infection and diabetes [22]. Some literature also suggests that the prenatal use of glucocorticoids may initiate, in the fetus, a program of physiological changes resulting in cardiovascular and metabolic disease in adulthood [23]. Therefore, in a morbidly nephrotic woman after 28 weeks' gestation, when fetal viability is likely to be good, delivery should be expedited and renal investigation pursued thereafter.

Acute kidney injury in pregnancy with no apparent cause may require renal biopsy. In some systemic disorders such as lupus, serological investigations may be helpful diagnostically, and elucidation of renal histopathology may be a key determinant of therapy. Indeed, prompt therapeutic intervention may be required to preserve renal function. Therefore, before 28 weeks, biopsy should be performed, but at later gestations, the pregnancy should be brought to an end to facilitate subsequent renal biopsy.

The finding in pregnancy of stable CKD and hypertension with an active urinary sediment suggestive of a renal parenchymal disease should provoke close supervision and blood pressure control, but not renal biopsy, which would be unlikely to alter management. A similar approach should be applied to non-nephrotic proteinuria, with or without renal functional impairment.

Overall renal biopsy in pregnancy appears safe. Definite indications for its use exist before 28 weeks' gestation, but are unusual. Thus renal biopsy should be needed only rarely in pregnancy, and not after 28 weeks' gestation.

References

1. Alwall N. Aspiration biopsy of the kidney, including a report of a case of amyloidosis diagnosed through aspiration biopsy of the kidney in 1944 and investigated at an autopsy in 1950. *Acta Med Scand* **143**, 420–435, 1952.

2. Topham PS. Renal biopsy. In *Comprehensive clinical nephrology*, edited by Johnson RJ, Floege J and Feehally J. Elsevier Health Sciences 2007, pp. 69–76.

3. Parrish AE. Complications of percutaneous renal biopsy: A review of 37 years' experience. *Clin Nephrol* **38**, 135–141, 1992.

4. Hergesell O, Felten H, Andrassy K, Kuhn K and Ritz E. Safety of ultrasound-guided percutaneous renal biopsy-retrospective analysis of 1090 consecutive cases. *Nephrol Dial Transplant* **13**, 975–977, 1998.

5. Manno C, Strippoli GF, Arnesano L, Bonifati C, Campobasso N, Gesualdo L and Schena FP. Predictors of bleeding complications in percutaneous ultrasound-guided renal biopsy. *Kidney Int* **66**, 1570–1577, 2004.

6. Eiro M, Katoh T and Watanabe T. Risk factors for bleeding complications in percutaneous renal biopsy. *Clin Exp Nephrol* **9**, 40–45, 2005.

7. Bennett AR and Wiener SN. Intrarenal arteriovenous fistula and aneurysm: A complication of percutaneous renal biopsy. *Am J Roentgenol Radium Ther Nucl Med* **95**, 372–382, 1965.

8. Jones DC and Hayslett JP. Outcome of pregnancy in women with moderate or severe renal insufficiency. *N Engl J Med* **335**, 226–232, 1996.

9. Fischer MJ, Lehnerz SD, Hebert JR and Parikh CR. Kidney disease is an independent risk factor for adverse fetal and maternal outcomes in pregnancy. *Am J Kidney Dis* **43**, 415–423, 2004.

10. McCartney CP. Pathological anatomy of acute hypertension of pregnancy. *Circulation* **30**: SUPPL 2, 37–42, 1964.

11. Schewitz LJ, Friedman IA and Pollak VE. Bleeding after renal biopsy in pregnancy. *Obstet Gynecol* **26**, 295–304, 1965.

12. Lindheimer MD, Spargo BH and Katz AI. Renal biopsy in pregnancy-induced hypertension. *J Reprod Med* **15**, 189–194, 1975.

13. Packham D and Fairley KF. Renal biopsy: Indications and complications in pregnancy. *Br J Obstet Gynaecol* **94**, 935–939, 1987.

14. Lindheimer MD and Davison JM. Renal biopsy during pregnancy: "To b ... or not to b ... ?" *Br J Obstet Gynaecol* **94**, 932–934, 1987.

15. Kuller JA, D'Andrea NM and McMahon MJ. Renal biopsy and pregnancy. *Am J Obstet Gynecol* **184**, 1093–1096, 2001.

16. Chen HH, Lin HC, Yeh JC and Chen CP. Renal biopsy in pregnancies complicated by undetermined renal disease. *Acta Obstet Gynecol Scand* **80**, 888–893, 2001.

17. Day C, Hewins P, Hildebrand S, Sheikh L, Taylor G, Kilby M and Lipkin G The role of renal biopsy in women with kidney disease identified in pregnancy. *Nephrol Dial Transplant* **23**, 201–206, 2008.

18. Strevens H, Wide-Swensson D, Hansen A, Horn T, Ingemarsson I, Larsen S, Willner J and Olsen S. Glomerular endotheliosis in normal pregnancy and pre-eclampsia. *Br J Obstet Gynaecol* **110**, 831–836, 2003.

19. Wide-Swensson D, Strevens H and Willner J. Antepartum percutaneous renal biopsy. *Int J Gynaecol Obstet*, **98**, 88–92, 2007.

20. Han L, Yang Z, Li K, Zon J, Han J, Zhou L, Liu X, Zhang X, Zheng Y, Yu L and Li L. Antepartum or immediate postpartum renal biopsies in preeclampsia/eclampsia of pregnancy: New morphologic and clinical findings. *Int J Clin Exp Pathol* 7, 5129–5143, 2014.

21. Piccoli GB, Daidola G, Attini R, Parisi S, Fassio F, Naretto C, Deagostini MC, Castellucia N, Ferraresi M, Roccatello D and Todros T. Kidney biopsy in pregnancy: Evidence for counselling? A systematic review. *BJOG* **120**, 412–427, 2013.

22. Petri M. Immunosuppressive drug use in pregnancy. *Autoimmunity* **36**, 51–56, 2003.

23. Seckl JR and Holmes MC. Mechanisms of disease: Glucocorticoids, their placental metabolism and fetal programming of adult pathophysiology. *Nat Clin Pract Endocrinol Metab* **3**, 479–488, 2007.

Appendix: Consensus Statements 2017

Matt Hall, Liz Lightstone, Catherine Nelson-Piercy, Kate Wiles, Jenny Myers, Louise Kenny, Lucy Mackillop, Graham Lipkin, Nadia Sarween, Ellen Knox, Sarah Winfield, Laura Baines, Andrea Goodlife, Floria Cheng, Nick Kametas, Kate Harding, Andrew McCarthy, Joyce Popoola, Michelle Hladunewich and Kate Bramham

Chronic Kidney Disease in Pregnancy – General

- Multidisciplinary teams (MDT) should be established to assess and care for pregnant women with chronic kidney disease (CKD), including women receiving dialysis and kidney transplant recipients.
- The MDT requires, as a minimum, an obstetrician, a renal/obstetric physician and a specialist midwife, all with expertise in the management of CKD in pregnancy.
- All women with CKD and any healthcare professionals looking after them should be able to access the MDT.
- Calculated GFR formulae, including estimated GFR (eGFR), are not valid for use in pregnancy, and monitoring of serum creatinine should be used in pregnancy.
- Women with CKD G1 and G2 can be advised that obstetric outcome is usually successful; however, there is an increased risk of antenatal complications including preeclampsia, preterm birth, fetal growth restriction, neonatal intensive care unit (NICU) admission and Caesarean delivery, such that consultant obstetrician-led care is advised with nephrology input as required.
- Women with CKD G3–G5 should be advised that risk of obstetric complications is substantial, including preeclampsia, preterm birth, fetal growth restriction, NICU admission, Caesarean delivery and temporary or permanent loss of renal function, such that management of the pregnancy should be by the MDT, with individualized plans for shared care.
- Women who have not had prepregnancy counseling by the MDT should be seen by the MDT in pregnancy.
- CKD is not a contraindication to vaginal delivery.

Prepregnancy Counseling

- Women of childbearing age with CKD should be made aware of implications regarding reproductive health and contraception.
- Women with CKD considering pregnancy, including women with lupus nephritis, recurrent urinary tract infection (UTI), stones, bladder reconstruction and living kidney donors, should be offered prepregnancy counseling by the MDT.
- Preparation for pregnancy should be individualized to each woman's needs and, where possible, should involve her partner.
- Prepregnancy counseling should allow discussion of and, where possible, modification of remediable risk factors, including disease activity, blood pressure control, weight management, stability of renal function, medication and familial conditions.
- Written information should be shared with the woman (and her referring clinician) to accompany the information shared at the clinic appointment.

General Antenatal Care

Proteinuria

- Proteinuria should not be assumed to be due to UTI.
- Women with greater than or equal to +1 dipstick positive proteinuria should have formal quantification of proteinuria.

- Baseline quantification of proteinuria may be undertaken by protein/creatinine ratio (PCR) or albumin:creatinine ratio (ACR). Twenty-four-hour collection for urine protein is not usually required.
- Newly detected persistent proteinuria (ACR > 20mg/mmol or PCR > 30mg/mmol) before 20 weeks of gestation warrants investigation for underlying renal disease.

Thromboprophylaxis

- Women with nephrotic syndrome should have thromboprophylaxis in pregnancy and for six weeks postpartum.
- Women with substantial proteinuria ACR > 70mg/mmol or PCR > 100mg/mmol) should be risk-assessed for venous thromboembolism and considered for thromboprophylaxis in pregnancy and for six weeks postpartum.
- In women with CKD, low molecular weight heparin dose should be adjusted for reduced kidney function (eGFR < 30mls/min/1.73 m^2) and body weight.

Blood Pressure

- In pregnant women with CKD and hypertension, blood pressure of < 120–139 / 70–85 mmHg should be the target.

Preeclampsia Prophylaxis

- Women with CKD stages G1–G5, including recipients of renal transplants, should be offered low-dose aspirin (75–150mg) as prophylaxis against preeclampsia.
- Women with CKD with low dietary calcium intake and/or low vitamin D levels should receive a calcium and/or vitamin D3 preparation during pregnancy.

Anemia and Bone Health

- Assessment of iron status should be performed in women with CKD at first antenatal visit and at 28 weeks, and more frequently if clinically indicated. Iron supplementation should be given if evidence exists of absolute or functional iron deficiency.
- Pregnant women with CKD who require rapid correction of anemia secondary to iron deficiency and who are intolerant of oral iron (or those who are unresponsive) can be given parental iron.

- Erythropoietin stimulating agents can be given if clinically indicated with appropriate monitoring of blood pressure in women with CKD.
- Women with CKD stages 3–5 should have mineral bone health surveillance and treatment during pregnancy by the MDT.

Urinary Tract Infection (UTI)

- Asymptomatic bacteriuria and urinary tract infection (UTI) in pregnancy should be treated.
- Antibiotic prophylaxis should be considered in women with structural renal abnormalities or recurrent bacteriuria/UTI.

Medication

Immunosuppression

- A drug passport should be provided for all women with CKD at the beginning of the pregnancy.
- Prednisolone, azathioprine, ciclosporin, tacrolimus and hydroxychloroquine are considered safe in pregnancy.
- Calcineurin inhibitor levels (i.e. ciclosporin and tacrolimus levels) should be performed more frequently in pregnancy and immediately postpartum, as doses required to achieve target blood levels are very likely to change.
- Certain medications (e.g. erythromycin) can interfere with calcineurin inhibitor metabolism and alternatives should be prescribed.
- Mycophenolate mofetil, mycophenolic acid, methotrexate and cyclophosphamide are teratogenic and should be avoided in pregnancy.
- Mycophenolate mofetil and mycophenolic acid are associated with an increased risk of spontaneous miscarriage and fetal abnormality and should be stopped before pregnancy. A three-month interval is advised before conception to allow conversion to a pregnancy-safe alternative and ensure stable disease/kidney function.
- The Rare Renal Disease Registry (RaDaR) Study Group recommends that potential fathers taking mycophenolate derivatives are informed of the theoretical risks of mycophenolate exposure to a fetus and be made aware of the contraceptive advice given by the Medicines and Healthcare Products Regulatory Agency (MHRA) and contained in the summary of product characteristics. They advise that these theoretical

risks should be balanced against the risks of conversion to alternative immunosuppressive regimes on their kidney transplant status in an individualized discussion.

- Rituximab does not appear to be teratogenic, but exposure in pregnancy can result in neonatal B cell depletion and the long-term outcome is unknown.
- The safety of sirolimus, everolimus and other biologics (including eculizumab) in pregnancy remains to be determined.
- Women should be reassured that they can breastfeed while taking prednisolone, hydroxychloroquine, azathioprine, ciclosporin and tacrolimus.
- Immunosuppressive treatment does not need to be empirically increased in the postpartum period to prevent reactivation of disease or graft rejection.

Antihypertensives

- Women with CKD should undergo a review of their antihypertensive therapy and the benefits and risks of specific drug treatment in pregnancy should be discussed.
- Labetalol, nifedipine and methyldopa are considered safe in pregnancy.
- Angiotensin-converting enzyme inhibitors (ACEis) or angiotensin receptor blockers (ARBs) are fetotoxic in the second and third trimesters.
- The use of ACEis or ARBs in women with non-proteinuric CKD should be discussed and conversion to alternative antihypertensive treatment known to be safe considered in advance of pregnancy.
- The use of ACEi or ARBs in women with proteinuric CKD should be discussed by the MDT in advance of pregnancy, and a plan made for timing of conversion to alternative treatment known to be safe in pregnancy, guided by the likelihood of early pregnancy confirmation.
- Women who conceive whilst taking ACEis or ARBs should stop taking these medications as soon as pregnancy is confirmed, and be offered alternative antihypertensives considered safe in pregnancy if necessary.

Oral Hypoglycemics

- Screening for gestational diabetes is recommended for all women taking prednisolone

and calcineurin inhibitors (ciclosporin and tacrolimus).
- Biguanides (metformin) and oral hypoglycemics should not be used in women with advanced CKD.

Fetal Monitoring

- First or second biochemistry screenings for aneuploidies have an increased false positive rate in advanced CKD. Screen positive results due to very high human chorionic gonadotrophin (hCG) concentrations should be treated with caution; however, negative predictive values are high. Screening alternatives include specialist ultrasound only screening or noninvasive prenatal testing.
- Fetal growth scans including umbilical artery Dopplers should be performed in women with CKD at 26–28 weeks and 32–34 weeks with additional scans considered for those with additional risk factors for growth restriction.
- Amniotic fluid index is not representative of placental health in women with advanced CKD and should not be relied upon for confirmation of fetal well-being.
- Continuous electronic fetal monitoring in labour should be considered for all women with CKD and is recommended for those with advanced CKD.

Specific Conditions

Transplant

- Women with renal transplants should have the same prepregnancy counseling and antenatal care as women with CKD – refer to earlier sections.
- Women should wait until their kidney function is stable on medications safe in pregnancy before conceiving, which is usually more than one year after transplantation.
- Clinicians caring for women who have undergone renal transplantation should liaise with the appropriate surgical team to advise on delivery plans if there are doubts about the transplant-related anatomy. Indications for Caesarean delivery in women with renal transplants are obstetric.
- Any Caesarean delivery in a transplant patient should be performed by the most senior obstetrician available, ideally a consultant. Consideration should be given to a vertical midline abdominal wall incision.

223

- Consider informing the on-call transplant surgical team if a woman with a renal transplant is admitted in established labor, or is having a planned delivery.
- All women with kidney pancreas transplants, dual kidney transplants or bladder reconstruction should be managed during pregnancy and delivery by the MDT at a transplant center.

Lupus

- Women with lupus nephritis should be advised to wait until their disease is quiescent for at least six months before conceiving.
- Early investigation of infertility should be considered for women who have had previous treatment with cyclophosphamide.
- All women with lupus nephritis should be managed in pregnancy by the MDT.
- Renal biopsy may be considered only if renal histology will change management during pregnancy.
- Activity of lupus should be monitored clinically and with serum complement, dsDNA, renal function, hematology and urine assessment.
- Women with antiphospholipid syndrome (with confirmed thromboembolic event, or adverse obstetric outcome – excluding recurrent early fetal loss) should receive low molecular weight heparin in pregnancy and for six weeks postpartum.
- Women with anti-Ro antibodies should have the fetal heart rate checked at every antenatal appointment from 18 weeks and fetal echocardiography is recommended.
- All women with lupus should be on hydroxychloroquine in pregnancy unless it is contraindicated.
- Steroids (including methyl-prednisolone), azathioprine, calcineurin inhibitors and IVIg can be used to treat lupus flares in pregnancy.

Diabetic Nephropathy

- Women with diabetic nephropathy benefit from optimization of blood pressure and blood glucose prior to conception.
- Women with diabetic nephropathy should be encouraged to consider continuation of ACEi/ARB treatment until conception.

Dialysis

- Renal units, in conjunction with obstetric units, should formulate a protocol for management of women receiving or starting dialysis in pregnancy to be activated when a dialysis patient becomes pregnant or a pregnant woman is started on dialysis.
- Women with advanced, deteriorating CKD during pregnancy may benefit from early initiation of hemodialysis before standard indications outside of pregnancy.
- Dialysis intensity should be prescribed accounting for residual renal function targeting a pre-dialysis urea < 10mmol/l.
- Women with preexisting end-stage renal disease should have an increased amount of dialysis in pregnancy to improve outcomes.

Acute Kidney Injury

- A rise in creatinine of ≥50 percent or a creatinine of ≥90μmol (if previous value unknown) should prompt investigation for acute kidney injury (AKI).
- The most common causes of AKI in pregnancy are preeclampsia, hypovolemia, sepsis and nephrotoxic medication.

Urological Disorders

- Imaging for loin pain or macroscopic hematuria in pregnancy should be performed by a clinician with uroradiology expertise. The first line of investigation is ultrasound with Doppler resistance indices. Magnetic resonance imaging and ultra-low-dose Computerized Tomography Kidney Ureter Bladder (CT-KUB) may be considered in selected cases.
- Management of stones should be conservative, but if necessary, nephrostomy with antegrade stenting or ureteroscopic stone extraction can be performed in pregnancy by an expert urologist/uroradiologist.
- Clinical suspicion of an infected obstructed kidney warrants emergency urological investigation and appropriate drainage.
- A pregnant woman with visible hematuria in the absence of a UTI should have urological investigation.
- Persistent, non-visible hematuria with structurally normal kidneys does not need investigation

during pregnancy, but the GP should be informed so the patient can be evaluated postpartum according to local guidelines.

- Pregnant women with previous reconstructive bladder surgery should have a urologist involved in planning delivery.

Postpartum Management

- Women with CKD in pregnancy should resume their established care with a planned early postpartum renal review.
- Women with newly diagnosed CKD in pregnancy need referral to nephrology for further evaluation and should be seen within an appropriate timescale decided by the MDT. A review within six weeks postpartum should be considered.
- A plan for postpartum management of hypertension in women with CKD should be made by the MDT.
- Postpartum evaluation of women with early-onset (necessitating delivery before 34 weeks of gestation) preeclampsia is important to identify women with underlying renal disease.
- NSAIDS should be avoided in women with AKI, CKD or hypertensive disorders of pregnancy.
- Women with CKD and an indication for ACEi or ARB treatment can be commenced on these medications in the postnatal period when serum creatinine is stable and serum potassium is within the normal range. Enalapril and captopril are compatible with breastfeeding, but other ACEi or ARB have not been studied. Appropriate monitoring of creatinine and potassium after commencing treatment should be arranged.

Contraception

- Contraceptive counseling should form part of the routine management of women with CKD.
- Advice on safe and effective contraception should be offered to all women with CKD, in particular women with advanced CKD, women with active glomerulonephritis, women taking teratogenic medication, women within one year of transplantation and women on dialysis.
- Safe and effective contraception for women with kidney disease includes the progesterone-only pill, a contraceptive implant or an intrauterine device.

Education

- Educational programs for healthcare professionals managing women of childbearing age with CKD should be developed, including education about contraception for nephrologists.
- Educational resources should be made available to women with CKD.

Assisted Conception

- Women with CKD considering assisted reproduction, including *in vitro* fertilization, should be referred for prepregnancy counseling by the MDT. Single-embryo transfer and frozen embryo transfer if IVF is required is highly recommended to reduce risk of complications of multifetal pregnancies.

Research

- Evaluate the role of prepregnancy counseling on pregnancy outcomes for women with CKD.
- Investigate the effect of health optimization before pregnancy for women with CKD.
- Establish and fund data collection and research on pregnancy and renal outcomes of women with CKD and their offspring.
- Define the time course and mechanism(s) of renal and systemic hemodynamic alterations and markers of renal function in health and disease during pregnancy.
- Investigate the altered gestational and postpartum natriuretic responses, and their relationship to plasma volume expansion, in normal pregnant women and in those with CKD.
- Define biomarkers that will effectively predict those women with CKD who are at particular risk of specific complications or poor maternal/fetal outcomes.
- Evaluation of serum screening for aneuploidy risk in women with CKD, including the use of free fetal DNA.
- Investigate the mechanisms that lead to pregnancy-associated decline in renal function.
- Develop strategies to prevent pregnancy-associated decline in renal function.
- Evaluate novel therapeutic strategies for preeclampsia in women with CKD.

- Establish the risk of venous thromboembolic disease associated with non-nephrotic range proteinuria in pregnancy.
- Evaluate the use of imaging modalities to improve differentiation of physiological hydronephrosis of pregnancy from urinary tract obstruction.
- Validate educational programs for patients and healthcare professionals managing women of childbearing age with CKD.
- Explore the interactions of women with CKD with multidisciplinary health professionals.
- Evaluate events during pregnancy that lead to sensitization relevant to future transplantation.

- Assess pregnancy outcomes in living kidney donors.
- Establish precisely how calcineurin inhibitor levels should be quantified in pregnancy (e.g. free serum or bound).
- Evaluate excretion into breast milk and the relevance to neonatal well-being of drugs used by women with CKD.
- Evaluate the maternal and neonatal outcomes of IVF pregnancies in women with CKD to establish optimal treatment.
- Assess long-term pediatric outcomes of women with CKD, including evaluation of *in utero* exposure to medication.

Index